Nutrigenetics

Nutrigenetics

Special Issue Editor

Dolores Corella

MDPI • Basel • Beijing • Wuhan • Barcelona • Belgrade

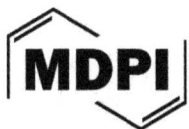

MDPI

Special Issue Editor
Dolores Corella
University of Valencia
Spain

Editorial Office
MDPI
St. Alban-Anlage 66
Basel, Switzerland

This is a reprint of articles from the Special Issue published online in the open access journal *Nutrients* (ISSN 2072-6643) from 2016 to 2017 (available at: http://www.mdpi.com/journal/nutrients/special_issues/nutrigenetics)

For citation purposes, cite each article independently as indicated on the article page online and as indicated below:

LastName, A.A.; LastName, B.B.; LastName, C.C. Article Title. *Journal Name* **Year**, *Article Number, Page Range.*

ISBN 978-3-03842-995-1 (Pbk)
ISBN 978-3-03842-996-8 (PDF)

Contents

About the Special Issue Editor vii

Preface to "Nutrigenetics" ix

Dolores Corella, Oscar Coltell, Jose V. Sorlí, Ramón Estruch, Laura Quiles,
Miguel Ángel Martínez-González, Jordi Salas-Salvadó, Olga Castañer, Fernando Arós,
Manuel Ortega-Calvo, Lluís Serra-Majem, Enrique Gómez-Gracia, Olga Portolés,
Miquel Fiol, Javier Díez Espino, Josep Basora, Montserrat Fitó, Emilio Ros and
José M. Ordovás
Polymorphism of the Transcription Factor 7-Like 2 Gene (TCF7L2) Interacts with Obesity on
Type-2 Diabetes in the PREDIMED Study Emphasizing the Heterogeneity of Genetic Variants
in Type-2 Diabetes Risk Prediction: Time for Obesity-Specific Genetic Risk Scores
Reprinted from: *Nutrients* **2016**, *8*, 793, doi: 10.3390/nu8120793   1

Nikul K. Soni, Alastair B. Ross, Nathalie Scheers, Otto I. Savolainen, Intawat Nookaew,
Britt G. Gabrielsson and Ann-Sofie Sandberg
Splenic Immune Response Is Down-Regulated in C57BL/6J Mice Fed Eicosapentaenoic Acid
and Docosahexaenoic Acid Enriched High Fat Diet
Reprinted from: *Nutrients* **2017**, *9*, 50, doi: 10.3390/nu9010050 19

Abraham Wall-Medrano, Laura A. de la Rosa, Alma A. Vázquez-Flores,
Gilberto Mercado-Mercado, Rogelio González-Arellanes, José A. López-Díaz,
Aarón F. González-Córdova, Gustavo A. González-Aguilar, Belinda Vallejo-Cordoba and
Francisco J. Molina-Corral
Lipidomic and Antioxidant Response to Grape Seed, Corn and Coconut Oils in Healthy
Wistar Rats
Reprinted from: *Nutrients* **2017**, *9*, 82, doi: 10.3390/nu9010082 36

Kaitlin J. Day, Melissa M. Adamski, Aimee L. Dordevic and Chiara Murgia
Genetic Variations as Modifying Factors to Dietary Zinc Requirements—A Systematic Review
Reprinted from: *Nutrients* **2017**, *9*, 148, doi: 10.3390/nu9020148 53

Kaitlin Roke, Kathryn Walton, Shannon L. Klingel, Amber Harnett, Sanjeena Subedi,
Jess Haines and David M. Mutch
Evaluating Changes in Omega-3 Fatty Acid Intake after Receiving Personal *FADS1* Genetic
Information: A Randomized Nutrigenetic Intervention
Reprinted from: *Nutrients* **2017**, *9*, 240, doi: 10.3390/nu9030240 69

Patrick Borel and Charles Desmarchelier
Genetic Variations Associated with Vitamin A Status and Vitamin A Bioavailability
Reprinted from: *Nutrients* **2017**, *9*, 246, doi: 10.3390/nu9030246 83

Juan J. Salinero, Beatriz Lara, Diana Ruiz-Vicente, Francisco Areces, Carlos Puente-Torres,
César Gallo-Salazar, Teodoro Pascual and Juan Del Coso
CYP1A2 Genotype Variations Do Not Modify the Benefits and Drawbacks of Caffeine during
Exercise: A Pilot Study
Reprinted from: *Nutrients* **2017**, *9*, 269, doi: 10.3390/nu9030269 100

You-Lin Tain, Yu-Ju Lin, Jiunn-Ming Sheen, Hong-Ren Yu, Mao-Meng Tiao, Chih-Cheng Chen, Ching-Chou Tsai, Li-Tung Huang and Chien-Ning Hsu
High Fat Diets Sex-Specifically Affect the Renal Transcriptome and Program Obesity, Kidney Injury, and Hypertension in the Offspring
Reprinted from: *Nutrients* **2017**, *9*, 357, doi: 10.3390/nu9040357 112

Chiara Murgia and Melissa M. Adamski
Translation of Nutritional Genomics into Nutrition Practice: The Next Step
Reprinted from: *Nutrients* **2017**, *9*, 366, doi: 10.3390/nu9040366 131

Min Yang, Min Xiong, Huan Chen, Lanlan Geng, Peiyu Chen, Jing Xie, Shui Qing Ye, Ding-You Li and Sitang Gong
Novel Genetic Variants Associated with Child Refractory Esophageal Stricture with Food Allergy by Exome Sequencing
Reprinted from: *Nutrients* **2017**, *9*, 390, doi: 10.3390/nu9040390 135

Josiane Steluti, Aline M. Carvalho, Antonio A. F. Carioca, Andreia Miranda, Gilka J. F. Gattás, Regina M. Fisberg and Dirce M. Marchioni
Genetic Variants Involved in One-Carbon Metabolism: Polymorphism Frequencies and Differences in Homocysteine Concentrations in the Folic Acid Fortification Era
Reprinted from: *Nutrients* **2017**, *9*, 539, doi: 10.3390/nu9060539 142

Brinda K. Rana, Shirley W. Flatt, Dennis D. Health, Bilge Pakiz, Elizabeth L. Quintana, Loki Natarajan and Cheryl L. Rock
The *IL6* Gene Promoter SNP and Plasma IL-6 in Response to Diet Intervention
Reprinted from: *Nutrients* **2017**, *9*, 552, doi: 10.3390/nu9060552 154

Frédéric Guénard, Annie Bouchard-Mercier, Iwona Rudkowska, Simone Lemieux, Patrick Couture and Marie-Claude Vohl
Genome-Wide Association Study of Dietary Pattern Scores
Reprinted from: *Nutrients* **2017**, *9*, 649, doi: 10.3390/nu9070649 159

Xingxing Song, Zongyao Li, Xinqiang Ji and Dongfeng Zhang
Calcium Intake and the Risk of Ovarian Cancer: A Meta-Analysis
Reprinted from: *Nutrients* **2017**, *9*, 679, doi: 10.3390/nu9070679 176

Kevin B. Comerford and Gonca Pasin
Gene–Dairy Food Interactions and Health Outcomes: A Review of Nutrigenetic Studies
Reprinted from: *Nutrients* **2017**, *9*, 710, doi: 10.3390/nu9070710 191

Janaina L. S. Donadio, Marcelo M. Rogero, Simon Cockell, John Hesketh and Silvia M. F. Cozzolino
Influence of Genetic Variations in Selenoprotein Genes on the Pattern of Gene Expression after Supplementation with Brazil Nuts
Reprinted from: *Nutrients* **2017**, *9*, 739, doi: 10.3390/nu9070739 208

About the Special Issue Editor

Dolores Corella, is Full Professor of Preventive Medicine and Public Health at the University of Valencia, Valencia, Spain. She has a background in Nutrition, Omics and Epidemiology. Since 1998, she has been the Director of the Genetic and Molecular Epidemiology Rresearch Unit. She focuses on the study of genetic determinants of disease and has developed research methodology for analyzing gene—environment interactions. Within In the a gene—environment interaction study, gene—diet interactions have constituted an important research line giving rise to the development of Nutritional Genomics, Nutrigenetics and Nutrigenomics. She has also been a principal investigator (PI) in the CIBER of Physiopathology of Obesity and Nutrition, a center of excellence for networking research in Spain. She has directed more than 23 PhD dissertations and has been the PI for more than 30 research projects. Currently, she is focused on omics (genomics, epigenomics, transcriptomics, metabolomics, proteomics, phenomics, etc.) integration into the field of diet, obesity, and cardiovascular-related diseases.

Preface to "Nutrigenetics"

In the new era of Precision Nutrition, it is crucial to provide scientific evidence of gene–diet interactions that can result in a practical application. Although enormous progress has been made in the development of omic technologies (genomics, epigenomics, transcriptomis, metabolomics, etc.), the integration of these technologies in the nutrition field is still scarce. Therefore, more studies are needed in Nutritional Genomics to provide the evidence required for Precision Nutrition. Moreover, Nutritional Genomics is a multidisciplinary field and both studies in humans and in animal models are required. In human studies, mainly epidemiological findings related to the associations between genetic variants and disease phenotypes have been published. Large cohorts have been analyzed and genome-wide association studies (GWAs) published. However, the dietary modulation of the reported genetic associations in the GWAs studies is largely unknown. Thus, both observational and experimental gene-diet interaction studies analyzing dietary modulations in determining the genetic risk of disease are needed. In this book, relevant epidemiological studies in the nutrigenetic field are included. These chapters analyze a wide range of study designs and clinical phenotypes, as well as dietary exposures and include, among others, a general overview of the translation of nutritional genomics into nutrition practice; a review of the nutrigenetic studies on gene–dairy food interactions and health outcomes; an analysis of the role of genetic variations associated with vitamin A status and bioavailability; the study of genetic variants involved in one-carbon metabolism and their effects; a meta-analysis of calcium intake and the risk of ovarian cancer; a systematic review of the effect of genetic variants as modifying factors to dietary zinc requirements; an analysis of the role of the genetic risk scores (GRS) derived from GWAs in determining disease risk taking into account their present limitations and the need of focusing on more novel trait-specific GRS; and a randomized nutrigenetic study aimed at evaluating changes in omega-3 fatty acid intake after receiving personal FADS1 genetic information. Likewise, in this book, several novel studies integrating the new omic technologies are included, both in human and in animal studies. These studies can help to look deeper into the molecular mechanisms behind the epidemiological gene–diet interactions. In several chapters, this book focuses on the effect of high fat diets on renal transcriptome and program obesity, kidney injury, and hypertension; the use of exome sequencing to investigate novel genetic variants associated with child refractory esophageal structure with food allergies; the lipidomic and antioxidant response to grape seed, corn and coconut oils in healthy Wistar rats and the analysis of the splenic immune response in C57BL/6J mice fed an eicosapentaenoic acid and docosahexaenoic acid-enriched high fat diet. Overall, this book provides the latest data on genetic variation and dietary response, nutrients and gene expression, and how other omics have adapted to Nutritional Genomics. This publication includes highly relevant information and will be an important tool for the future work of nutritionists, dietitians, food technologists, geneticists, bioinformatics, epidemiologists, educators, policy makers and other health-related professionals.

Dolores Corella
Special Issue Editor

nutrients

MDPI

Article

Polymorphism of the Transcription Factor 7-Like 2 Gene (TCF7L2) Interacts with Obesity on Type-2 Diabetes in the PREDIMED Study Emphasizing the Heterogeneity of Genetic Variants in Type-2 Diabetes Risk Prediction: Time for Obesity-Specific Genetic Risk Scores

Dolores Corella [1,2,*], Oscar Coltell [2,3], Jose V. Sorlí [1,2], Ramón Estruch [2,4], Laura Quiles [1,2], Miguel Ángel Martínez-González [2,5], Jordi Salas-Salvadó [2,6], Olga Castañer [2,7], Fernando Arós [2,8], Manuel Ortega-Calvo [2,9], Lluís Serra-Majem [2,10], Enrique Gómez-Gracia [2,11], Olga Portolés [1,2], Miquel Fiol [2,12], Javier Díez Espino [2,13], Josep Basora [2,6], Montserrat Fitó [2,7], Emilio Ros [2,14] and José M. Ordovás [2,15,16]

1   Department of Preventive Medicine and Public Health, School of Medicine, University of Valencia, 46010 Valencia, Spain; jose.sorli@uv.es (J.V.S.); laura.quiles@uv.es (L.Q.); olga.portoles@uv.es (O.P.)
2   CIBER Fisiopatología de la Obesidad y Nutrición, Instituto de Salud Carlos III, 28029 Madrid, Spain; oscar.coltell@uji.es (O.C.); RESTRUCH@clinic.cat (R.E.); mamartinez@unav.es (M.Á.M.-G.); jordi.salas@urv.cat (J.S.-S.); ocastaner@imim.es (O.C.); aborau@secardiologia.es (F.A.); 106mayorque104@gmail.com (M.O.-C.); lluis.serra@ulpgc.es (L.S.-M.); egomezgracia@uma.es (E.G.-G.); miguel.fiol@ssib.es (M.F.); javierdiezesp@ono.com (J.D.E.); jbasora.tarte.ics@gencat.cat (J.B.); MFito@imim.es (M.F.); EROS@clinic.ub.es (E.R.); jose.ordovas@tufts.edu (J.M.O.)
3   Department of Computer Languages and Systems, School of Technology and Experimental Sciences, Universitat Jaume I, 12071 Castellón, Spain
4   Department of Internal Medicine, Hospital Clinic, IDIBAPS, 08036 Barcelona, Spain
5   Department of Preventive Medicine and Public Health, University of Navarra—Navarra Institute for Health Research (IdisNa), 31009 Pamplona, Spain
6   Human Nutrition Unit, Biochemistry and Biotechnology Department, IISPV, University Rovira i Virgili, 43003 Reus, Spain
7   Cardiovascular Risk and Nutrition Research Group, Hospital del Mar Medical Research Institute (IMIM), 08003 Barcelona, Spain
8   Department of Cardiology, Hospital Txagorritxu, 01009 Vitoria, Spain
9   Department of Family Medicine, Distrito Sanitario Atención Primaria Sevilla, Centro de Salud Las Palmeritas, 41003 Sevilla, Spain
10   Research Institute of Biomedical and Health Sciences, University of Las Palmas de Gran Canaria, 35001 Las Palmas de Gran Canaria, Spain
11   Department of Epidemiology, School of Medicine, University of Malaga, 29071 Malaga, Spain
12   Palma Institute of Health Research (IdISPa), Hospital Son Espases, 07014 Palma de Mallorca, Spain
13   Department of Preventive Medicine and Public Health, University of Navarra—Navarra Institute for Health Research (IdisNA)—Servicio Navarro de Salud-Osasunbidea, 31009 Pamplona, Spain
14   Lipid Clinic, Endocrinology and Nutrition Service, Institut d'Investigacions Biomèdiques August Pi Sunyer (IDIBAPS), Hospital Clinic, 08036 Barcelona, Spain
15   Nutrition and Genomics Laboratory, JM-USDA Human Nutrition Research Center on Aging at Tufts University, Boston, MA 02111, USA
16   Department of Cardiovascular Epidemiology and Population Genetics, Centro Nacional de Investigaciones Cardiovasculares (CNIC), Madrid 28029—IMDEA Alimentación, 28049 Madrid, Spain
*   Correspondence: dolores.corella@uv.es; Tel.: +34-963-864-800

Received: 23 September 2016; Accepted: 17 November 2016; Published: 6 December 2016

Abstract: Nutrigenetic studies analyzing gene–diet interactions of the TCF7L2-rs7903146 C > T polymorphism on type-2 diabetes (T2D) have shown controversial results. A reason contributing to this may be the additional modulation by obesity. Moreover, TCF7L2-rs7903146 is one of the most influential variants in T2D-genetic risk scores (GRS). Therefore, to increase the predictive value (PV) of GRS it is necessary to first see whether the included polymorphisms have heterogeneous effects. We comprehensively investigated gene-obesity interactions between the TCF7L2-rs7903146 C > T polymorphism on T2D (prevalence and incidence) and analyzed other T2D-polymorphisms in a sub-sample. We studied 7018 PREDIMED participants at baseline and longitudinally (8.7 years maximum follow-up). Obesity significantly interacted with the TCF7L2-rs7903146 on T2D prevalence, associations being greater in non-obese subjects. Accordingly, we prospectively observed in non-T2D subjects (n = 3607) that its association with T2D incidence was stronger in non-obese (HR: 1.81; 95% CI: 1.13–2.92, p = 0.013 for TT versus CC) than in obese subjects (HR: 1.01; 95% CI: 0.61–1.66; p = 0.979; p-interaction = 0.048). Accordingly, TCF7L2-PV was higher in non-obese subjects. Additionally, we created obesity-specific GRS with ten T2D-polymorphisms and demonstrated for the first time their higher strata-specific PV. In conclusion, we provide strong evidence supporting the need for considering obesity when analyzing the TCF7L2 effects and propose the use of obesity-specific GRS for T2D.

Keywords: TCF7L2; type-2 diabetes; obesity; T2D-genetic risk scores; TCF7L2-predictive value; PREDIMED study

1. Introduction

It is common knowledge that obesity is associated with an increased risk of developing type 2 diabetes (T2D) [1–3]. However, current genetic information adds some heterogeneity to this notion [4]. Thus, whereas some genetic variants may appear to be associated with T2D mainly in obese subjects [5–7], others may show such association primarily in non-obese individuals [5,6,8]. Understanding these differences is crucial to improving the predictive value of genetic variants when investigating T2D as well as gene–diet interactions. Currently, the rs7903146 C > T Single nucleotide polymorphism (SNP) in the Transcription Factor 7-Like 2 (TCF7L2) gene is the locus most strongly associated with T2D risk at the population level [9–11]. However, despite the strong overall association of this SNP with higher T2D risk, various studies have suggested a modulation of this association by obesity [6,12–15].

Cauchi et al. [6] first reported that the association between the TCF7L2-rs7903146 SNP and prevalent T2D in Europeans was stronger in non-obese subjects. These findings were observed in other populations [12–15]. Nevertheless, this potential heterogeneity by obesity has not been widely reflected in the analytical approaches of subsequent investigations, and most of them have not formally tested the interaction between the TCF7L2-rs7903146 polymorphism and obesity status in determining T2D risk. A contributory factor is that previous findings were mainly based on cross-sectional or case-control studies [5,6,9,12–14] with a strong likelihood of being affected by potential biases, more prospective studies being required to assess this interaction on T2D incidence. Moreover, in addition to the TCF7L-2-rs7903146 SNP, other SNPs have been associated with T2D risk [10,16–18]. These SNPs are combined and analyzed together in the so-called genetic risk scores (GRS) to predict T2D [16–18]. However, simply summing up the number of risk alleles (unweighted or weighted) associated with T2D obtained from non-stratified genome-wide association studies (GWAS) in conventional GRS calculations may overlook important obesity-specific associations in T2D. Although the GRS usually include dozens of SNPs associated with T2D, one of the most important SNPs is the rs7903146 C > T in the TCF7L2 gene [9–11,16]. Recently, large prospective studies have focused on the interaction between some multi-SNP GRS and BMI on T2D incidence [16–19], among them, that of Langerberg et al. [16], employing a case-cohort design in the EPIC interact study. The authors found a statistically significant interaction between a GRS comprising 49 SNPs associated with T2D and BMI (three categories) in determining T2D incidence, the genetic risk being greater in lean subjects. However, on examining the interaction of each SNP of the GRS with BMI on T2D incidence, no statistically significant interaction with BMI was found for the TCF7L2-rs7903146 SNP [16]. This could be because they did not specifically test the interaction with obesity and made a strict correction for multiple comparisons due to the simultaneous analyses of 7 phenotypes and 49 SNPs in the same study. Bearing the results of the result in EPIC cohort in mind, this interaction, therefore, must be prospectively validated in studies focusing on the TCF7L2-rs7903146 polymorphism (to avoid the need of correction for multiple SNP comparisons) and obesity.

Furthermore, the heterogeneity of associations related to this locus also extends to BMI. The T-allele, conferring higher T2D risk, has been associated with lower BMI in some studies [20–23], but not in others [24–26]. A modulation of this association by T2D was first suggested by Helgason et al. [27] who showed that the TCF7L2-T2D risk allele was correlated with decreased BMI in T2D cases but not in controls. Similar results were observed both by Cauchi et al. [21] and in a meta-analysis including more than 300,000 individuals [28], but further studies are required to explore this interaction prospectively. Moreover, as previous findings come from studies focusing on either obesity or T2D, it is necessary to obtain comprehensive evidence of the interplay between both interactions prospectively in the same population. Therefore, our main aims were: (1) To investigate the interaction between the TCF7L2-rs7903146 polymorphism and obesity status in determining T2D prevalence as well as T2D incidence after a median ~6-year follow-up and (2) to examine whether the association of the TCF7L2-rs7903146 SNP with obesity-related parameters depends on T2D status both at baseline and prospectively in the PREvención con DIeta MEDiterránea (PREDIMED) study. In addition, a secondary aim was to construct obesity-specific GRS (analyzing 10 T2D-SNPs previously characterized [16]) in determining T2D prevalence in a sub-sample of PREDIMED participants in order to extend the findings to other T2D-SNPs.

2. Materials and Methods

The present study was conducted within the framework of the PREDIMED trial, the design of which has been described in detail elsewhere [29]. Briefly, the PREDIMED study is a multicenter, randomized, and controlled clinical trial aimed at assessing the effects of the Mediterranean diet (MedDiet) on the primary cardiovascular prevention [30]. This study was registered at controlled-trials.com (http://www.controlledtrials.com/ISRCTN35739639). Here we included 7018 participants from whom DNA was isolated, the TCF7L2-rs7903146 determined, and who had valid data for the main clinical and lifestyle variables analyzed. From October 2003 physicians in Primary Care Centers selected high cardiovascular risk participants. Eligible were community-dwelling persons (55–80 years for men; 60–80 years for women) who met at least one of two criteria: T2D or three or more cardiovascular risk factors [29]. The Institutional Review Board of each participating center approved the study protocol, and all participants provided written informed consent. The trial was stopped following the statistical analysis of data obtained up to December 2010 (median follow-up of 4.8 years), due to early evidence of the benefit of the MedDiet on the prevention of major cardiovascular events [30]. However, the ascertainment of endpoints was extended. The present study is based on the extended follow-up (until 30 June 2012) using the same methods to obtain updated information on clinical events, including T2D. The median follow-up time in this extended follow-up was 5.7 years (maximum: 8.7 years). The present study was mainly conducted as an observational prospective cohort design with adjustment for the nutritional intervention in the longitudinal analyses. In addition, some association analyses were carried out at baseline.

2.1. Demographic, Clinical, Anthropometric, and Dietary Measurements

The baseline examination included assessment of standard cardiovascular risk factors, medication use, socio-demographic factors, and lifestyle variables by validated questionnaires [29,30]. Weight and height were measured with calibrated scales and a wall-mounted stadiometer, respectively. BMI and the waist-to-height ratio were calculated. Obesity was defined as BMI $\geq$30 kg/m^2. Percentage of body fat was evaluated by using a validated equation [31].

2.2. Biochemical Determinations, DNA Extraction and Genotyping

At baseline, blood samples were obtained after overnight fasting. Fasting glucose and lipids were measured as previously described [30,32]. Genomic DNA was extracted from buffy-coat and the TCF7L2-rs7903146, was genotyped in the whole cohort on a 7900 HT Sequence Detection System (Applied Biosystems, Foster City, CA, USA) using a fluorescent allelic discrimination TaqManTM assay as previously reported [33]. Genotype frequencies did not deviate from Hardy–Weinberg equilibrium expectations.

For the secondary outcome focused on the predictive value of the obesity-specific GRSs, in addition to the TCF7L2-rs7903146 SNP, nine previously described SNPs associated with T2D, and included in a 49-SNP T2D-GRS [16], were selected and genotyped. The selected SNPs were: PRC1 (Protein Regulator of Cytokinesis 1)-rs12899811, ZFAND6 (Zinc Finger AN1-Type Containing 6)-rs11634397, CDC123_CAMK1D (Cell Division Cycle Protein 123 Homolog_Calcium/Calmodulin Dependent Protein Kinase ID)-rs11257655, KCNQ1 (Potassium Voltage-Gated Channel Subfamily Q Member 1)-rs163184, ADYC5 (adenylyl cyclase 6)-rs6798189, IGF2BP2 (Insulin Like Growth Factor 2 MRNA Binding Protein 2)-rs4402960, SLC30A8 (Solute Carrier Family 30 Member 8)-rs3802177, KLHDC5 (Kelch Domain-Containing Protein 5)-rs10842994, and HMGA2 (High Mobility Group AT-Hook 2)-rs2261181. Genotyping was carried out with the HumanOmniExpress Illumina array in a sub-sample (all the participants from one of the PREDIMED field centers, the PREDIMED-Valencia center; n = 1055 subjects), as it was not possible to genotype the whole cohort. Genotype frequencies did not deviate from Hardy–Weinberg equilibrium expectations.

2.3. Outcomes and Follow-Up

Clinical diagnosis of T2D was an inclusion criterion of the PREDIMED study [29], and these subjects were considered as prevalent cases of T2D. Incidence of T2D was a pre-specified secondary outcome of the PREDIMED trial [30]. New-onset diabetes during follow-up was diagnosed using the American Diabetes Association criteria, namely fasting plasma glucose levels $\geq$7.0 mmol/L ($\geq$126.1 mg/dL) or 2-h plasma glucose levels $\geq$11.1 mmol/L ($\geq$200.0 mg/dL) after a 75-g oral glucose load, as previously reported [32]. A review of all medical records of participants was completed yearly in each center by physician-investigators who were blinded to the intervention. When new-onset diabetes cases were identified on the basis of a medical diagnosis reported in the medical charts or on a glucose test during routine biochemical analyses (conducted at least once per year), these reports were sent to the PREDIMED Clinical Events Committee [32]. When a new case of T2D was detected, the glucose analysis was repeated within the next three months, so that the new case of diabetes could be confirmed by the adjudication committee. Cases that occurred between 1 October 2003 and 30 June 2012 (maximum: 8.7 years; median: 5.7 years) were included in the present analysis (n = 312).

Given that the study involved an open cohort, in which the inclusion of participants lasted from 1 October 2003 to 1 December 2009, not all participants had the same length of follow-up period [29]. Hence for the longitudinal analyses of BMI in relation to the polymorphism and T2D, two follow-up periods were selected; one of up to four years and the other up to six years. There were a greater number of participants in the first period (n = 3141), as most of the cohort completed this follow-up period. A lower number of participants had anthropometric measurements at six years (n = 1750), but this group was considered to be of interest both for the internal replication of the finding and for providing more evidence of the interaction. Only participants whose anthropometric data had been directly measured were included.

2.4. Statistical Analyses

The present analysis was mainly conducted as an observational prospective cohort study with adjustment for the nutritional intervention in longitudinal analyses. In addition, some analyses were carried out cross-sectionally at baseline (*n* = 7018). Prevalence of diagnosed T2D was analyzed as the dependent variable at baseline. In the longitudinal analysis, incidence of T2D was considered as the end-point in non-diabetic subjects (*n* = 3607). Moreover, baseline and annual BMI evolution was considered as the dependent variable for evaluating the interaction of the polymorphism with T2D in determining BMI.

2.4.1. Baseline Association and Interaction Analyses in Determining T2D Prevalence and Obesity-Related Variables

Chi-square tests were used to test differences in percentages. We first tested the polymorphism by considering the 3 genotypes. The interactions between the TCF7L2-rs7903146 polymorphism and obesity in determining T2D prevalence at baseline was tested by multivariable logistic regression models including main effect and interaction terms. Models were adjusted for basic potential confounders (age, gender, and center) (Model 1). Afterwards, an additional control for more potential confounders such as alcohol consumption, physical activity, adherence to the MedDiet, total energy intake, hypertension, and dyslipidemias was undertaken (Model 2). Analyses stratified by obesity status were also undertaken for models 1 and 2. CC subjects were considered as the reference category and the effect in CT and TT was estimated. Odds ratios (OR) and 95% Confidence intervals (CI) were estimated. Likewise, the interaction between the TCF7L2 polymorphism and T2D in determining obesity prevalence at baseline was evaluated by multivariable logistic regression models (model 1 and model 2), and stratified analysis by T2D status undertaken. In addition, associations between the TCF7L2 polymorphism and baseline BMI and other obesity-related variables were analyzed by linear regression models including main effects and interaction terms. Multivariable adjustments for potential confounding variables were carried out as indicated above. Analyses stratified by T2D were also undertaken.

2.4.2. Interaction Analysis between the TCF7L2-rs7903146 Polymorphism and Obesity in Determining T2D Incidence

This analysis was carried out in non-T2D subjects at baseline. We used Cox regression models with the length of follow-up as the primary time variable. Follow-up time was calculated from the date of enrollment to the date of diagnosis of T2D for cases, and to the date of the last visit or the end of the follow-up period (30 June 2012 for non-cases), or the date at death, whichever came first. Hazard ratios (HR) with 95% CI for the TCF7L2-rs7903146 genotypes (three categories), stratified by obesity were computed. Afterwards, C-allele carriers were grouped together and compared with C-carriers (recessive model). Multivariable Cox regression models with main effects and interaction terms were computed. In multivariable Model 1 (basic model) we adjusted for sex, age, center, and intervention group. In multivariable Model 2 additional adjustments were undertaken as previously described. Stratified analyses by obesity were carried out. In addition, Kaplan–Meier survival curves (one minus the cumulative T2D free survival) were plotted to estimate the probability of remaining free of T2D during follow-up depending on the TCF7L2 genotype and obesity status.

2.4.3. Predictive Value Calculations for the TCF72-rs7903146 Polymorphism on T2D Incidence and Prevalence in the Whole PREDIMED Participants

To estimate the predictive ability of the genetic models depending on the obesity status, we used two approaches: (a) In non-T2D subjects, we estimated its sensitivity, specificity, positive predictive value (PPV), negative predictive value (NPV) for two categories (recessive model) in predicting T2D incidence taking into account obesity status; (b) At baseline, we estimated the area under the receiver operating characteristic curve (AUC) [19] of the TCF7L2-rs7903146 (as 0, 1 and 2) to predict T2D prevalence depending on obesity status (we selected the recessive and additive models for T2D incidence and prevalence prediction based on the observed association results).

2.4.4. Construction of Obesity-Specific GRS with the TCF7L2 and Other T2D-SNPs; Association and Evaluation of the PV for T2D Prevalence

Taking into account the obesity-specific association of the TCF7L2 polymorphism with T2D, our secondary aim was to extend this analysis to more T2D SNPs. This was considered a pilot study as we only have genotype data from one of the PREDIMED field centers (PREDIMED-Valencia participants with complete data; n = 1000 participants; 46% T2D prevalence). These SNPs were selected from the list of 49 SNPs associated with T2D that were used in the EPIC-InterAct study for the multi-SNP GRS construction and T2D association [16]. From the list of the 49 T2D-SNP, in addition to the TCF7L2-SNP, we selected those included in our genotyping array (n = 27) and specifically tested the association between the corresponding SNP and T2D by obesity status. Those SNPs showing suggestive heterogeneity in the associations in our population were included in the obesity-specific GRS analyses (PRC1-rs12899811, ZFAND6-rs11634397, CDC123_CAMK1D-rs11257655, KCNQ1-rs163184, ADYC5-rs6798189, IGF2BP2-rs4402960, SLC30A8-rs3802177, KLHDC5-rs10842994, and HMGA2-rs2261181). For some of these SNPs (in the ZFAND6, ADYC5, IGF2BP2, SLC30A8, KLHDC5, and HMGA2 genes), statistically significant or borderline significant interactions with BMI (or with waist circumference) in determining T2D were reported in the EPIC-InterAct study (p = 0.055, p < 0.01; p = 0.034; p = 0.099; p = 0.10, respectively) [16]. However, the authors did not construct obesity-specific GRS. Depending on the results obtained in the stratified analysis, SNPs were grouped in two obesity-specific GRS. One GRS included five T2D-SNPs more associated with T2D in obese subjects (obGRS); and the other GRS included five T2D-SNPs more associated with T2D in non-obese subjects (nobGRS). nobGRS: TCF7L2-rs7903146, PRC1-rs12899811, ZFAND6-rs11634397, CDC123_CAMK1D-rs11257655 and KCNQ1-rs163184; obGRS: ADYC5-rs6798189, IGF2BP2-rs4402960, SLC30A8-rs3802177, KLHDC5-rs10842994 and HMGA2-rs2261181. SNPs in these GRS were considered as additive (0, 1, or 2 risk alleles). Multivariable logistic regression models with prevalent T2D as dependent variable and the obesity-specific GRS (as continuous) as independent variables, adjusted for age, sex, and obesity were fitted for the total and for obese and non-obese subjects; OR and 95% CI were calculated to estimate the association between the GRS and T2D.

Finally; the AUC of the two GRS predicting T2D at baseline in the PREDIMED-Valencia subsample by obesity status (obesity-specific GRS) in the whole population and in obese and non-obese subjects were calculated.

2.4.5. Longitudinal Association and Interaction Analysis between the TCF7L2-rs7903146 Polymorphism and T2D in Determining BMI

The longitudinal influence of the TCF7L2-rs7903146 polymorphism and T2D on BMI was analyzed by multivariable-ANCOVA of repeated measures including those subjects having complete data at baseline, 1, 2, 3, and 4 years (first four-year period) and at baseline, 1, 2, 3, 4, 5, and 6 years (second six-year period).

2.4.6. Power Calculations

Sample size in the PREDIMED study (n = 7447 participants) was estimated taking into account the expected incidence of the primary outcome (incidence of cardiovascular diseases) and the differences in the effects of the dietary interventions to be detected among groups [30]. In the present study, we focused on T2D prevalence and T2D incidence in PREDIMED participants with the TCF7L2-*rs7903146* data available (n = 7018). At baseline our study (including n = 3607 non-T2D and n = 3411 T2D subjects), had a large statistical power (>80%) to detect associations (OR >1.2) at alpha = 5% between the TCF7L2 polymorphism and T2D prevalence in obese and non-obese subjects. Taking into account the similar sample size of T2D and non-T2D subjects at baseline, as well as the %

of obese and non-obese subjects, our study has the strong advantage of having comparable statistical power to detect a similar association in both groups. Therefore, the lack of association between the TCF7L2-rs7903146 polymorphism and T2D risk in the stratified analyses in obese or non-obese subjects is not due to the lack of power in one of the groups. At baseline, our sample size was adequately powered (power >80%) to detect statistically significant TCF7L2-obesity interactions (at alpha <5%) in determining T2D prevalence (>40%) at an interaction effect of OR for interaction >1.21 (co-dominant model). Similar estimations in sample size and effects were computed for the interaction between the TC7L2 polymorphism and T2D in determining obesity risk. For continuous variables our sample size at baseline was adequately powered (power >80%) to detect statistically significant interactions and associations in the effect strata. In the longitudinal analysis, taking into account that the number of incident cases of T2D was small (n = 312) and that only non-T2D subjects at baseline were considered (n = 3607), the power to detect statistically significant interactions and association was lower than in the baseline analysis. Therefore, at alpha = 5% and beta = 20%, our sample size was adequately powered (>80%) to detected interaction effects (recessive model) of HR >1.75. Statistical analyses were performed with the IBM SPSS Statistics version 22, NY. All tests were two-tailed and p values < 0.05 were considered statistically significant.

3. Results

Table 1 shows the characteristics of the studied population (n = 7018 subjects) as a whole and depending on the T2D status at baseline.

Table 1. Demographic, clinical, lifestyle, and genetic characteristics of the study participants at baseline according to the diabetes status.

	Total (n = 7018)		Non-Diabetic Subjects (n = 3607)		T2D Subjects (n = 3411)		p
Age (years)	67.0	±6.2	66.6	±6.1	67.4	±6.3	<0.001
Weight (Kg)	76.8	±11.9	76.7	±11.7	76.9	±12.2	0.476
BMI (Kg/m^2)	30.0	±3.8	30.1	±3.7	29.9	±4.0	0.042
Waist circumference (cm)	100.4	±10.6	99.7	±10.6	101.2	±10.5	<0.001
Body fat (%)	39.3	±7.4	39.9	±7.2	38.7	±7.7	<0.001
Female sex: n, %	4025	(57.4)	2232	(61.9)	1793	(52.6)	<0.001
Current smokers: n, %	989	(14.1)	581	(16.1)	408	(12.0)	<0.001
TCF7L2-rs7903146: n, %							<0.001
CC	2770	(39.5)	1612	(44.7)	1158	(33.9)	
CT	3249	(46.3)	1569	(43.5)	1680	(49.3)	
TT	999	(14.2)	426	(11.8)	573	(16.8)	
Intervention groups: n, %							0.059
MedDiet + EVOO	2411	(34.4)	1204	(33.4)	1207	(35.4)	
MedDiet + nuts	2316	(33.0)	1235	(34.2)	1081	(31.7)	
Control group	2291	(32.6)	1168	(32.4)	1123	(32.9)	
Energy intake (kcal/day)	2276	±607	2322	±603	2228	±607	<0.001
Total fat (% energy)	39.2	±6.8	38.5	±6.5	39.9	±7.0	<0.001
Saturated fat (% energy)	10.0	±2.3	9.7	±2.2	10.2	±2.3	<0.001
MUFA (% energy)	19.5	±4.6	19.2	±4.3	19.7	±4.8	<0.001
Carbohydrates (% energy)	41.9	±7.2	42.8	±6.9	40.9	±7.3	<0.001
Adherence to the MedDiet	8.7	±2.0	8.7	±2.0	8.6	±2.0	0.003
Alcohol consumption (g/day)	8.4	±14.2	9.1	±14.8	7.6	±13.5	<0.001
Physical activity (MET.min/day)	231.6	±240.4	225.5	±226.8	238.0	±253.8	0.030
SBP (mm·Hg)	149.3	±20.8	149.0	±20.6	149.7	±21.0	0.187
DBP (mm·Hg)	83.4	±11.0	84.5	±11.0	82.2	±10.9	<0.001
Total cholesterol (mg/dL)	211.0	±39.4	220.0	±39.8	201.4	±36.6	<0.001
LDL-C (mg/dL)	130.3	±35.1	137.9	±36.2	122.1	±31.8	<0.001
HDL-C (mg/dL)	53.8	±14.1	55.8	±14.6	51.7	±13.2	<0.001
Triglycerides (mg/dL)	137.4	±79.7	132.6	±73.9	142.4	±85.2	<0.001
Fasting glucose (mg/dL)	122.2	±41.6	98.2	±16.4	147.4	±45.1	<0.001

Values are mean ± SD for continuous variables and number (%) for categorical variables. T2D indicates Type 2 diabetes. BMI indicates body mass index, MUFA, Monounsaturated fatty acids; MedDiet, Mediterranean diet; EVOO, extra virgin olive oil, SPB: Systolic blood pressure, DBP: Diastolic blood pressure. p: p-value for the comparisons (means or %) between non-diabetic and type 2 diabetic subjects.

3.1. Interaction between the TCF7L2-rs7903146 Polymorphism and Obesity in Determining T2D at Baseline

Even though the TCF7L2-rs7903146 polymorphism was significantly associated with a higher T2D prevalence in the whole population ($p = 3.1 \times 10^{-21}$), this association was of greater magnitude (OR: 2.26; 95% CI: 1.84–2.78 for TT compared to CC homozygotes; $p = 1.6 \times 10^{-14}$) in non-obese ($n = 3739$) than in obese ($n = 3279$) subjects (OR: 1.51; 95% CI: 1.22–1.92 for TT compared to CC homozygotes; $p = 0.0002$) even after multivariable adjustment (Table 2).

Table 2. Association between the TCF7L2-rs7903146 polymorphism and prevalence of T2D depending on the obesity status at baseline. Stratified logistic regression analysis.

		Non-Obese			p[3] for Interaction			Obese		
	n	OR	95% CI	p-Value	Genotype × Obesity	n	OR	95% CI	p-Value
Model 1[1]					0.002				
TCF7L2									
CC	1424	1.00	(reference)			1346	1.00	(reference)	
CT	1742	1.79	(1.55–2.08)	5.5×10^{-15}		1507	1.28	(1.10–1.49)	0.0012
TT	573	2.32	(1.90–2.85)	5.4×10^{-16}		426	1.51	(1.21–1.89)	0.0003
		p[4]: 2.5×10^{-20}						p[4]: 0.0002		
Model 2[2]									
TCF7L2									
CC		1.00	(reference)				1.00	(reference)	
CT		1.78	(1.54–2.09)	1.4×10^{-14}	0.003		1.27	(1.09–1.48)	0.0020
TT		2.26	(1.84–2.78)	1.6×10^{-14}			1.53	(1.22–1.92)	0.0002
		p[4]: 4.3×10^{-19}						p[4]: 0.00017		

[1] Model 1: adjusted for sex, age, and field center; [2] Model 2: adjusted for sex, age, field center, total energy intake, adherence to the Mediterranean diet, alcohol intake, smoking, physical activity, dyslipidemia, and hypertension; [3] p-value obtained for the interaction term between the TCF7L2 genotype and obesity in the corresponding multivariable logistic regression model; [4] p-value obtained for the global TCF7L2 polymorphism in the multivariable logistic regression model.

3.2. Interaction between the TCF7L2-rs7903146 Polymorphism and T2D in Determining Obesity-Related Measures at Baseline

At baseline, the T2D risk allele was significantly associated with lower averages for BMI, body fat, waist-to-height ratio, and lower prevalence of obesity (BMI $\geq$30 kg/m^2) (Supplementary Materials Table S1). However, we detected a strong heterogeneity in these associations depending on T2D status. Figure 1 shows these interactive effects on BMI (A) and % body fat (B), the TCF7L2-rs7903146 polymorphism being inversely associated with these traits only in T2D subjects (p-interactions < 0.05). Likewise, the inverse association between the TCF7L2-rs7903146 polymorphism and obesity at baseline (Table 3) was statistically significant in T2D ($p = 0.0002$) but not in non-T2D subjects ($p = 0.737$). Accordingly, the multivariable adjusted OR for obesity in TT subjects compared to CC individuals was 0.63; 95% CI 0.51–0.78; $p = 1.63 \times 10^{-5}$ in T2D, showing a reduced risk, and no association (0.93; 95% CI: 0.74–1.16; $p = 0.493$) in non-diabetic subjects.

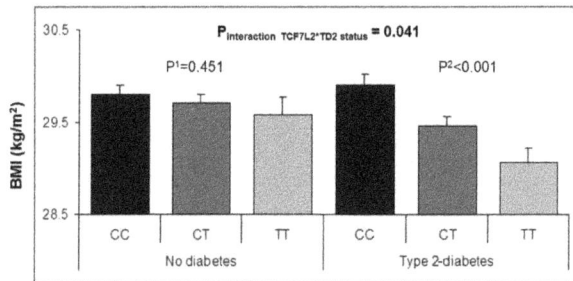

(a)

Figure 1. *Cont.*

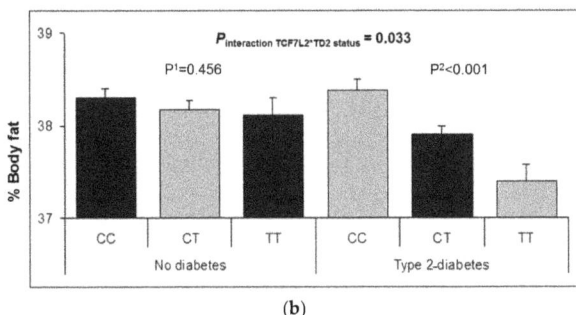

(b)

Figure 1. Adjusted means of BMI (**a**) and % body fat (**b**) at baseline depending on the TCF7L2-rs7903146 polymorphism and T2D diabetes status (*n* = in 7018 PREDIMED participants at baseline. Means were adjusted for age, sex, center, total energy intake, physical activity, smoking, drinking, adherence to the Mediterranean diet, dyslipidemia, and hypertension. The *p*-values for the interaction terms were obtained in the corresponding multivariable adjusted models. p^1 and p^2 values were obtained for the multivariable comparison of means between depending on the T2D strata in non-diabetic (*n* = 3607) subjects and T2D (*n* = 3411) subjects, respectively. Error bars: SE of means.

Table 3. Association between the TCF7L2-rs7903146 polymorphism and obesity depending on T2D status. Stratified logistic regression analysis.

		Non-Diabetic			p^3 for Interaction		T2D Subjects		
	n	OR	95% CI	*p*-Value	Genotype × T2D	*n*	OR	95% CI	*p*-Value
Model 1 [1]									
TCF7L2					0.008				
CC	1612	1.00	(reference)			1158	1.00	(reference)	
CT	1569	1.05	(0.91–1.20)	0.544		1680	0.78	(0.67–0.91)	0.001
TT	426	0.96	(0.77–1.19)	0.694		573	0.64	(0.52–0.78)	2.0×10^{-5}
			p^4: 0.685					p^4: 3.90×10^{-5}	
Model 2 [2]									
TCF7L2									
CC		1.00	(reference)				1.00	(reference)	
CT		1.05	(0.91–1.21)	0.529	0.014		0.77	(0.66–0.90)	0.001
TT		0.93	(0.74–1.16)	0.493			0.63	(0.51–0.78)	1.6×10^{-5}
			p^4: 0.528					p^4: 3.02×10^{-5}	

[1] Model 1: adjusted for sex, age, and field center; [2] Model 2: adjusted for sex, age, field center, total energy intake, adherence to the Mediterranean diet, alcohol intake, smoking, physical activity, dyslipidemia, and hypertension; [3] *p*-value obtained for the interaction term between the TCF7L2 genotype and type-2 diabetes in the corresponding multivariable logistic regression model; [4] *p*-value obtained for the global TCF7L2 polymorphism in the multivariable logistic regression model.

3.3. Interaction between the TCF7L2-rs7903146 Polymorphism and Obesity in the Incidence of T2D

We analyzed the interaction between the TCF7L2-rs7903146 polymorphism and obesity status in determining the incidence of T2D in non-diabetic subjects (*n* = 3607) over the extended follow-up period (with median 5.7 years) (Table 4). We observed that the association between the TCF7L2-rs7903146 and T2D incidence only was statistically significant in obese subjects (*p* = 0.035 in the basic model and *p* = 0.045 in the additionally adjusted model). Thus, we observer a significantly stronger association in non-obese (HR: 1.81; 95% CI: 1.13–2.92, *p* = 0.013 for TT versus CC) than in obese individuals (HR: 1.01; 95% CI: 0.61–1.66; *p* = 0.979); *p*-interaction = 0.048. A recessive effect was found in agreement with results obtained in previous studies [20]. Figure 2 shows T2D-free survival Kaplan–Meier curves in non-obese (A) and obese subjects (B). Taking into account that a recessive effect was noted, homozygous subjects for the risk allele (TT) were also compared with C-allele carriers.

Furthermore, we estimated the influence of obesity status on T2D incidence over the 5.7-year median follow-up period in this population in the whole sample and depending on the TCF7L2-rs7903146 polymorphism. Although for the whole population of T2D-free subjects at baseline obesity was significantly associated with higher TD2 risk (HR: 1.44; 95% CI: 1.14–1.82; p = 0.002), this association was heterogeneous in the different genotypes (Supplementary Materials Figure S1). Thus, in CC subjects, obesity was strongly associated with T2D incidence (HR: 1.75; 95% CI: 1.22–2.51; p = 0.002 in obese compared with non-obese). This significant association decreased in CT subjects (HR: 1.45; 95% CI: 102–2.07; p = 0.041 in obese versus non-obese subjects). No significant association between obesity status and T2D incidence was found in subjects with the TT genotype (HR: 0.79; 95% CI: 0.43–1.46; p = 0.454).

Table 4. Incidence and hazard ratios (HR) for T2D depending on the TCF7L2-rs7903146 polymorphism and stratified by obesity after 5.7 years of median follow-up.

	Cases	Non-Cases	Person-Years	Incidence Rate [4]	Model 1 [2]			Model 2 [3]		
					HR	95% CI	p-Value	HR	95% CI	p-Value
					**Obese Subjects [1]** (n = 1693)					
TCF7L2 genotypes							0.960			0.965
CC	73	677	4117.5	17.7	1.00	(reference)		1.00	(reference)	
CT	79	669	4203.8	18.8	1.04	(0.76–1.44)	0.777	1.05	(0.76–1.46)	0.750
TT	21	174	1094.0	19.2	1.01	(0.62–1.65)	0.957	1.01	(0.61–1.66)	0.979
					Non-Obese Subjects (n = 1904)					
					Model 1 [2]			Model 2 [3]		
TCF7L2 genotypes							0.035			0.045
CC	56	803	4819.0	11.6	1.00	(reference)		1.00	(reference)	
CT	57	758	4661.8	12.2	1.08	(0.75–1.57)	0.671	1.14	(0.79–1.66)	0.531
TT	26	204	1285.7	20.2	1.82	(1.14–2.92)	0.012	1.81	(1.13–2.92)	0.013

[1] Obesity: BMI $\geq$ 30 kg/m^2; [2] Model 1: Adjusted for sex, age, field center, and dietary intervention group; [3] Model 2: Adjusted for variables in model 1 plus total energy intake, adherence to the Mediterranean diet, alcohol intake, smoking, physical activity, dyslipidemia, and hypertension at baseline; [4] Crude incidence rates are expressed per 1000 person-years of follow-up.

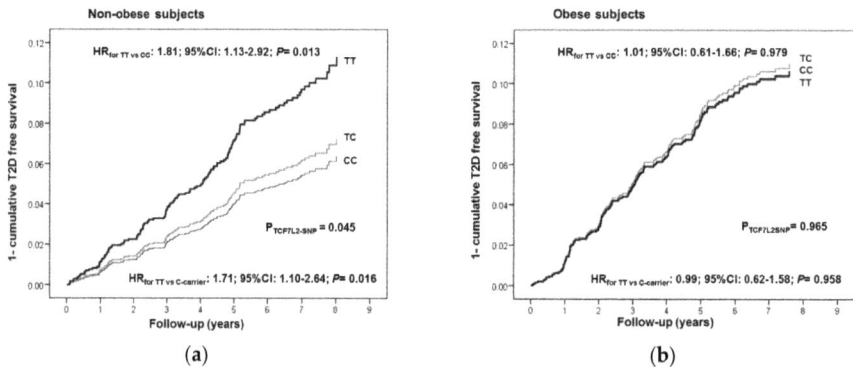

Figure 2. One minus the cumulative T2D-free survival by TCF7L2-rs7903146 genotypes in non-diabetic subjects at baseline (n = 3607) depending of the obesity status: non-obese subjects (**a**) and obese subjects (**b**). Cox regression models with outcome of T2D incidence by the TCF7L2-rs7903146 polymorphism (CC, CT and TT) were adjusted for sex, age, center, intervention group, alcohol, smoking, total energy intake and adherence to the Mediterranean diet, physical activity, smoking, drinking, dyslipidemia, and hypertension at baseline. HR and 95% CI were obtained in the multivariable adjusted model. The p-values for the TCF7L2 polymorphism and for the corresponding genotypes (TT versus CC or TT versus C-carriers) were obtained in the multivariable adjusted models.

3.4. Predictive Ability of the TCF7L2-rs7903146 on T2D Incidence and Prevalence Depending on Obesity Status

Supplementary Materials Table S2 shows the sensitivity, specificity, PPV, and NPV for the TCF7L2-SNP (as recessive according to the observed association effect) on predicting T2D incidence in non-TD2 PREDIMED participants. Significantly better parameters were obtained in non-obese subjects ($p = 0.03$) than in obese subjects ($p = 0.787$).

Likewise, in the ROC analysis, the AUC for the TCF7L2 SNP (additive model) for T2D prevalence in PREDIMED participants was higher in non-obese (AUC: 0.58; $p = 1.37 \times 10^{-17}$) than in obese subjects (AUC: 0.53; $p = 1.4 \times 10^{-4}$) (Supplementary Materials Figure S2).

3.5. Obesity Specific-GRS Construction, Association with T2D Prevalence and Estimations of the Predictive Value of These GRS in a Subsample of Participants

Our secondary aim was to extend the TCF7L2 analysis to more T2D SNPs. This was considered a pilot study as we only have genotype data from one of the PREDIMED field centers ($n = 1000$ PREDIMED-Valencia participants with complete data). In addition to the TCF7L2-rs7903146 SNP, we selected nine T2D-SNPs from the list of the 49 SNPs included in the T2D-GRS used in the EPIC-Interact Study [16] (see statistical analysis for the SNP selection) and tested their association with T2D prevalence by obesity strata in our sample. Those SNPs showing significant (or near significance) associations in one of the obesity strata were selected for combination in the corresponding obesity-specific GRS (nobGRS and obGRS). Five SNPs in each score were combined (nobGRS: TCF7L2-rs7903146, PRC1-rs12899811, ZFAND6-rs11634397, CDC123_CAMK1D-rs11257655 and KCNQ1-rs163184; obGRS: ADYC5-rs6798189, IGF2BP2-rs4402960, SLC30A8-rs3802177, KLHDC5-rs10842994, and HMGA2-rs2261181 as indicated in methods). Supplementary Materials Figure S3 shows frequency distribution of nobGRS (A) and obGRS (B) in the whole sample ($n = 1000$). First, we tested the association of these obesity-specific GRS with T2D prevalence in obese and non-obese subjects (Supplementary Materials Table S3). As expected, the nobGRS was significantly associated with T2D in non-obese subjects ($p = 0.006$). No significant association was found for the nobGRS in obese subjects ($p = 0.535$). Likewise, the obGRS was significantly associated with T2D in obese subjects ($p < 0.001$), and not associated in non-obese subjects ($p = 0.130$). We also estimated the predictive value for these obesity-specific GRS for T2D in the whole sample (Supplementary Materials Figure S4) and by obesity strata (Figure 3). When we consider the obesity-specific GRS in their specific strata, we observed that the nobGRS had greater and significantly AUC in non-obese (AUC: 0.581; $p = 0.002$) than in obese subjects (AUC: 0.522; $p = 0.384$). Likewise, the obGRS had higher AUC in obese (0.591; $p = 0.004$) than in non-obese subjects (0.531; $p = 0.239$), thus supporting our hypothesis.

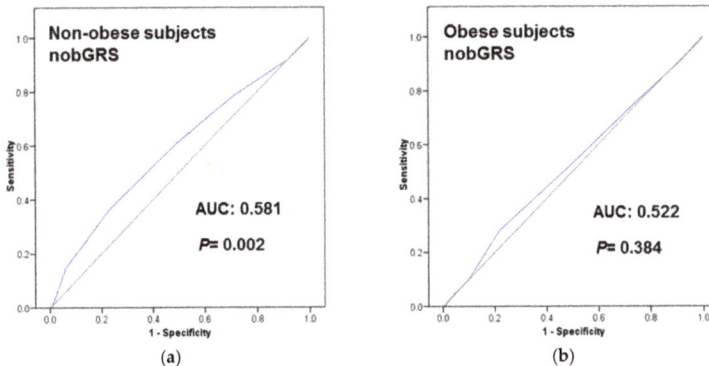

(a) (b)

Figure 3. *Cont.*

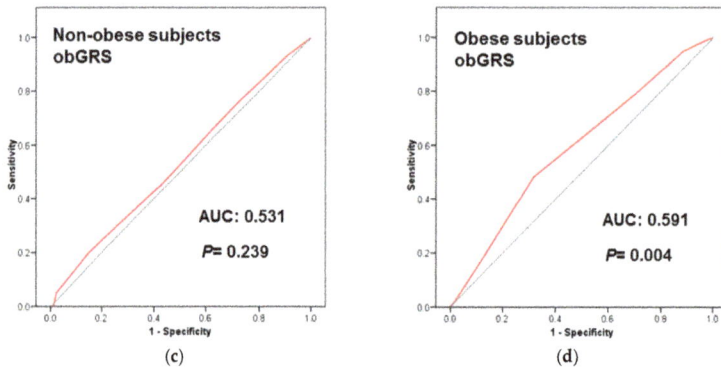

(c)   (d)

Figure 3. Receiver operating curves (ROC) of the two Genetic Risk Scores (GRS) [One including T2D-SNPs more associated in obese subjects (obGRS); and the other including T2D-SNPs more associated in non-obese subjects (nobGRS)] to predict T2D (prevalent) at baseline in the PREDIMED-Valencia participants (*n* = 1000): (**a**) nobGRS in non-obese subjects; (**b**) nobGRS in obese subjects; (**c**) obGRS in non-obese subjects; (**d**) obGRS in obese subjects. Areas under the curves (AUC) and *p*-values are indicated. The straight line represents the ROC expected by chance only. *n* = 493 non-obese and *n* = 507 obese with genotype data for all the SNPs included in the GRS were analyzed. Five SNPs were included in each unweighted additive (risk allele) GRS as follows: nobGRS: TCF7L2-rs7903146, PRC1-rs12899811, ZFAND6-rs11634397, CDC123-CAMK1D-rs11257655 and KCNQ1-rs163184; obGRS: ADYC5-rs6798189, IGF2BP2-rs4402960, SLC30A8-rs3802177, KLHDC5-rs10842994, and HMGA2-rs2261181.

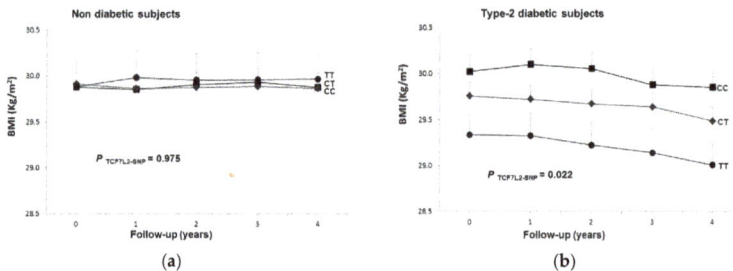

(a)   (b)

Figure 4. Longitudinal effect of the TCF7L2-rs7903146 polymorphism on BMI over a 4-year follow-up period in *n* = 3141 subjects depending on T2D status: (**a**) non-diabetic; (**b**) T2D subjects. Adjusted means BMI depending on the polymorphism (co-dominant model) and T2D at baseline and 1, 2, 3 and 4 years of follow-up in all subjects having data for all the five measurements were estimated from a repeated-measures ANOVA model with interaction terms adjusted for dietary intervention (MedDiet versus control), sex, age, center, BMI, adherence to the Mediterranean diet (AdMedDiet), smoking, drinking, and physical activity at baseline. Adjusted *p* values for the overall effect of the polymorphism and for the interaction among the polymorphism and T2D, were obtained in the multivariable model.

3.6. Longitudinal Interaction between the TCF7L2-rs7903146 Polymorphism and T2D in BMI

At baseline, we have observed a shared interactive effect between the FCF7L2-rs7903146 polymorphism and T2D in determining BMI. Here we tested whether this shared interactive effect is also observed longitudinally. We analyzed two periods based on the inclusion of a larger number of participants (at four-year follow-up, with 3141 participants) or on a longer follow-up period (at six-year follow-up, with 1750 participants). Figure 4 shows the association between the TCF7L2-SNP and BMI longitudinally for every year of the four-year follow-up period. We observed a significant heterogeneity (*p*-interaction: 0.041) in non-diabetic (A) and in T2D (B) subjects. In T2D subjects the association between the SNP and lower BMI was detected yearly (*p*-for the average inter-subjects effects: 0.02), whereas in non-diabetic subjects no significant association with BMI was observed over the follow-up period (*p*: 0.975). The later analysis, including participants with six years of follow-up, confirmed these results (Supplementary Materials Figure S5).

4. Discussion

Combining longitudinal and cross-sectional analyses in a well-characterized population [30], we have obtained new epidemiological evidence to unravel the complex relationship between the TCF7L2-rs7903146 polymorphism, obesity, and T2D. At the population level, we have obtained consistent results showing that, on the one hand, the TCF7L2-rs7903146 polymorphism significantly interacts with obesity to determine the prevalence and incidence of T2D, and, on the other, that T2D interacts with the TCF7L2-rs7903146 in BMI both at baseline and prospectively. As these three variables are so closely interrelated [1,2] it is very difficult to distinguish cause from effect. According to previous investigations [5,6,8], it seems most plausible that obesity status interacts with the TCF7L2 gene, prompting the TT risk genotype to associate itself with a higher incidence of T2D in lean subjects; perhaps the effect we observed of the T-allele being associated with lower obesity risk in T2D subjects is a secondary observation to the primary one. However, we cannot discard the real influence of the T-allele on body weight. Despite this SNP being one of the strongest common genetic determinant of T2D yet described [9–11,34], there is still much controversy over the molecular mechanisms involved in how this genetic variation of TCF7L2 gene leads to altered biological function [35–38].

Although some previous studies [5,6,12–14] have described that the TCF7L2-rs7903146 polymorphism was more strongly associated with T2D in non-obese subjects, most of these studies have been retrospective and prone to potential bias. Only one study has prospectively and specifically analyzed the interaction between the TCF7L2-rs7903146 SNP and BMI in determining T2D incidence [15]. However, this study included only men. Thus, our study, including both men and women, is the first prospective report showing that at the population level (analyzing both men and women) the TCF7L2 polymorphism is more associated with T2D incidence in non-obese subjects. Our results support and extend the findings, adding more prospective evidence to the heterogeneity in the association. Recent prospective studies [16–19] have analyzed the interaction between genetic variants and BMI on T2D using multi-SNP GRS [39] rather than focusing specifically on the TCF7L2-SNP (which was only one of the loci in the GRS). In the EPIC-InterAct study [16], where they analyzed the interaction between each of the SNPs of the GRS and BMI on T2D, despite the fact that they found that the global GRS significantly interacted with BMI, these authors did not find any significant interaction of BMI with the TCF7L2 SNP after correction for multiple comparisons. These results may be due to the fact that they undertook multiple comparisons and the statistical significance was set at $p < 0.05/343$. These results could be considered as a false negative and so clearly show the need to continue investigating this interaction in more depth. Several studies have examined the effect of other T2D-SNPs integrated in GRSs, among them that from Talmud et al. [19], including seven prospective studies and using a T2D 65-SNP GRS. They showed heterogeneity on the effects of the GRS by BMI in determining T2D (the 65-SNP GRS being associated with higher T2D incidence in leaner individuals). Talmud et al. [19] also evaluated the predictive value of the GRS and showed heterogeneity by BMI [19]. In our study, we have found better results for the TCF7L2-rs7903146 in predicting T2D in non-obese than in obese subjects. In addition to the TCF7L2, other genes [8,40,41] could be associated with higher T2D risk in non-obese individuals. Moreover a recent study carried out in Chinese subjects [42] investigated the association between a 25-SNP GRS (global and by SNP) and T2D prevalence in obese and non-obese subjects separately, concluding that some SNP were strongly associated with T2D in non-obese subjects, whereas others were specific for obese subjects. However, the authors did not construct obesity-specific GRS.

An important finding of our study is that, unlike previous studies, we have constructed obesity-specific GRS by combining in the specific score only those SNPs more associated with T2D in the specific obesity strata. Thus we constructed an obGRS (including the T2D-SNPs more associated with T2D in obese subjects) and a nobGRS (including the T2D-SNPs more associated with T2D in non-obese subjects, such as the TCF7L2). As far as we know, this is the first time that the use of obesity-specific GRS has been tested. Our results show that, consistent with our hypothesis, a GRS including the TCF7L2 polymorphism and others in a nobGRS present greater AUC for T2D prevalence in non-obese than in obese subjects. Likewise, the obGRS presented greater AUC for T2D in obese subjects. These results support the desirability of taking stratification by obesity into account on analyzing the genetic influence in T2D. One limitation of our results is that we only have tested these GRS in a subsample of the PREDIMED study (all the subjects in a field center with genetic data available). Additional replication in the whole cohort or in another population, also using T2D incidence, will be needed to establish the concept of obesity-specific GRS. However, our preliminary results are important for this upcoming work and will improve the predictive values of the obesity-specific GRS. Thus, whereas two SNPs may present similar overall significant association with T2D incidence, this significance could be driven in one case by obesity and in the other by leanness, making it inappropriate to combine them in the same GRS.

Moreover, our results will be highly relevant for future nutrigenetic studies, taking into account that currently heterogeneity by obesity is not evaluated when analyzing gene–diet interactions in determining T2D risk. Controversial results have been reported regarding the protective effects of fiber intake depending on the TCF7L2 polymorphism [43]. According to our results, in studies aimed at analyzing gene–diet interactions involving the TCF7L2 polymorphism in the determination of T2D, stratification by obesity status should be needed. Likewise, much more investigation regarding gene–diet interactions in lean subjects with the high-risk TCF7L2-rs7903146-genotype is needed to better characterize the potential dietary modulations for T2D prevention.

Overall, these data support the need to carry out analyses stratified by obesity when evaluating genetic associations and gene–diet interactions in determining T2D. This will be key when examining the sensitivity and specificity of genetic analyses to predict T2D risk, as these parameters may vary substantially depending on the obesity status of the person submitted to the test. Along these lines, some studies examining the potential utility of the TCF7L2 gene variant for the prediction of T2D have produced disappointing results [44,45]. Assessing heterogeneity by obesity and other factors may help to fill the gap that exists between genetic discoveries and their practical applications to T2D prevention [46,47].

In terms of obesity as an outcome, our results also suggest an inverse association of the TCF7L2 polymorphism with BMI in T2D subjects. In agreement with us, a meta-analysis of GWAs [28] detected such heterogeneity at the cross-sectional level but did not explore this association longitudinally, with stronger effects in T2D case/control studies (the T2D-risk allele associated with lower BMI) than in population-based studies. As far as we know, our study is the first to show a prospective interaction between the TCF7L2-rs7903146 polymorphism and T2D in determining BMI (up to six years). This is also important as other studies have focused on gene–diet interactions on weight changes involving the TCF7L2 polymorphism [48]. In these studies stratification by T2D status should be considered to reduce the confounding effect of this heterogeneity. Our interaction results will be highly relevant for upcoming nutrigenetic studies focusing on the influence of the TCF7L2 polymorphism on BMI.

5. Conclusions

In conclusion, we have comprehensively demonstrated that the TCF7L2-rs7903146 polymorphism interacts with obesity status in determining T2D risk, emphasizing the heterogeneity of genetic variants' T2D risk prediction. We support stratified analysis by obesity or by T2D, depending on whether the association of the TCF7L2 polymorphism with T2D or with BMI is being investigated. We suggest that taking into account this heterogeneity by obesity will improve the predictive value of this SNP in

Nutrients **2016**, *8*, 793

determining T2D risk. Moreover, this heterogeneity of the TCF7L2-rs7903146 effects on T2D can be extended to other T2D SNPs and we have created for the first time the concept of obesity-specific GRS. We have tested two obesity-specific GRS, showing an increase in the predictive value of the GRS in the corresponding strata. The creation and validation of the proposed obesity-specific GRS, including more SNPs, will be important in the new era of personalized genetic risk prediction for T2D as well as in nutrigenetic studies for more accurate testing of gene–diet interactions.

Supplementary Materials: The following are available online at http://www.mdpi.com/2072-6643/8/12/793/s1.

Acknowledgments: This study was funded by the Spanish Ministry of Health (Instituto de Salud Carlos III) and the Ministerio de Economía y Competitividad-Fondo Europeo de Desarrollo Regional (projects PI051839, PI070240, PI1001407, G03/140, CIBER 06/03, RD06/0045 PI07-0954, CNIC-06, PI11/02505, SAF2009-12304, AGL2010-22319-C03-03, and PRX14/00527; contract JR14/00008), by the University Jaume I (Project P1-1B2013-54) and by the Generalitat Valenciana (AP111/10, AP-042/11, BEST/2015/087, GVACOMP2011-151, ACOMP/2011/145, ACOMP/2012/190, and ACOMP/2013/159). CIBEROBN is an initiative of Institute of Health Carlos III of Spain which is supported by FEDER funds (CB06/03).This material is based upon work supported by the U.S. Department of Agriculture—Agricultural Research Service (ARS), under Agreement No. 58-1950-4-003. Dolores Corella acknowledges the collaboration of the Real Colegio Complutense at Harvard University, Cambridge. MA, USA. The PREDIMED study was registered at controlled-trials.com (http://www.controlledtrials.com/ISRCTN35739639; ethics approval by the Institutional Review Board of the Hospital Clinic at Barcelona, Spain, 16/07/2002, under the protocol number "G03/140"). The Institutional Review Board of each participating center approved the study protocol, and all participants provided written informed consent. The Institutional Review Board of the Valencia University (protocol number "G03/140", 22/05/2003) approved the PREDIMED-Valencia study protocol, and all participants provided written informed consent.

Author Contributions: Dolores Corella, José V. Sorlí, Ramón Estruch, Miguel Ángel Martínez-González, Jordi Salas-Salvadó, Fernando Arós, Manuel Ortega-Calvo, Lluís Serra-Majem, Enrique Gómez-Gracia, Miquel Fiol, Montserrat Fitó, Emilio Ros and José M. Ordovás conceived the study concept and design, obtained funding, and reviewed the manuscript. Laura Quiles, Olga Castañer, Olga Portolés, Javier Díez Espino and Josep Basora acquired data and reviewed the manuscript. Oscar Coltell designed and developed the data management system and managed all submission procedures. Dolores Corella, Oscar Coltell and José M. Ordovás analyzed and interpreted data, wrote the manuscript, and reviewed/edited the manuscript. Dolores Corella is the guarantor of this work and, as such, had full access to all the data in the study and takes responsibility for the integrity of the data and the accuracy of the data analysis.

Conflicts of Interest: The authors declare no conflict of interest. The founding sponsors had no role in the design of the study; in the collection, analyses, or interpretation of data; in the writing of the manuscript, and in the decision to publish the results.

References

1. Jaacks, L.M.; Siegel, K.R.; Gujral, U.P.; Narayan, K.M. Type 2 diabetes: A 21st century epidemic. *Best Pract. Res. Clin. Endocrinol. Metab.* **2016**, *30*, 331–343. [CrossRef] [PubMed]

2. Kahn, S.E.; Cooper, M.E.; Del Prato, S. Pathophysiology and treatment of type 2 diabetes: Perspectives on the past, present, and future. *Lancet* **2014**, *383*, 1068–1083. [CrossRef]

3. Huang, T.; Qi, Q.; Zheng, Y.; Ley, S.H.; Manson, J.E.; Hu, F.B.; Qi, L. Genetic predisposition to central obesity and risk of type 2 diabetes: Two independent cohort studies. *Diabetes Care* **2015**, *38*, 1306–1311. [CrossRef] [PubMed]

4. Tuomi, T.; Santoro, N.; Caprio, S.; Cai, M.; Weng, J.; Groop, L. The many faces of diabetes: A disease with increasing heterogeneity. *Lancet* **2014**, *383*, 1084–1094. [CrossRef]

5. Timpson, N.J.; Lindgren, C.M.; Weedon, M.N.; Randall, J.; Ouwehand, W.H.; Strachan, D.P.; Rayner, N.W.; Walker, M.; Hitman, G.A.; Doney, A.S.; et al. Adiposity-related heterogeneity in patterns of type 2 diabetes susceptibility observed in genome-wide association data. *Diabetes* **2009**, *58*, 505–510. [CrossRef] [PubMed]

6. Cauchi, S.; Nead, K.T.; Choquet, H.; Horber, F.; Potoczna, N.; Balkau, B.; Marre, M.; Charpentier, G.; Froguel, P.; Meyre, D. The genetic susceptibility to type 2 diabetes may be modulated by obesity status: Implications for association studies. *BMC. Med. Genet.* **2008**, *9*, 45. [CrossRef] [PubMed]

7. Manning, A.K.; Hivert, M.F.; Scott, R.A.; Grimsby, J.L.; Bouatia-Naji, N.; Chen, H.; Rybin, D.; Liu, C.T.; Bielak, L.F.; Prokopenko, I.; et al. A genome-wide approach accounting for body mass index identifies genetic variants influencing fasting glycemic traits and insulin resistance. *Nat. Genet.* **2012**, *44*, 659–669. [CrossRef] [PubMed]

8. Perry, J.R.; Voight, B.F.; Yengo, L.; Amin, N.; Dupuis, J.; Ganser, M.; Grallert, H.; Navarro, P.; Li, M.; Qi, L.; et al. Stratifying type 2 diabetes cases by BMI identifies genetic risk variants in LAMA1 and enrichment for risk variants in lean compared to obese cases. *PLoS Genet.* **2012**, *8*, e1002741. [CrossRef] [PubMed]

9. Grant, S.F.; Thorleifsson, G.; Reynisdottir, I.; Benediktsson, R.; Manolescu, A.; Sainz, J.; Helgason, A.; Stefansson, H.; Emilsson, V.; Helgadottir, A.; et al. Variant of transcription factor 7-like 2 (TCF7L2) gene confers risk of type 2 diabetes. *Nat. Genet.* **2006**, *38*, 320–323. [CrossRef] [PubMed]

10. Voight, B.F.; Scott, L.J.; Steinthorsdottir, V.; Morris, A.P.; Dina, C.; Welch, R.P.; Zeggini, E.; Huth, C.; Aulchenko, Y.S.; Thorleifsson, G.; et al. Twelve type 2 diabetes susceptibility loci identified through large-scale association analysis. *Nat. Genet.* **2010**, *42*, 579–589. [CrossRef] [PubMed]

11. Peng, S.; Zhu, Y.; Lü, B.; Xu, F.; Li, X.; Lai, M. TCF7L2 gene polymorphisms and type 2 diabetes risk: A comprehensive and updated meta-analysis involving 121,174 subjects. *Mutagenesis* **2013**, *28*, 25–37. [CrossRef] [PubMed]

12. Bouhaha, R.; Choquet, H.; Meyre, D.; Abid Kamoun, H.; Ennafaa, H.; Baroudi, T.; Sassi, R.; Vaxillaire, M.; Elgaaied, A.; Froguel, P.; et al. TCF7L2 is associated with type 2 diabetes in nonobese individuals from Tunisia. *Pathol. Biol. (Paris)* **2010**, *58*, 426–429. [CrossRef] [PubMed]

13. Lukacs, K.; Hosszufalusi, N.; Dinya, E.; Bakacs, M.; Madacsy, L.; Panczel, P. The type 2 diabetes-associated variant in TCF7L2 is associated with latent autoimmune diabetes in adult Europeans and the gene effect is modified by obesity: A meta-analysis and an individual study. *Diabetologia* **2012**, *55*, 689–693. [CrossRef] [PubMed]

14. Kalnina, I.; Geldnere, K.; Tarasova, L.; Nikitina-Zake, L.; Peculis, R.; Fridmanis, D.; Pirags, V.; Klovins, J. Stronger association of common variants in TCF7L2 gene with nonobese type 2 diabetes in the Latvian population. *Exp. Clin. Endocrinol. Diabetes* **2012**, *120*, 466–468. [CrossRef] [PubMed]

15. Salpea, K.D.; Gable, D.R.; Cooper, J.A.; Stephens, J.W.; Hurel, S.J.; Ireland, H.A.; Feher, M.D.; Godsland, I.F.; Humphries, S.E. The effect of WNT5B IVS3C > G on the susceptibility to type 2 diabetes in UK Caucasian subjects. *Nutr. Metab. Cardiovasc. Dis.* **2009**, *19*, 140–145. [CrossRef] [PubMed]

16. Langenberg, C.; Sharp, S.J.; Franks, P.W.; Scott, R.A.; Deloukas, P.; Forouhi, N.G.; Froguel, P.; Groop, L.C.; Hansen, T.; Palla, L.; et al. Gene-lifestyle interaction and type 2 diabetes: The EPIC interact case-cohort study. *PLoS Med.* **2014**, *11*, e1001647. [CrossRef] [PubMed]

17. Vassy, J.L.; Hivert, M.F.; Porneala, B.; Dauriz, M.; Florez, J.C.; Dupuis, J.; Siscovick, D.S.; Fornage, M.; Rasmussen-Torvik, L.J.; Bouchard, C.; et al. Polygenic type 2 diabetes prediction at the limit of common variant detection. *Diabetes* **2014**, *63*, 2172–2182. [CrossRef] [PubMed]

18. Scott, R.A.; Fall, T.; Pasko, D.; Barker, A.; Sharp, S.J.; Arriola, L.; Balkau, B.; Barricarte, A.; Barroso, I.; Boeing, H.; et al. Common genetic variants highlight the role of insulin resistance and body fat distribution in type 2 diabetes, independent of obesity. *Diabetes* **2014**, *63*, 4378–4387. [CrossRef] [PubMed]

19. Talmud, P.J.; Cooper, J.A.; Morris, R.W.; Dudbridge, F.; Shah, T.; Engmann, J.; Dale, C.; White, J.; McLachlan, S.; Zabaneh, D.; et al. Sixty-five common genetic variants and prediction of type 2 diabetes. *Diabetes* **2015**, *64*, 1830–1840. [CrossRef] [PubMed]

20. Florez, J.C.; Jablonski, K.A.; Bayley, N.; Pollin, T.I.; de Bakker, P.I.; Shuldiner, A.R.; Knowler, W.C.; Nathan, D.M.; Altshuler, D. Diabetes Prevention Program Research Group. TCF7L2 polymorphisms and progression to diabetes in the Diabetes Prevention Program. *N. Engl. J. Med.* **2006**, *355*, 241–250. [CrossRef] [PubMed]

21. Cauchi, S.; Choquet, H.; Gutiérrez-Aguilar, R.; Capel, F.; Grau, K.; Proença, C.; Dina, C.; Duval, A.; Balkau, B.; Marre, M.; et al. Effects of TCF7L2 polymorphisms on obesity in European populations. *Obesity (Silver Spring)* **2008**, *16*, 476–482. [CrossRef] [PubMed]

22. Peter, I.; McCaffery, J.M.; Kelley-Hedgepeth, A.; Hakonarson, H.; Reis, S.; Wagenknecht, L.E.; Kopin, A.S.; Huggins, G.S.; Genetics Subgroup of the Look AHEAD Study. Association of type 2 diabetes susceptibility loci with one-year weight loss in the look AHEAD clinical trial. *Obesity (Silver Spring)* **2012**, *20*, 1675–1682. [CrossRef] [PubMed]

23. Lyssenko, V.; Lupi, R.; Marchetti, P.; Del Guerra, S.; Orho-Melander, M.; Almgren, P.; Sjögren, M.; Ling, C.; Eriksson, K.F.; Lethagen, A.L.; et al. Mechanisms by which common variants in the TCF7L2 gene increase risk of type 2 diabetes. *J. Clin. Investig.* **2007**, *117*, 2155–2163. [CrossRef] [PubMed]

24. Pecioska, S.; Zillikens, M.C.; Henneman, P.; Snijders, P.J.; Oostra, B.A.; van Duijn, C.M.; Aulchenko, Y.S. Association between type 2 diabetes loci and measures of fatness. *PLoS ONE* **2010**, *5*, e8541. [CrossRef] [PubMed]

25. Stolerman, E.S.; Manning, A.K.; McAteer, J.B.; Fox, C.S.; Dupuis, J.; Meigs, J.B.; Florez, J.C. TCF7L2 variants are associated with increased proinsulin/insulin ratios but not obesity traits in the Framingham Heart Study. *Diabetologia* **2009**, *52*, 614–620. [CrossRef] [PubMed]

26. Gupta, V.; Vinay, D.G.; Sovio, U.; Rafiq, S.; Kranthi Kumar, M.V.; Janipalli, C.S.; Evans, D.; Mani, K.R.; Sandeep, M.N.; Taylor, A.; et al. Association study of 25 type 2 diabetes related Loci with measures of obesity in Indian sib pairs. *PLoS ONE* **2013**, *8*, e53944. [CrossRef] [PubMed]

27. Helgason, A.; Pálsson, S.; Thorleifsson, G.; Grant, S.F.; Emilsson, V.; Gunnarsdottir, S.; Adeyemo, A.; Chen, Y.; Chen, G.; Reynisdottir, I.; et al. Refining the impact of TCF7L2 gene variants on type 2 diabetes and adaptive evolution. *Nat. Genet.* **2007**, *39*, 218–225. [CrossRef] [PubMed]

28. Locke, A.E.; Kahali, B.; Berndt, S.I.; Justice, A.E.; Pers, T.H.; Day, F.R.; Powell, C.; Vedantam, S.; Buchkovich, M.L.; Yang, J.; et al. Genetic studies of body mass index yield new insights for obesity biology. *Nature* **2015**, *518*, 197–206. [CrossRef] [PubMed]

29. Martínez-González, M.A.; Corella, D.; Salas-Salvadó, J.; Ros, E.; Covas, M.I.; Fiol, M.; Wärnberg, J.; Arós, F.; Ruíz-Gutiérrez, V.; Lamuela-Raventós, R.M.; et al. Cohort profile: Design and methods of the PREDIMED study. *Int. J. Epidemiol.* **2012**, *41*, 377–385. [CrossRef] [PubMed]

30. Estruch, R.; Ros, E.; Salas-Salvadó, J.; Covas, M.I.; Corella, D.; Arós, F.; Gómez-Gracia, E.; Ruiz-Gutiérrez, V.; Fiol, M.; Lapetra, J.; et al. Primary prevention of cardiovascular disease with a Mediterranean diet. *N. Engl. J. Med.* **2013**, *368*, 1279–1290. [CrossRef] [PubMed]

31. Gómez-Ambrosi, J.; Silva, C.; Catalán, V.; Rodríguez, A.; Galofré, J.C.; Escalada, J.; Valentí, V.; Rotellar, F.; Romero, S.; Ramírez, B.; et al. Clinical usefulness of a new equation for estimating body fat. *Diabetes Care* **2012**, *35*, 383–388. [CrossRef] [PubMed]

32. Salas-Salvadó, J.; Bulló, M.; Estruch, R.; Ros, E.; Covas, M.I.; Ibarrola-Jurado, N.; Corella, D.; Arós, F.; Gómez-Gracia, E.; Ruiz-Gutiérrez, V.; et al. Prevention of diabetes with Mediterranean diets: A subgroup analysis of a randomized trial. *Ann. Intern. Med.* **2014**, *160*, 1–10. [CrossRef] [PubMed]

33. Corella, D.; Carrasco, P.; Sorlí, J.V.; Estruch, R.; Rico-Sanz, J.; Martínez-González, M.Á.; Salas-Salvadó, J.; Covas, M.I.; Coltell, O.; Arós, F.; et al. Mediterranean diet reduces the adverse effect of the TCF7L2-rs7903146 polymorphism on cardiovascular risk factors and stroke incidence: A randomized controlled trial in a high-cardiovascular-risk population. *Diabetes Care* **2013**, *36*, 3803–3811. [CrossRef] [PubMed]

34. Florez, J.C. Leveraging genetics to advance type 2 diabetes prevention. *PLoS Med.* **2016**, *13*, e1002102. [CrossRef] [PubMed]

35. Xia, Q.; Chesi, A.; Manduchi, E.; Johnston, B.T.; Lu, S.; Leonard, M.E.; Parlin, U.W.; Rappaport, E.F.; Huang, P.; Wells, A.D.; et al. The type 2 diabetes presumed causal variant within TCF7L2 resides in an element that controls the expression of ACSL5. *Diabetologia* **2016**, *59*, 2360–2368. [CrossRef] [PubMed]

36. Zhou, Y.; Park, S.Y.; Su, J.; Bailey, K.; Ottosson-Laakso, E.; Shcherbina, L.; Oskolkov, N.; Zhang, E.; Thevenin, T.; Fadista, J.; et al. TCF7L2 is a master regulator of insulin production and processing. *Hum. Mol. Genet.* **2014**, *23*, 6419–6431. [CrossRef] [PubMed]

37. Mitchell, R.K.; Mondragon, A.; Chen, L.; Mcginty, J.A.; French, P.M.; Ferrer, J.; Thorens, B.; Hodson, D.J.; Rutter, G.A.; Da Silva Xavier, G. Selective disruption of TCF7L2 in the pancreatic β cell impairs secretory function and lowers β cell mass. *Hum. Mol. Genet.* **2015**, *24*, 1390–1399. [CrossRef] [PubMed]

38. Dimas, A.S.; Lagou, V.; Barker, A.; Knowles, J.W.; Mägi, R.; Hivert, M.F.; Benazzo, A.; Rybin, D.; Jackson, A.U.; Stringham, H.M.; et al. Impact of type 2 diabetes susceptibility variants on quantitative glycemic traits reveals mechanistic heterogeneity. *Diabetes* **2014**, *63*, 2158–2171. [CrossRef] [PubMed]

39. Bailey, K.A.; Savic, D.; Zielinski, M.; Park, S.Y.; Wang, L.J.; Witkowski, P.; Brady, M.; Hara, M.; Bell, G.I.; Nobrega, M.A. Evidence of non-pancreatic beta cell-dependent roles of TCF7L2 in the regulation of glucose metabolism in mice. *Hum. Mol. Genet.* **2015**, *24*, 1646–1654. [CrossRef] [PubMed]

40. Läll, K.; Mägi, R.; Morris, A.; Metspalu, A.; Fischer, K. Personalized risk prediction for type 2 diabetes: The potential of genetic risk scores. *Genet. Med.* **2016**. [CrossRef] [PubMed]

41. Gamboa-Meléndez, M.A.; Huerta-Chagoya, A.; Moreno-Macías, H.; Vázquez-Cárdenas, P.; Ordóñez-Sánchez, M.L.; Rodríguez-Guillén, R.; Riba, L.; Rodríguez-Torres, M.; Guerra-García, M.T.; Guillén-Pineda, L.E.; et al. Contribution of common genetic variation to the risk of type 2 diabetes in the Mexican Mestizo population. *Diabetes* **2012**, *61*, 3314–3321. [CrossRef] [PubMed]

42. Brito, E.C.; Lyssenko, V.; Renström, F.; Berglund, G.; Nilsson, P.M.; Groop, L.; Franks, P.W. Previously associated type 2 diabetes variants may interact with physical activity to modify the risk of impaired glucose regulation and type 2 diabetes: A study of 16,003 Swedish adults. *Diabetes* **2009**, *58*, 1411–1418. [CrossRef] [PubMed]

43. Kong, X.; Xing, X.; Hong, J.; Zhang, X.; Yang, W. Genetic variants associated with lean and obese type 2 diabetes in a Han Chinese population: A case-control study. *Medicine (Baltimore)* **2016**, *95*, e3841. [CrossRef] [PubMed]

44. Palomaki, G.E.; Melillo, S.; Marrone, M.; Douglas, M.P. Use of genomic panels to determine risk of developing type 2 diabetes in the general population: A targeted evidence-based review. *Genet. Med.* **2013**, *15*, 600–601. [CrossRef] [PubMed]

45. Evaluation of Genomic Applications in Practice and Prevention (EGAPP) Working Group. Recommendations from the EGAPP Working Group: Does genomic profiling to assess type 2 diabetes risk improve health outcomes? *Genet. Med.* **2013**, *15*, 612–617.

46. Fox, C.S.; Hall, J.L.; Arnett, D.K.; Ashley, E.A.; Delles, C.; Engler, M.B.; Freeman, M.W.; Johnson, J.A.; Lanfear, D.E.; Liggett, S.B.; et al. Future translational applications from the contemporary genomics era: A scientific statement from the American Heart Association. *Circulation* **2015**, *131*, 1715–1736. [CrossRef] [PubMed]

47. Keating, B.J. Advances in risk prediction of type 2 diabetes: Integrating genetic scores with Framingham risk models. *Diabetes* **2015**, *64*, 1495–1497. [CrossRef] [PubMed]

48. Roswall, N.; Ängquist, L.; Ahluwalia, T.S.; Romaguera, D.; Larsen, S.C.; Østergaard, J.N.; Halkjaer, J.; Vimaleswaran, K.S.; Wareham, N.J.; Bendinelli, B.; et al. Association between Mediterranean and Nordic diet scores and changes in weight and waist circumference: Influence of FTO and TCF7L2 loci. *Am. J. Clin. Nutr.* **2014**, *100*, 1188–1197. [CrossRef] [PubMed]

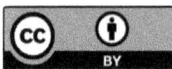

nutrients

Article

Splenic Immune Response Is Down-Regulated in C57BL/6J Mice Fed Eicosapentaenoic Acid and Docosahexaenoic Acid Enriched High Fat Diet

Nikul K. Soni [1,*], Alastair B. Ross [1], Nathalie Scheers [1], Otto I. Savolainen [1], Intawat Nookaew [2,3], Britt G. Gabrielsson [1] and Ann-Sofie Sandberg [1]

[1] Division of Food and Nutrition Science, Department of Biology and Biological Engineering, Chalmers University of Technology, SE-41296 Gothenburg, Sweden; alastair.ross@chalmers.se (A.B.R.); nathalie.scheers@chalmers.se (N.S.); otto.savolainen@chalmers.se (O.I.S.); brittg@chalmers.se (B.G.G.); ann-sofie.sandberg@chalmers.se (A.-S.S.)

[2] Division of Systems and Synthetic Biology, Department of Biology and Biological Engineering, Chalmers University of Technology, SE-41296 Gothenburg, Sweden; intawat@chalmers.se or INookaew@uams.edu

[3] Department of Biomedical Informatics, College of Medicine, University of Arkansas for Medical Science, Little Rock, AR 72205, USA

* Correspondence: soni@chalmers.se; Tel.: +46-31-772-3816

Received: 8 November 2016; Accepted: 5 January 2017; Published: 10 January 2017

Abstract: Dietary *n*-3 fatty acids eicosapentaenoic acid (EPA) and docosahexaenoic acid (DHA) are associated with reduction of inflammation, although the mechanisms are poorly understood, especially how the spleen, as a secondary lymphoid organ, is involved. To investigate the effects of EPA and DHA on spleen gene expression, male C57BL/6J mice were fed high fat diets (HFD) differing in fatty acid composition, either based on corn oil (HFD-CO), or CO enriched with 2 g/100 g EPA and DHA (HFD-ED), for eight weeks. Spleen tissue was analyzed using transcriptomics and for fatty acids profiling. Biological processes (BPs) related to the immune response, including T-cell receptor signaling pathway, T-cell differentiation and co-stimulation, myeloid dendritic cell differentiation, antigen presentation and processing, and the toll like receptor pathway were downregulated by HFD-ED compared with control and HFD-CO. These findings were supported by the down-regulation of NF-κB in HFD-ED compared with HFD-CO fed mice. Lower phospholipid arachidonic acid levels in HFD-ED compared with HFD-CO, and control mice suggest attenuation of pathways via prostaglandins and leukotrienes. The HFD-ED also upregulated BPs related to erythropoiesis and hematopoiesis compared with control and HFD-CO fed mice. Our findings suggest that EPA and DHA down-regulate the splenic immune response induced by HFD-CO, supporting earlier work that the spleen is a target organ for the anti-inflammatory effects of these *n*-3 fatty acids.

Keywords: eicosapentaenoic acid (EPA)/docosahexaenoic acid (DHA); spleen transcriptomics; inflammation and immunity; NF-κB; arachidonic acid

1. Introduction

Inflammation is an important biological process for the maintenance of tissue homeostasis. However, sustained inflammation could lead to certain diseases [1]. Chronic low-grade inflammation and immune system activation are observed in abdominal obesity and may have a role in the pathogenesis of obesity related diseases such as type-2 diabetes (T2D) and cardiovascular diseases (CVD) [2,3], and therefore is one of the main threats to health with increased risk of mortality and morbidity [4]. The World Health Organization reports that chronic diseases kills more than 38 million people worldwide [5]. Thus, resolution of low-grade inflammation has become a therapeutic target for preventing CVD and may have wider application in the prevention of chronic diseases.

The spleen is a secondary lymphoid organ, with the primary function to filtrate the blood from damaged or senescent erythrocytes and antigens. During filtration, blood is exposed to mature lymphocytes leading to the production of new immune cells and antibodies. The spleen contains high levels of specialized T-cells and B-cells [6], and is therefore a suitable choice, e.g., for studies of the immune response during chronic inflammation. Inflammation is characterized by increase in white blood cell count [7,8], pro-inflammatory cytokines [9], and chemokines [10]. Diets high in saturated fatty acids are thought to stimulate chronic low-grade inflammation [11], whereas replacing saturated fatty acids with unsaturated fatty acids reduces the risk of inflammation [12]. Cell culture, animal studies, human trials and epidemiological studies have shown the potential preventive effects of *n*-3 polyunsaturated fatty acids in reducing inflammation [13–16].

The main polyunsaturated *n*-3 fatty acids in marine oils, eicosapentaenoic acid (EPA) and docosahexaenoic acid (DHA), are widely used as supplements and are purported to have a wide range of effects. It is unclear how *n*-3 fatty acids may reduce risk of inflammation, though there have been many mechanistic studies on *n*-3 fatty acids [17]. Although several studies have investigated the effects of *n*-3 fatty acids in spleen or splenocytes [18–20], few studies have investigated the effects of *n*-3 fatty acids on the spleen transcriptome [21]. We recently found that the innate and adaptive immune system in spleen was down-regulated by menhaden fish oil [21], a mix of fatty acids and other lipophilic compounds, including EPA and DHA. To explore the effects and understand the underlying mechanisms of pure EPA and DHA on the splenic immune response, we used transcriptomics to measure the response in gene-expression in spleen from mice who were fed a high-fat diet based on corn oil, partly replaced by EPA and DHA. Direct effects of the difference in fat intake on spleen fatty acid composition were also measured.

2. Materials and Methods

2.1. Animals and Ethical Declaration

Six-week-old male C57BL/6J mice were purchased from the Harlan Laboratories (Envigo, Horst, The Netherlands). They were caged 5–6 per group with ad libitum access to food and water throughout the study and were acclimatized in temperature and humidity controlled environment with 12-h dark/light cycle for three-weeks at a certified animal facility in Gothenburg, Sweden [22]. After acclimatization, the mice were fed either a HFD or normal diets (see Diets for details) for 8 weeks thereafter. Upon termination with intraperitoneal sodium barbital injection followed by cervical dislocation, spleen was dissected, weighed and snap-frozen in liquid nitrogen and stored at −80 °C until further use. The animal study was approved by the Animal Ethical Committee at Gothenburg University (Approval # 253-2009).

2.2. Diet

During the three-week acclimatization period, the mice were fed a standard control chow (based on AIN93m) [23]. There were no measured differences in mice body weight at the start of study (Table 1), and their body weights were measured weekly during the 8-week intervention study. Two mice from the control group were removed due to unsocial behavior, leaving *n* = 10 mice in control and *n* = 12 mice in each of the two HFD groups. HFD were used to induce obesity in the mice. In the two HFD groups, the HFD were matched for macronutrient content. The HFD was prepared either with 5% (*w/w*) corn oil, while the EPA and DHA enriched HFD was prepared with 3% (*w/w*) corn oil and 2% (*w/w*) EPA and DHA triglycerides (EPAX AS, Lysaker, Norway). The content of EPA and DHA in HFD-ED diet was 8 g/kg [24,25]. The control diet provided 24% energy (E%) as protein, 12 E% as fat and 65 E% as carbohydrates, whereas the two HFD contained 25 E% as protein, 32 E% as fat and 44 E% as carbohydrates (Table 1). The diets were prepared by Lantmännen AB

(Kimstad, Sweden). Mice had ad libitum access to water and diet, and the diets were changed three times per week during the study.

Table 1. The composition of the different diets used in this study. Data are adapted from [22]. Control = control chow; HFD-ED = high fat diet—eicosapentaenoic acid and docosahexaenoic acid; HFD-CO = high fat diet—corn oil.

Ingredient (g/100 g Diet)		Control	HFD-ED	HFD-CO
Protein	Casein	22.20	25.60	25.60
Carbohydrates	Sucrose	5.00	10.00	10.00
	Corn starch	56.00	34.80	34.80
	Cellulose	5.00	5.80	5.80
Fat	Total	5.00	15.00	15.00
	Corn oil	2.50	3.00	5.00
	Coconut oil	2.50	10.00	10.00
	EPAX oils [a]	0.00	2.00	0.00
Minerals [b]		2.00	2.50	2.50
Miconutrients [c]		3.00	3.00	3.00
Choline bitartrate		1.60	2.00	2.00
Cholesterol		0.00	1.00	1.00
Methionine		0.20	0.30	0.30
Energy content (kJ/100 g)		1599	1752	1752
	Protein E%	24	25	25
	Carbohydrate E%	65	44	44
	Fat E%	12	32	32
Fatty acid composition [d] (mg/g diet)				
	C10:0	0.20	1.47	1.33
	C12:0	2.37	7.58	7.72
	C14:0	1.54	4.58	4.78
	C16:0	1.90	3.44	3.59
	C18:0	0.68	2.26	2.49
	SFA	6.70	19.33	19.91
	C18:1 *n*-9	2.82	4.80	5.26
	MUFA	2.82	4.80	5.26
	C18:2 *n*-6	3.62	5.03	7.36
	C18:3 *n*-6	0.12	0.22	0.26
	Total *n*-6 PUFA	3.74	5.26	7.62
	C20:5 *n*-3 (EPA)	0.00	2.03	0.01
	C22:6 *n*-3 (DHA)	0.00	4.58	0.01
	Total *n*-3 PUFA	0.00	6.61	0.02

[a] EPAX 1050. EPAX 6015. [b] $CaCO_3$ (57.7%); KCl (19.9%); KH_2PO_4 (11.9%); $MgSO_4$ (10.4%). [c] Corn starch (98.22%); $Ca(IO_3)_2$ (0.0007%); $CoCO_3$ (0.064%); CuO (0.02%); $FeSO_4$ (0.5%); MnO_2 (0.035%); Na_2MoO_4 (0.001%); $NaSeO_3$ (0.0007%); ZnO (0.1%); Vitamin A (0.013%); B_2 (Riboflavin-5-phosphate sodium; 0.027%); B_3 (0.1%); B_5 (Ca Pantothenate; 0.057%); B_6 (0.023%); B_7 (0.0007%); B_9 (0.007%); B_{12} (0.00008%); D_3 (0.007%); E (0.25%); K (0.003%). [d] Diet analyses were performed in triplicates, and the data were obtained by Gas chromatography mass spectroscopy.

2.3. Splenic Fatty Acid Profiling

Approximately 100 mg spleen tissue was weighed, freeze-dried and extracted using the Folch total lipid extraction method [26]. Internal phospholipids (C17:0) and triglyceride (C19:0) standards (Nu-Chek prep, Inc., Elysian, MN, USA) were added to the samples prior to the separation of neutral fatty acids, free fatty acids and phospholipids fractions using solid phase extraction. The fatty acids profiles in each fraction was quantified by gas chromatography mass spectroscopy (GC-MS) as previously described [27].

2.4. RNA Isolation, Quality Assurance and Microarray Analysis

Spleen from four different mice from each group was selected for total RNA isolation on the basis of their body weight, plasma triglyceride and plasma cholesterol levels. Total RNA was purified using the RNeasy® Plus Universal Mini kit (Qiagen Nordic, Sollentuna, Sweden). RNA integrity was estimated using RNA 6000 Nano LabChip for Agilent 2100 Bioanalyzer (Agilent Technologies, Santa Clara, CA, USA). RNA was quantified by NanoDrop 2000c UV-Vis Spectrophotometer (Thermo Scientific, Wilmington, NC, USA).

Microarray experiments were run at the Swegene Centre for Integrative Biology at Lund University Genomics core facility. Briefly, total RNA was labeled and hybridized to MouseWG-6_V2.0 Expression BeadChip (MouseWG-6_V2.0_R3_11278593_A; Illumina, CA, USA) containing 45,281 transcripts. The BeadChip content is derived from the National Center for Biotechnology Information Reference Sequence (NCBI RefSeq) database (Build 36, Release 22). The chip is supplemented with probes derived from the Mouse Exonic Evidence Based Oligonucleotide (MEEBO) set as well as examples protein-coding sequences from RIKEN FANTOM2 database. The data (raw and normalized) are deposited in SOFT-format at Gene Expression Omnibus (GEO) database under the accession number GSE76622.

The fluorescence intensities (raw signals), for the mean intensities of arrays were extracted from illumina bead array files using GenomeStudio Gene Expression software (GSGX v1.9.0, Illumina, San Diego, CA, USA). The data were quantile normalized, and variance-stabilizing transformation (VST) was performed using the default setting of lumiExpresso function from lumi package [28]. Empirical Bayes method from the Linear Models for Microarray Data (limma) package was then applied to the signals to calculate moderated t- and F-statistics, log odds and differential expression for comparisons between the diets [29].

Platform for integrative analysis of omics data (Piano) Bioconductor package was used for gene-set enrichment analysis (GSEA) for functional inference [30]. Before implementing the gene-set enrichment function from Piano, gene-set collection (gsc) files were prepared for gene ontologies (GO) related to biological processes (BPs), molecular function (MF) and cellular components (CC) and the other gsc file contains subset for BPs related to immune system process (GO:0002376). Furthermore, canonical signaling and metabolic pathways from the KEGG database was used for pathway analysis. Pathview function from the Pathview package was used to visualize the data, which renders KEGG pathway based on the experimental results [31]. As spleen is considered an important immunological tissue, we ran Piano for both, global and immune related changes in spleen for all diet combinations. In both gene-set analyses, gene-sets with less than 10 or more than 500 genes were excluded. For gene-expression analysis, a Benjamini–Hochberg corrected p-value < 0.001 for at least one diet comparison was considered significant.

2.5. Quantitative Real-Time PCR (qRT-PCR)

RNA of genes that were identified as being of especial interested based on the transcriptomics analysis was quantified to confirm the transcriptomics findings. Briefly, total RNA was isolated from selected mice spleen tissue and 10 ng/μL of total RNA were used for cDNA synthesis using universal cDNA synthesis kit to make the final reaction volume up to 10 μL (ExiLERATE LNA™ qPCR, Exiqon Inc., Woburn, MA, USA). Then, 1 μL of cDNA solution was diluted with 79 μL of nuclease free water. From this reaction, 4 μL of diluted cDNA was used for the qRT-PCR using the PCR starter kit (ExiLERATE LNA™ qPCR, Exiqon). The plate was run on Bio-Rad CFX96 (Bio-Rad Laboratories Inc., Hercules, CA, USA) real time detection system for 40 cycles following the manufacturers protocol. The KiCqStart™ SYBR green primers used were as follows: (a) Adipoq: *for*—CCACTTTCTCCTCATTTCTG, *rev*—CTAGCTCTTCAGTTGTACTAAC; (b) Ltf: *for*—CAAAAGGATAGATTCCCCAAC, *rev*—GTAACTCCTCAAATACCGTGC; (c) Ccl19: *for*—TTCTT AATGAAGATGGCTGC, *rev*—CTTTGTTCTTGGCAGAAGAC; and (d) Ubc: *for*—GAGACGATGCAG ATCTTTG, *rev*—ATGTTGTAGTCTGACAGGG. Data analyses were performed by comparing ΔΔCt values exported from the CFX manager software (BIORAD), using *Ubiquitin (Ubc)* as the reference gene and expressing changes relative to the control group.

2.6. Statistical Analysis

Differences due to diet in the physiological parameters and fatty acid concentrations measured were tested using one-way Anova followed by post-hoc Tukey-Honest significant difference test (Tukey-HSD). A p-value < 0.05 was considered significant unless otherwise stated. Statistical and sequencing data were analyzed in R Studio interface (Version 0.99.902—© 2009–2016 RStudio Inc., Boston, MA, USA) and packages from Bioconductor. The data are presented as mean $\pm$ SEM.

3. Results

3.1. Physiological Changes in Mice—Effects of High Fat Diets Differing in Their Fat Composition

No difference was observed in absolute spleen weight between the diet groups, though the HFD-CO fed animals had a lower spleen to body weight ratio (17%) compared with HFD-ED (p-value = 0.02) (Table 2). After eight-week intervention, the body weight gain was slightly higher in HFD-CO fed mice compared with HFD-ED fed mice (Table 2). We have previously reported higher plasma triglycerides and lower hepatic total lipids in the HFD-ED fed mice compared with HFD-CO fed mice [22].

Table 2. Changes in body weight composition and plasma lipid composition.

Parameter	Control	HFD-ED	HFD-CO
Total number of animals; n	9	12	12
Initial body weight (g)	27.50 ± 0.80	28.60 ± 0.80	24.30 ± 0.50
Final body weight (g)	31.40 ± 1.00	33.80 ± 0.80	36.20 ± 0.90
Change in body weight (g)	3.90 ± 0.50 [a]	5.20 ± 0.30 [a]	8.60 ± 0.50 [b]
Absolute spleen weight (g)	0.09 ± 0.01	0.10 ± 0.00	0.09 ± 0.00
Spleen/body weight ratio (g/100 g)	0.29 ± 0.02 [a,b]	0.29 ± 0.01 [a]	0.24 ± 0.01 [b]

The data are shown as mean $\pm$ SEM; different letters show significant different tested by ANOVA followed by Tukey's multiple comparison test. To calculate the changes in body weight (g), initial body weight values from individual animals was subtracted from the final body weight measurement.

3.2. Spleen Fatty Acid Profiles

Neutral lipids: The amount of total neutral lipid was higher in HFD-CO fed mice compared with HFD-ED but the amounts did not differ between control and HFD-ED fed mice (Table 3). The amount of saturated fatty acid (SFA) C14:0 was higher in HFD-CO compared with HFD-ED fed mice. The amount of C20:3 *n*-6 was lower in HFD-ED fed mice compared with control diet fed mice. C20:4 *n*-6 (arachidonic acid) did not differ between any compared diet groups. As expected, the amount of C22:6 *n*-3 (DHA) was higher in HFD-ED fed mice compared with mice fed HFD-CO (Table 3), whereas no C20:5 *n*-3 (EPA) was detected in the neutral lipid fraction.

Free fatty acids: Total free fatty acids (FFA) did not significantly differ between groups (Table 3). The amounts of C18:1 *n*-9 and C20:3 *n*-6 were higher in HFD-CO fed mice compared with the mice fed HFD-ED, whereas they did not differ between control fed mice compared with either HFD. The amount of C22:6 *n*-3 (DHA) was higher in HFD-ED fed mice compared with both control and HFD-CO fed animals (Table 3).

Phospholipids: The total phospholipids amount was lower in the mice fed HFD-ED compared with either control or HFD-CO fed mice (Table 3), though *n*-3 PUFAs including C20:5 *n*-3 (EPA), C22:5 *n*-3 (DPA) and C22:6 *n*-3 (DHA) were higher in HFD-ED fed mice. The amount of C18:2 *n*-6 (linoleic acid) was higher in HFD-ED fed mice compared with either control or HFD-CO fed animals whereas the amount of C20:3 *n*-6 and C20:4 *n*-6 (arachidonic acid) was higher in HFD-CO fed mice compared with the mice fed HFD-ED. The amount of SFA C12:0 was higher in HFD-CO fed mice compared with the mice fed control diet but did not differ from HFD-ED fed mice. No differences were observed for SFA including C14:0, C16:0, and C18:0 between any of the diet groups (Table 3).

Table 3. The fatty acid profiles of different lipid fractions in spleen tissues (mg/g dry spleen biomass).

Neutral Lipids	Control $n = 5$	HFD-ED $n = 8$	HFD-CO $n = 8$
C12:0	0.00 ± 0.00	0.01 ± 0.00	0.06 ± 0.02
C14:0	0.01 ± 0.00	0.01 ± 0.00 [a]	0.14 ± 0.06 [b]
C16:0	1.03 ± 0.20	1.46 ± 0.22	3.34 ± 1.05
C18:0	0.21 ± 0.02	0.19 ± 0.04	0.13 ± 0.03
C18:1 *n*-9	1.78 ± 0.46	1.05 ± 0.17	1.43 ± 0.33
C18:2 *n*-6	0.03 ± 0.02 [a]	0.2 ± 0.08 [a]	0.86 ± 0.25 [b]
C20:3 *n*-6	0.11 ± 0.01 [a]	0.03 ± 0.01 [b]	0.05 ± 0.02
C20:4 *n*-6	0.00 ± 0.00	0.00 ± 0.00	0.24 ± 0.14
C22:6 *n*-3	0.00 ± 0.00 [a]	0.16 ± 0.04 [b]	0.00 ± 0.00 [a]
Total	3.16 ± 0.58	3.12 ± 0.43	6.25 ± 1.37
Free fatty acids			
C12:0	0.01 ± 0.00 [a]	0.02 ± 0.00	0.04 ± 0.01 [b]
C14:0	0.01 ± 0.00	0.02 ± 0.00	0.05 ± 0.01
C16:0	0.20 ± 0.02	0.20 ± 0.01	0.35 ± 0.07
C18:1 *n*-9	0.05 ± 0.00	0.05 ± 0.00 [a]	0.06 ± 0.00 [b]
C18:3 *n*-3	0.02 ± 0.00	0.02 ± 0.00	0.03 ± 0.00
C20:3 *n*-6	0.06 ± 0.01	0.02 ± 0.00 [a]	0.07 ± 0.01 [b]
C22:6 *n*-3	0.00 ± 0.00 [a]	0.05 ± 0.00 [b]	0.00 ± 0.00 [a]
Total	0.35 ± 0.03	0.38 ± 0.02	0.60 ± 0.11
Phospholipids			
C12:0	0.00 ± 0.00 [a]	0.01 ± 0.00	0.01 ± 0.00 [b]
C14:0	0.07 ± 0.00 [a]	0.15 ± 0.01 [b]	0.13 ± 0.00 [c]
C16:0	1.69 ± 0.05	1.70 ± 0.03	1.69 ± 0.05
C18:0	0.61 ± 0.02	0.59 ± 0.01	0.67 ± 0.04
C18:1 *n*-9	0.32 ± 0.01 [a]	0.28 ± 0.01 [b]	0.31 ± 0.01 [a]
C18:2 *n*-6	0.12 ± 0.00 [a]	0.22 ± 0.02 [b]	0.14 ± 0.01 [a]
C20:0	0.00 ± 0.00	0.01 ± 0.00	0.00 ± 0.00
C20:1 *n*-7	0.02 ± 0.00	0.02 ± 0.00	0.02 ± 0.00
C20:2 *n*-6	0.02 ± 0.00 [a]	0.05 ± 0.01 [b]	0.03 ± 0.00 [a]
C20:3 *n*-6	0.17 ± 0.01 [a]	0.18 ± 0.01 [a]	0.25 ± 0.02 [b]
C20:4 *n*-6	4.41 ± 0.10 [a]	1.92 ± 0.05 [b]	4.33 ± 0.08 [a]
C20:5 *n*-3	0.00 ± 0.00 [a]	0.41 ± 0.01 [b]	0.00 ± 0.00 [a]
C22:0	0.02 ± 0.01	0.02 ± 0.00	0.01 ± 0.00
C22:5 *n*-3	0.00 ± 0.00 [a]	0.34 ± 0.01 [b]	0.00 ± 0.00 [a]
C22:6 *n*-3	0.20 ± 0.02 [a]	0.82 ± 0.02 [b]	0.19 ± 0.01 [a]
Total	7.67 ± 0.19 [a]	6.71 ± 0.13 [b]	7.78 ± 0.22 [a]

The fatty acid profiles from the mice fed either control, HFD-ED or HFD-CO are shown as mean ± SEM and as a proportion of total fatty acid fraction; different letters show statistical difference tested by ANOVA followed by Tukey's multiple comparison test. For details see methods section.

3.3. Global Gene Expression Analysis of the Spleen Transcriptome

Changes in splenic gene expression were most obvious in response to HFD-ED compared to control or HFD-CO diets (Supplementary Materials Figure S1a). Principle component analysis of the spleen transcriptome did not detect any outliers in the data (Supplementary Materials Figure S1b) indicating good analytical reproducibility. At a stringent cutoff of p_{adj}-value < 0.001, there were 1372 differentially expressed genes (DEGs) in splenic RNA from mice fed HFD-ED and 285 DEGs in the RNA from mice fed HFD-CO compared with control diet. Furthermore, to scrutinize dietary effects on the spleen transcriptome, GSEA on biological processes (BP) without immune system processes (GO:0002376) was implemented. For assessment of regulated BPs, p-value $< 10 \times 10^9$ for at least one comparison of HFD-ED, HFD-CO and control was considered significant. At this *p*-value cutoff, there were 110 BPs identified as differentially expressed (Supplementary Materials Figure S1c). Furthermore, KEGG pathway analysis of the spleen transcriptome for the comparison of HFD-ED vs. HFD-CO effects in mice, revealed down-regulation of arachidonic acid and linoleic acid pathways. For the arachidonic acid pathway in particular, HFD-ED down-regulated genes belonging to the cytochrome P450 superfamily, including the cytochrome P450 family 4 subfamily f polypeptide 14 (*Cyp4f14*), prostaglandin I2 (prostacyclin) synthase (*Ptgis* or *Cyp8a1*), and phospholipase A2 group IB pancreas (*Pla2g1b*), compared to HFD-CO group. Moreover, the glutathione peroxidase 1 (*Gpx1*) gene was up-regulated in the mice spleen, after ingesting a HFD-ED compared with a HFD-CO (Supplementary Materials Figure S1d). Given the role of the spleen as a secondary lymphoid organ [32], we further investigated the effects of EPA and DHA on the regulation of immune related BPs.

3.4. Immune System Related Gene Expression in the Spleen

To study the effect of including EPA and DHA in a HFD on immune system gene expression, we ran gene-set enrichment analysis on BP "immune system process" (GO:0002376). The resultant cluster analysis of 75 significantly different changes of immune related BPs (*p*-value < 0.001 in at least one comparison) can be classified into three clusters, which we have named I–III (Figure 1). Cluster I represent up-regulation of the BPs related to erythrocyte development and differentiation, hematopoiesis, negative regulation of megakaryocyte differentiation, and innate immune response in the mucosa, in the mice fed HFD-ED compared with control and HFD-CO, whereas these same BPs were down-regulated in the mice fed HFD-CO vs. control diet. Cluster IIa represents down-regulation of BPs related to both the innate and adaptive immune responses including T-cell signaling, T-helper cell 1 and 2 differentiation and T-cell co-stimulation, humoral immune response, interferon-gamma and an adaptive immune process such as α-β T cell differentiation in the mice fed HFD-ED compared with control and HFD-CO. Cluster IIb represents down-regulation of BPs related to T- and B-cell homeostasis, natural killer cell differentiation, antigen processing and presentation via MHC class I, and T-cell cytokine production by HFD-ED compared with the other two diets. These processes in cluster IIa and IIb were up-regulated by HFD-CO compared with control fed animals. Cluster IIIa represents down-regulation of BPs in both of the comparisons between HFD and the control diet. This included BPs mostly related to T- and B-cell activation and differentiation. Cluster IIIb represents pronounced down-regulation of BPs in the mice fed HFD-ED compared with HFD-CO, and included toll-like receptor 3 and receptor 4 signaling pathway, MyD88-dependent toll-like receptor signaling pathway, adaptive and innate immune response. These processes were also down-regulated by HFD-CO compared with control fed mice but were less pronounced compared to HFD-ED (Figure 1).

3.5. Modulation of NF-κB Related Gene Expression

As a broad range of BPs related to immunity were affected by HFD-ED, we hypothesized that expression of NF-κB, a transcription factor that appears to link chronic low-grade inflammation and immunity to insulin resistance [2] and may influence obesity and related disorders, was accordingly affected. We compared the genes involved in the modulation of NF-κB for all three diets (Figure 2a). HFD-ED down-regulated genes, in comparison to either control or HFD-CO, that were involved in activation of the NF-κB signaling pathway directly or indirectly including Adiponectin C1Q and collagen domain containing (*Adipoq*), Gremlin 1 DAN family BMP antagonist (*Grem1*), Tumor necrosis factor receptor superfamily, member 11a NF-κB activator (*Tnfrsf11a*), Chemokine (C-C motif) ligand 19 (*Ccl19*), Nucleotide-binding oligomerization domain containing 1 (*Nod1*) a NOD-like receptor family of pattern recognition receptor, Protein kinase C beta (*Prkcb*), and NLR family CARD domain containing 4 (*Nlrc4*). The remaining 5 genes were up-regulated by HFD-ED compared with either control or HFD-CO and includes Peroxiredoxin 3 (*Prdx3*), Coagulation factor II (thrombin) receptor-like 2 (*F2rl2*), Extracellular matrix protein 1 (*Ecm1*), Lactotransferrin (*Ltf*), Heme oxygenase 1 (*Hmox1*). Relative expression of mRNA involved directly and indirectly involved in modulation of NF-κB including *Adipoq, Ltf, Ccl19* and *Tnfrsf11a* (*p*-value = 0.059; data not shown) verifies our transcriptome data (Figure 2b).

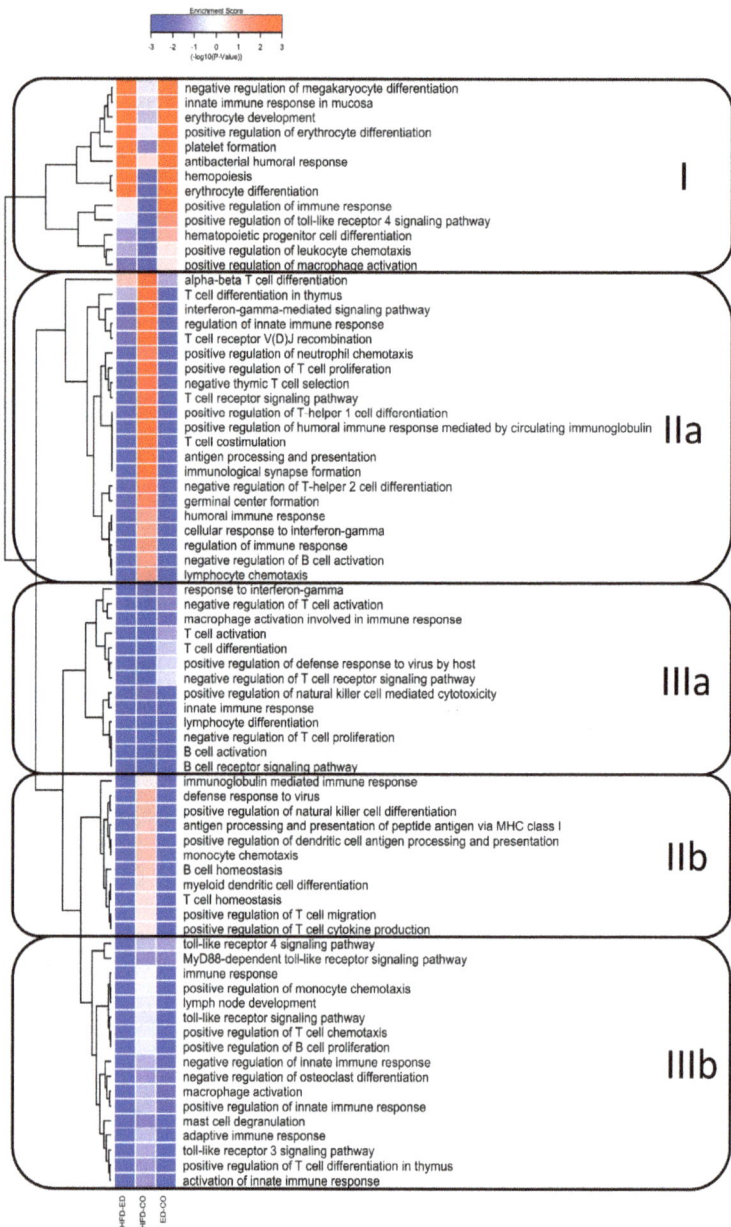

Figure 1. A hierarchical clustering and gene ontology (GO) enrichment analysis of DEGs showing 76 significantly regulated BPs (*p*-value < 0.001) related to immune system process for every diet comparison after eight weeks. The heat map is divided into four main clusters according to the regulation pattern and discussed in detail in results section. Color patterns indicate the direction of regulation, where red indicates up-regulation and blue indicates down-regulation of immune specific GO-terms. HFD-ED = HFD-ED vs. control diet; HFD-CO = HFD-corn oil vs. control diet; ED-CO = HFD-ED vs. HFD-CO.

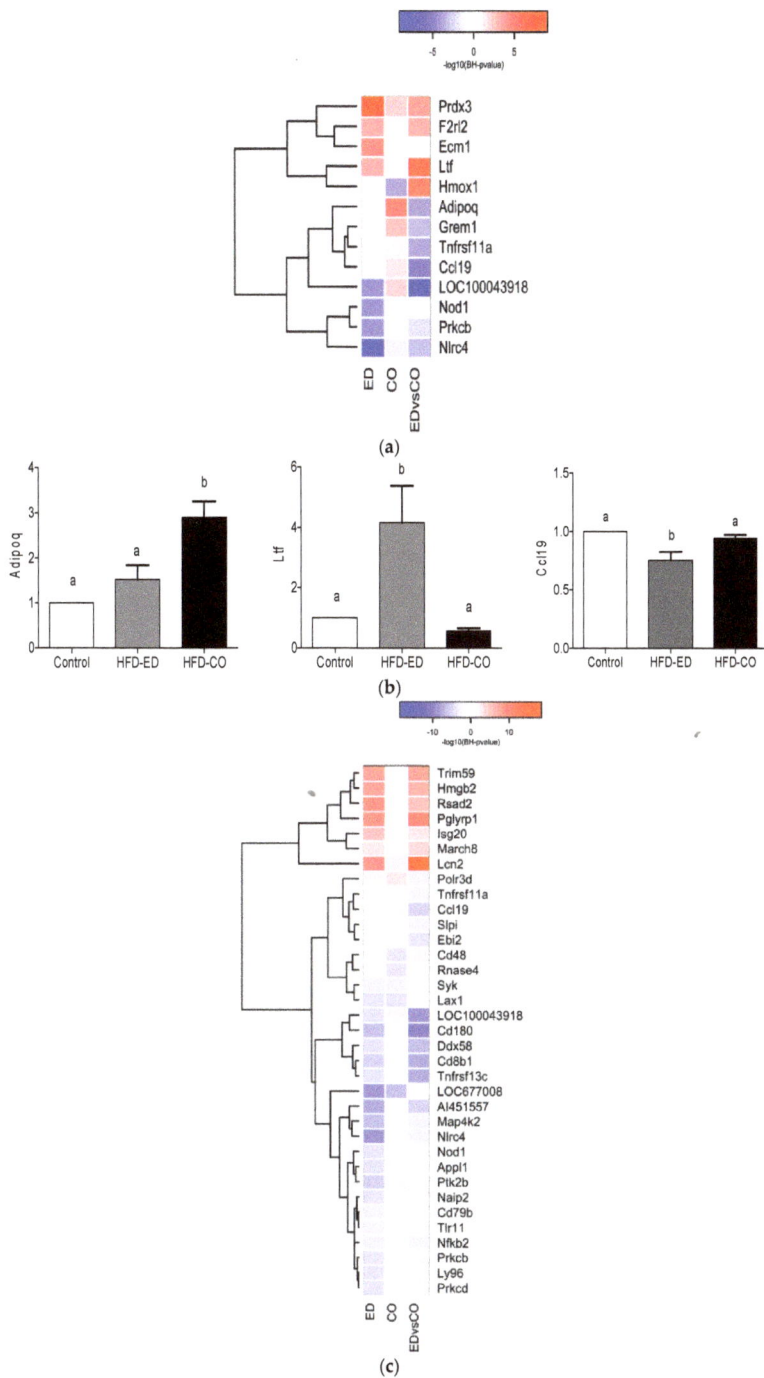

Figure 2. *Cont.*

(d)

(e)

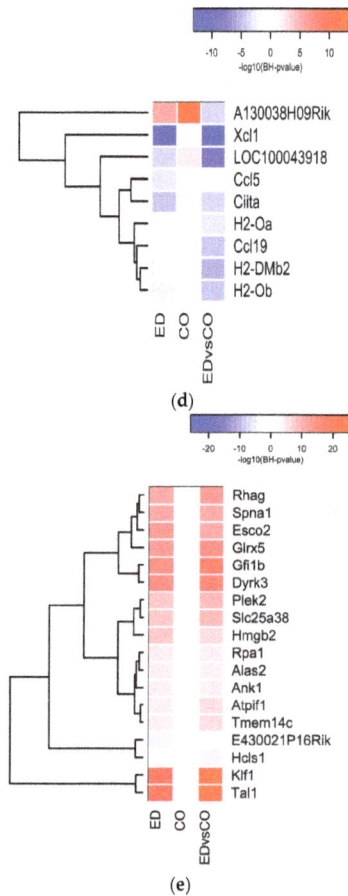

Figure 2. Heat map showing gene-expression patterns for any diet comparison i.e., HFD-ED vs. control; HFD-CO vs. control; HFD-ED vs. HFD-CO. for atleast one comparison BH-*p* value < 0.001 was considered significant. (**a**) Heat map showing group of genes regulated in NF-κB regulation, in BP GO:0043123 positive regulation of I-κB kinase/NF-κB signaling, BP GO:0051092 positive regulation of NF-κB transcription factor activity, and BP GO:0042346 positive regulation of NF-κB import into nucleus; (**b**) Relative expression of different genes involved in modulation of NF-κB in mouse spleen. Each gene is normalized against the house-keeping gene Ubiquitin (*Ubc*), and expression level shown as relative to the control diet; (**c**) Heat map showing groups of genes regulated in immune-related processes, including BP GO:0045087 innate immune response, BP GO:0002250 adaptive immune response, BP GO:0006959 humoral immune response, BP GO:0016064 immunoglobulin mediated immune response, BP GO:0001771 immunological synapse formation, BP GO:0042116 macrophage activation, BP GO:0002224 toll-like receptor signaling pathway, and BP GO:0002755 MyD88-dependent toll-like receptor signaling pathway; (**d**) Heat map showing groups of genes regulated in interferon-gamma regulation, including BP GO:0060333 interferon gamma mediated signaling pathway, BP GO:0019882 antigen processing and presentation, and BP GO:0071346 cellular response to interferon-gamma; (**e**) Heat map showing groups of genes regulated in erythrocyte turnover, including BP GO:0030218erythrocyte differentiation, BP GO:0048821 erythrocyte development, BP GO:0045648 positive regulation of erythrocyte differentiation, BP GO:0030097 hemopoieses, and BP GO:0002244 hematopoietic progenitor cell differentiation.

To observe the effects of dietary response on regulation of genes involved in innate, humoral and adaptive immune response including Toll-like receptors (Tlrs), the expression of immune-related genes was determined. Among the genes down-regulated by HFD-ED compared with the other two diets were Toll-like receptor 11 (*Tlr11*), Nucleotide-binding oligomerization domain containing 1 (*Nod1*), Mitogen-activated protein kinase kinase kinase kinase 2 (*Map4k2*), Nuclear factor of kappa light polypeptide gene enhancer in B cells 2, p49/p100 (*Nfkb2*), PTK2 protein tyrosine kinase 2 β (*Ptk2b*), CD180 antigen (*Cd180*) (Figure 2c). Cytokines and chemokines involved in the regulation of interferon-gamma mediated inflammation including Chemokine (C motif) ligand 1 (*Xcl1*), Chemokine (C-C motif) ligand 5 (*Ccl5*), Chemokine (C-C motif) ligand 19 (*Ccl19*), Histocompatibility 2, O region α/β locus (H2-Oa; H2-Ob) and Histocompatibility 2 class II locus Mb2 (*H2-DMb2*) were down-regulated in the mice fed HFD-ED, compared with the other two diets, while no changes were seen in the mice fed HFD-CO compared with control (Figure 2d). Genes associated with erythrocyte differentiation and development, and hematopoiesis were up-regulated in the mice fed HFD-ED compared with either diet but no changes were observed in HFD-CO fed mice compared with the control animals (Figure 2e). Plasma erythrocyte concentrations were not measured due to limited sample volume, but it has previously been shown that these genes may reflect increased turnover of erythrocytes without changing erythrocyte concentration in blood [33].

4. Discussion

We have investigated changes in the transcriptome profiles of mouse spleen tissue after an eight-week dietary intervention with control, HFD-ED or HFD-CO diets, the HFD-ED diet differing from the HFD-CO diet by the replacement of 40% of the corn oil (2% out of 5% CO) with purified triglycerides of EPA and DHA. We found that the gene coding for the lipid mediators of both the innate and adaptive immune response were markedly downregulated by the HFD-ED diet. The extensive down-regulation of the innate and adaptive immune system in mice spleen found in this study is in agreement with our previous study of spleen tissues from HFD-fish oil (menhaden oil) fed mice, compared to mice fed HFD-lard [21]. Several other rodent studies using splenic T-cells [18,34–36] also suggesting that EPA and DHA are the components in fish oil responsible for this effect.

In the present study, the spleen transcriptome was extensively influenced by EPA and DHA in the mice fed HFD-ED compared with the mice fed HFD-CO or control diet. Immune system related BPs including T- and B-cell activation and NF-κB related processes were down-regulated in the mice fed HFD-ED compared with either diets suggesting anti-inflammatory effects of a relatively low level of EPA and DHA enrichment of the diet. Contrary to our results, some other studies have found that B-cell response is enhanced in obesity when exposed to EPA and DHA [20,37]. These studies have been conducted in isolated murine B-cells, which may explain the divergent results. Moreover, BPs related to erythropoiesis were up-regulated in mice fed HFD-ED compared with either diets despite similar fat content, indicating possible increased turnover of red blood cells. Again, these data are supported by the previous study of spleen tissues from mice fed HFD-fish oil (menhaden oil) compared to HFD-lard [21].

Diets high in saturated fatty acids may contribute to greater serum levels of inflammatory mediators [11], though these results vary widely in humans [38,39]. Substituting saturated for unsaturated fatty acids can reduce the risk of inflammation [21]. However, the mechanism by which EPA and DHA impact the immune system and especially in spleen is not fully understood. Several hypotheses for how marine fatty acids, EPA and DHA in particular, may be protective against inflammatory disease have been proposed. These include alteration of cell membranes [40], modulation of NF-κB suppression [41,42], and altering of lipid rafts involved in T-lymphocyte signaling in immunological synapses [19]. A role for EPA and DHA in modulating the spleen-inflammatory response is well established [18–20,43], and our transcriptomics results support this role. Moreover, EPA and DHA derived resolvins, the E-series and D-series have chemically unique structural forms. A member of E-series, namely resolvin E1 reduces inflammation in vivo, and blocks human neutrophil transendothelial migration [44]. The DHA derived D-series resolvins, 17S and 17R D-series, are produced during the resolution of inflammation [45]. Thus, the difference in lipid mediators formed from the different fatty acid compositions in the diet may play an important role in effects on the spleen.

NF-κB is a transcription factor that regulates transcription of pro-inflammatory cytokines such as interleukin 6 and 12, interferon-gamma, and tumor necrosis factor [17,46]. Our study shows that HFD-ED can down-regulate certain tumor necrosis factors, as well as toll-like and nod-like receptors that are involved in activation of NF-κB transcription factor compared with the HFD-CO and control diets (Figure 2a,b). In addition, HFD-ED up-regulates the gene for peroxiredoxin 3 (*Prdx3*) involved in mitochondrial homeostasis [47]. This gene has been shown to be up-regulated in adipocyte oxidative stress, mitochondrial biogenesis and adipokines expression [48].

In addition, we found a pronounced decrease in the amount of phospholipid arachidonic acid in the spleen of HFD-ED mice compared to both HFD-CO and the control animals, showing down-regulation of the arachidonic acid pathway leading to the production of lipid mediators [49]. Lipid mediators from arachidonic acid have many functions, and can be both inflammatory and anti-inflammatory [49]. Due to insufficient tissue, further measurement of these lipid mediators was not conducted and should be measured in future studies to confirm this finding, and nor were there measurements of inflammation markers which would have indicated if the effect on phospholipid arachidonic acid concentrations had any effect on inflammation [49]. Linoleic acid, a precursor of arachidonic acid, was nearly two fold higher in the spleen phospholipids of HFD-ED fed mice compared to the other two groups, despite higher amounts of linoleic acid in the HFD-CO diets. One reason behind higher linoleic acid could be due to the fact that, dietary n-3 fatty acids down regulates the gene coding for desaturase [22,25,50], or another reason could be that linoleic acid competes with alpha linolenic acid for the same enzyme system for desaturation and elongation, and is likely that alpha linolenic acid would be preferentially desaturated and elongated to EPA and DHA [50]. However, the corn oil contains quite low-amounts of alpha linolenic acid, which make the latter suggestion less likely. Furthermore, we observed that HFD-ED down-regulated different chemokines such as Xcl1, Ccl5, and Ccl19 when compared with control or HFD-CO (Figure 2c). Disturbed cytokine and chemokine levels may lead to elevated inflammatory conditions [51]. Increased accumulation of the chemokines chemokine (C motif) ligand 1 (*Xcl1*) [52], chemokine (C-C motif) ligand 5 (*Ccl5*), and chemokine (C-C motif) ligand 19 (*Ccl19*) have been observed in infection [53]. Why the dietary enrichment with EPA and DHA has this effect is not clear, and we presume that the effect on phospholipid fatty acid composition may be in part responsible.

HFD-ED down-regulated mitogen-activated protein kinase 2 (*Map4k2*) which is known to have similarity with other serine/threonine kinases found in human lymphoid tissue and are activated in stress response [54]. Different *Mapk* such as Extracellular signal-regulated kinase 1/2 (*Erk1/2*), C-Jun N-terminal kinase (Jnk) and p38 are upregulated in obesity-induced inflammation [55]. Moreover, down-regulation of Protein kinase C β, and δ (*Prkcb* and *Prkcd*) contributes to improved insulin resistance in HFD fed mice [56,57]. Our data show down-regulation of these protein kinases in HFD-ED fed animals compared with control but no changes were seen in HFD-CO compared with control fed animals suggesting that this may mediate lower HFD-induced insulin resistance in HFD-ED fed animals. Although circulating glucose and insulin concentrations were not measured in this study, liver fat and triglycerides were increased by 1.75 and 3 fold, respectively in the HFD-CO compared to HFD-ED [22]. Furthermore, Nuclear factor of κ light polypeptide gene enhancer in B cells 2, p49/p100 (*Nfkb2*) up-regulation is seen in inflammation and activation of the immune response [46], a gene that was down-regulated in HFD-ED fed mice. Nevertheless, a reduced immune response does not indicate a reduced capability to defend against bacterial infection. In a study using menhaden oil, Svahn et al. reported that this led to increased survival and decreased bacterial load in mice with septic infection, even though regulation of the splenic immune response was down-regulated [43].

By studying the effects of EPA and DHA on spleen, we have gained global insight that a relatively small change in dietary fat may have profound effects on spleen metabolism in the context of a HFD. Given the important role of the spleen as a secondary lymphoid organ in immune function and signaling, further research needs to determine if the observed downregulation of immune system related genes has an effect on other tissues, especially those that are known to be adversely affected by inflammation such as adipose tissue or vice-versa and most importantly, if the effects can be translated into humans. The amount of EPA and DHA fed to the mice was about 377 mg EPA and 577 mg DHA/kg per day, respectively. When converted to an equivalent dose in humans [58–60] approximately 9.5 mg/kg and 25 mg/kg was fed. This is somewhat higher relative to what a human would expect to get from eating fatty fish and similar to eating 3 g of fish oil capsules, suggesting that based on dose alone, these results may have relevance for humans. Future dose response studies are needed to establish whether the effects on transcriptomics and fatty acids are reproducible across a wider range of doses, and studies looking at the transcriptome effects across different ages are needed to establish whether long-term supplementation is required to observe the changes in gene-expression. Replication studies in humans are not feasible due to the need to get spleen biopsies from healthy subjects, though measuring work on immune markers and lipid meditators related to our findings may help to confirm that the spleen is affected by supplementation with EPA and DHA.

5. Conclusions

Overall, our data provide a novel insight into the regulation of the splenic transcriptome by EPA and DHA suggesting that EPA and DHA enriched corn oil down-regulate the splenic immune response induced by HFD. EPA and DHA also upregulated hematopoiesis. Furthermore, EPA and DHA decreased splenic phospholipid arachidonic acid concentrations, which could lead to reduced production of inflammatory mediators such as prostaglandins and leukotrienes.

Supplementary Materials: The following are available online at http://www.mdpi.com/2072-6643/9/1/50/s1, Figure S1: (a) Venn diagram depicting overlaps among differentially expressed genes upon dietary intervention. Most regulation can be seen for comparison HFD-ED vs. control diet (ED vs. CD), and HFD-ED vs. HFD-corn oil (ED vs. CO). HFD-corn oil vs. control diet (CO vs. CD) shows comparatively less bidirectional differentially regulated genes; (b) Principle Component Analysis (PCA) plot based on the normalized gene expression from the spleen tissue fed control, HFD-ED and HFD-corn oil is plotted for assessing the quality of the datasets. No animals or any related data was excluded from further assessment; (c) A heatmap showing significantly regulated BPs (p-value $< 10 \times 10^9$) without immune system process for every diet comparison after 8 weeks. Changes in the diet, especially HFD-ED positively regulate BPs mostly related to DNA repair and cell cycle down-regulates NF-κB, interleukin-12 and interferon-gamma related processes. HFD-ED = HFD-ED vs. control diet; HFD-CO = HFD-corn oil vs. control diet; ED-CO = HFD-ED vs. HFD-corn oil; (d) Illustration of linoleic acid and arachidonic acid signaling pathway analysis of the splenic transcriptome for the comparison HFD-ED vs. HFD-CO fed mice. The genes highlighted in red including *Gpx1* (glutathione peroxidase 1) and *Alox12* (arachidonate 12-lipoxigenase) are up-regulated and the genes in green including *Pla2g1b* (phospholipase A2 group IB), *Cyp4f14* (cytochrome P450 family 4 subfamily f polypeptide 14) and *Ptgis* (prostaglandin 12 synthase) are down-regulated. In black are the lipid mediators and synthetic intermediates including prostaglandins, prostacyclins, leukotrienes, 5-oxo-eicosatetraenoic acid, 15-oxo-eicosatetraenoic acid, 12-hydroxy-eicosatetraenoic acid, 20-hydroxy-eicosatetraenoic acid.

Acknowledgments: The study was supported by grants from the Swedish Research Council for Environment, Agricultural Sciences and Spatial Planning (222-2011-1322); the Region of Västra Götaland (VGR; RUN 612-0959-11); and Swedish Research Council (VR-2013-4504). We would like to acknowledge SCIBLU, Lund University for the labelling of RNA and hybridization to the Illumina microarrays chips, and CBI, University of Gothenburg, for their assistance with the animal experiments. We also acknowledge Chalmers Mass Spectrometry Infrastructure (CMSI), Chalmers University of Technology for their help with fatty acid profiling. We would like to thank Taral R Lunavat, Krefting Research Center, Department of Internal Medicine and Clinical Nutrition, University of Gothenburg, for his help with qRT-PCR experiments. We also gratefully acknowledge the kind gifts of the EPAX oils from EPAX AS, Norway (now FMC Corporation, Philadelphia, PA 19104, USA).

Author Contributions: B.G.G., I.N., and A.-S.S. designed the study. B.G.G. performed the animal experiments. B.G.G. and N.K.S. conducted the RNA isolation and microarray data collection. I.N. coordinated microarray experiment and analysis. N.K.S. and O.I.S. performed fatty acid analysis. N.K.S. performed statistical analyses and wrote the manuscript. A.B.R. and N.S. aided in the interpretation of the data and gave their input during the preparation of manuscript. All authors reviewed and approved the final version of manuscript.

Conflicts of Interest: The authors declare no conflict of interest.

References

1. Nathan, C. Points of control in inflammation. *Nature* **2002**, *420*, 846–852. [CrossRef] [PubMed]
2. Shoelson, S.E.; Lee, J.; Goldfine, A.B. Inflammation and insulin resistance. *J. Clin. Investig.* **2006**, *116*, 1793–1801. [CrossRef] [PubMed]
3. Chawla, A.; Nguyen, K.D.; Goh, Y.P. Macrophage-mediated inflammation in metabolic disease. *Nat. Rev. Immunol.* **2011**, *11*, 738–749. [CrossRef] [PubMed]
4. Sowers, J.R. Obesity as a cardiovascular risk factor. *Am. J. Med.* **2003**, *115*, 37S–41S. [CrossRef] [PubMed]
5. World Health Organization. Noncommunicable Diseases. Fact Sheet fs355. 2015. Available online: http://www.who.int/mediacentre/factsheets/fs355/en/ (accessed on 6 September 2016).
6. Mebius, R.E.; Kraal, G. Structure and function of the spleen. *Nat. Rev. Immunol.* **2005**, *5*, 606–616. [CrossRef] [PubMed]
7. Duncan, B.B.; Schmidt, M.I.; Pankow, J.S.; Ballantyne, C.M.; Couper, D.; Vigo, A.; Hoogeveen, R.; Folsom, A.R.; Heiss, G.; Atherosclerosis Risk in Communities Study. Low-grade systemic inflammation and the development of type 2 diabetes: The atherosclerosis risk in communities study. *Diabetes* **2003**, *52*, 1799–1805. [CrossRef] [PubMed]
8. Vozarova, B.; Weyer, C.; Lindsay, R.S.; Pratley, R.E.; Bogardus, C.; Tataranni, P.A. High white blood cell count is associated with a worsening of insulin sensitivity and predicts the development of type 2 diabetes. *Diabetes* **2002**, *51*, 455–461. [CrossRef] [PubMed]
9. Spranger, J.; Kroke, A.; Mohlig, M.; Hoffmann, K.; Bergmann, M.M.; Ristow, M.; Boeing, H.; Pfeiffer, A.F. Inflammatory cytokines and the risk to develop type 2 diabetes: Results of the prospective population-based European Prospective Investigation into Cancer and Nutrition (EPIC)-Potsdam Study. *Diabetes* **2003**, *52*, 812–817. [CrossRef] [PubMed]
10. Herder, C.; Baumert, J.; Thorand, B.; Koenig, W.; de Jager, W.; Meisinger, C.; Illig, T.; Martin, S.; Kolb, H. Chemokines as risk factors for type 2 diabetes: Results from the MONICA/KORA Augsburg study, 1984–2002. *Diabetologia* **2006**, *49*, 921–929. [CrossRef] [PubMed]
11. Lee, J.Y.; Sohn, K.H.; Rhee, S.H.; Hwang, D. Saturated fatty acids, but not unsaturated fatty acids, induce the expression of cyclooxygenase-2 mediated through Toll-like receptor 4. *J. Biol. Chem.* **2001**, *276*, 16683–16689. [CrossRef] [PubMed]
12. Nagakura, T.; Matsuda, S.; Shichijyo, K.; Sugimoto, H.; Hata, K. Dietary supplementation with fish oil rich in omega-3 polyunsaturated fatty acids in children with bronchial asthma. *Eur. Respir. J.* **2000**, *16*, 861–865. [CrossRef] [PubMed]
13. Anderson, B.M.; Ma, D.W. Are all *n*-3 polyunsaturated fatty acids created equal? *Lipids Health Dis.* **2009**, *8*, 33. [CrossRef] [PubMed]
14. Duda, M.K.; O'Shea, K.M.; Stanley, W.C. Omega-3 polyunsaturated fatty acid supplementation for the treatment of heart failure: Mechanisms and clinical potential. *Cardiovasc. Res.* **2009**, *84*, 33–41. [CrossRef] [PubMed]
15. Saremi, A.; Arora, R. The utility of omega-3 fatty acids in cardiovascular disease. *Am. J. Ther.* **2009**, *16*, 421–436. [CrossRef] [PubMed]
16. Yashodhara, B.M.; Umakanth, S.; Pappachan, J.M.; Bhat, S.K.; Kamath, R.; Choo, B.H. Omega-3 fatty acids: A comprehensive review of their role in health and disease. *Postgrad. Med. J.* **2009**, *85*, 84–90. [CrossRef] [PubMed]
17. Calder, P.C. Marine omega-3 fatty acids and inflammatory processes: Effects, mechanisms and clinical relevance. *Biochim. Biophys. Acta* **2015**, *1851*, 469–484. [CrossRef] [PubMed]
18. Fan, Y.Y.; McMurray, D.N.; Ly, L.H.; Chapkin, R.S. Dietary (*n*-3) polyunsaturated fatty acids remodel mouse T-cell lipid rafts. *J. Nutr.* **2003**, *133*, 1913–1920. [PubMed]
19. Fan, Y.Y.; Ly, L.H.; Barhoumi, R.; McMurray, D.N.; Chapkin, R.S. Dietary docosahexaenoic acid suppresses T cell protein kinase C theta lipid raft recruitment and IL-2 production. *J. Immunol.* **2004**, *173*, 6151–6160. [CrossRef] [PubMed]

20. Teague, H.; Harris, M.; Fenton, J.; Lallemand, P.; Shewchuk, B.M.; Shaikh, S.R. Eicosapentaenoic and docosahexaenoic acid ethyl esters differentially enhance B-cell activity in murine obesity. *J. Lipid Res.* **2014**, *55*, 1420–1433. [CrossRef] [PubMed]

21. Svahn, S.L.; Varemo, L.; Gabrielsson, B.G.; Peris, E.; Nookaew, I.; Grahnemo, L.; Sandberg, A.S.; Wernstedt Asterholm, I.; Jansson, J.O.; Nielsen, J.; et al. Six Tissue Transcriptomics Reveals Specific Immune Suppression in Spleen by Dietary Polyunsaturated Fatty Acids. *PLoS ONE* **2016**, *11*, e0155099. [CrossRef] [PubMed]

22. Soni, N.K.; Nookaew, I.; Sandberg, A.S.; Gabrielsson, B.G. Eicosapentaenoic and docosahexaenoic acid-enriched high fat diet delays the development of fatty liver in mice. *Lipids Health Dis.* **2015**, *14*, 74. [CrossRef] [PubMed]

23. Reeves, P.G.; Nielsen, F.H.; Fahey, G.C., Jr. AIN-93 purified diets for laboratory rodents: Final report of the American Institute of Nutrition ad hoc writing committee on the reformulation of the AIN-76A rodent diet. *J. Nutr.* **1993**, *123*, 1939–1951. [PubMed]

24. Nookaew, I.; Gabrielsson, B.G.; Holmäng, A.; Sandberg, A.-S.; Nielsen, J. Identifying Molecular Effects of Diet through Systems Biology: Influence of Herring Diet on Sterol Metabolism and Protein Turnover in Mice. *PLoS ONE* **2010**, *5*, e12361. [CrossRef] [PubMed]

25. Gabrielsson, B.G.; Wikstrom, J.; Jakubowicz, R.; Marmon, S.K.; Carlsson, N.G.; Jansson, N.; Gan, L.M.; Undeland, I.; Lonn, M.; Holmang, A.; et al. Dietary herring improves plasma lipid profiles and reduces atherosclerosis in obese low-density lipoprotein receptor-deficient mice. *Int. J. Mol. Med.* **2012**, *29*, 331–337. [CrossRef] [PubMed]

26. Folch, J.; Lees, M.; Stanley, G.H.S. A simple method for the isolation and purification of total lipides from animal tissues. *J. Biol. Chem.* **1957**, *226*, 497–509. [PubMed]

27. Soni, N.; Ross, A.; Scheers, N.; Savolainen, O.; Nookaew, I.; Gabrielsson, B.; Sandberg, A.-S. Eicosapentaenoic and Docosahexaenoic Acid-Enriched High Fat Diet Delays Skeletal Muscle Degradation in Mice. *Nutrients* **2016**, *8*, 543. [CrossRef] [PubMed]

28. Du, P.; Kibbe, W.A.; Lin, S.M. Lumi: A pipeline for processing Illumina microarray. *Bioinformatics* **2008**, *24*, 1547–1548. [CrossRef] [PubMed]

29. Ritchie, M.E.; Phipson, B.; Wu, D.; Hu, Y.; Law, C.W.; Shi, W.; Smyth, G.K. Limma powers differential expression analyses for RNA-sequencing and microarray studies. *Nucleic Acids Res.* **2015**, *43*, e47. [CrossRef] [PubMed]

30. Varemo, L.; Nielsen, J.; Nookaew, I. Enriching the gene set analysis of genome-wide data by incorporating directionality of gene expression and combining statistical hypotheses and methods. *Nucleic Acids Res.* **2013**, *41*, 4378–4391. [CrossRef] [PubMed]

31. Luo, W.; Brouwer, C. Pathview: An R/Bioconductor package for pathway-based data integration and visualization. *Bioinformatics* **2013**. [CrossRef] [PubMed]

32. Cesta, M.F. Normal structure, function, and histology of the spleen. *Toxicol. Pathol.* **2006**, *34*, 455–465. [CrossRef] [PubMed]

33. Oarada, M.; Furukawa, H.; Majima, T.; Miyazawa, T. Fish oil diet affects on oxidative senescence of red blood cells linked to degeneration of spleen cells in mice. *Biochim. Biophys. Acta* **2000**, *1487*, 1–14. [CrossRef]

34. Fowler, K.H.; Chapkin, R.S.; McMurray, D.N. Effects of purified dietary *n*-3 ethyl esters on murine T lymphocyte function. *J. Immunol.* **1993**, *151*, 5186–5197. [PubMed]

35. Yaqoob, P.; Newsholme, E.A.; Calder, P.C. The effect of dietary lipid manipulation on rat lymphocyte subsets and proliferation. *Immunology* **1994**, *82*, 603–610. [PubMed]

36. Yaqoob, P.; Calder, P. Effects of dietary lipid manipulation upon inflammatory mediator production by murine macrophages. *Cell. Immunol.* **1995**, *163*, 120–128. [CrossRef] [PubMed]

37. Teague, H.; Fhaner, C.J.; Harris, M.; Duriancik, D.M.; Reid, G.E.; Shaikh, S.R. N-3 PUFAs enhance the frequency of murine B-cell subsets and restore the impairment of antibody production to a T-independent antigen in obesity. *J. Lipid Res.* **2013**, *54*, 3130–3138. [CrossRef] [PubMed]

38. Gordon, T.; Kannel, W.B.; Castelli, W.P.; Dawber, T.R. Lipoproteins, cardiovascular disease, and death. The Framingham study. *Arch. Intern. Med.* **1981**, *141*, 1128–1131. [CrossRef] [PubMed]

39. Rahilly-Tierney, C.R.; Lawler, E.V.; Scranton, R.E.; Michael Gaziano, J. Low-density lipoprotein reduction and magnitude of cardiovascular risk reduction. *Prev. Cardiol.* **2009**, *12*, 80–87. [CrossRef] [PubMed]

40. Wassall, S.R.; Stillwell, W. Docosahexaenoic acid domains: The ultimate non-raft membrane domain. *Chem. Phys. Lipids* **2008**, *153*, 57–63. [CrossRef] [PubMed]

41. Mullen, A.; Loscher, C.E.; Roche, H.M. Anti-inflammatory effects of EPA and DHA are dependent upon time and dose-response elements associated with LPS stimulation in THP-1-derived macrophages. *J. Nutr. Biochem.* **2010**, *21*, 444–450. [CrossRef] [PubMed]

42. Mishra, A.; Chaudhary, A.; Sethi, S. Oxidized omega-3 fatty acids inhibit NF-kappaB activation via a PPARalpha-dependent pathway. *Arterioscler. Thromb. Vasc. Biol.* **2004**, *24*, 1621–1627. [CrossRef] [PubMed]

43. Svahn, S.L.; Grahnemo, L.; Palsdottir, V.; Nookaew, I.; Wendt, K.; Gabrielsson, B.; Schele, E.; Benrick, A.; Andersson, N.; Nilsson, S.; et al. Dietary polyunsaturated fatty acids increase survival and decrease bacterial load during septic Staphylococcus aureus infection and improve neutrophil function in mice. *Infect. Immun.* **2015**, *83*, 514–521. [CrossRef] [PubMed]

44. Serhan, C.N.; Clish, C.B.; Brannon, J.; Colgan, S.P.; Chiang, N.; Gronert, K. Novel functional sets of lipid-derived mediators with antiinflammatory actions generated from omega-3 fatty acids via cyclooxygenase 2-nonsteroidal antiinflammatory drugs and transcellular processing. *J. Exp. Med.* **2000**, *192*, 1197–1204. [CrossRef] [PubMed]

45. Serhan, C.N.; Hong, S.; Gronert, K.; Colgan, S.P.; Devchand, P.R.; Mirick, G.; Moussignac, R.L. Resolvins: A family of bioactive products of omega-3 fatty acid transformation circuits initiated by aspirin treatment that counter proinflammation signals. *J. Exp. Med.* **2002**, *196*, 1025–1037. [CrossRef] [PubMed]

46. Kumar, A.; Takada, Y.; Boriek, A.M.; Aggarwal, B.B. Nuclear factor-kappaB: Its role in health and disease. *J. Mol. Med.* **2004**, *82*, 434–448. [CrossRef] [PubMed]

47. Lee, K.P.; Shin, Y.J.; Cho, S.C.; Lee, S.M.; Bahn, Y.J.; Kim, J.Y.; Kwon, E.S.; Jeong do, Y.; Park, S.C.; Rhee, S.G.; et al. Peroxiredoxin 3 has a crucial role in the contractile function of skeletal muscle by regulating mitochondrial homeostasis. *Free Radic Biol. Med.* **2014**, *77*, 298–306. [CrossRef] [PubMed]

48. Huh, J.Y.; Kim, Y.; Jeong, J.; Park, J.; Kim, I.; Huh, K.H.; Kim, Y.S.; Woo, H.A.; Rhee, S.G.; Lee, K.J.; et al. Peroxiredoxin 3 is a key molecule regulating adipocyte oxidative stress, mitochondrial biogenesis, and adipokine expression. *Antioxid. Redox Signal.* **2012**, *16*, 229–243. [CrossRef] [PubMed]

49. Calder, P.C. Polyunsaturated fatty acids and inflammatory processes: New twists in an old tale. *Biochimie* **2009**, *91*, 791–795. [CrossRef] [PubMed]

50. Vessby, B. Dietary fat, fatty acid composition in plasma and the metabolic syndrome. *Curr. Opin. Lipidol.* **2003**, *14*, 15–19. [CrossRef] [PubMed]

51. Brydon, E.W.; Morris, S.J.; Sweet, C. Role of apoptosis and cytokines in influenza virus morbidity. *FEMS Microbiol. Rev.* **2005**, *29*, 837–850. [CrossRef] [PubMed]

52. Lei, Y.; Takahama, Y. XCL1 and XCR1 in the immune system. *Microbes Infect.* **2012**, *14*, 262–267. [CrossRef] [PubMed]

53. Mantovani, A. The chemokine system: Redundancy for robust outputs. *Immunol. Today* **1999**, *20*, 254–257. [CrossRef]

54. Ren, M.; Zeng, J.; De Lemos-Chiarandini, C.; Rosenfeld, M.; Adesnik, M.; Sabatini, D.D. In its active form, the GTP-binding protein rab8 interacts with a stress-activated protein kinase. *Proc. Natl. Acad. Sci. USA* **1996**, *93*, 5151–5155. [CrossRef] [PubMed]

55. Kushiyama, A.; hojima, N.; Ogihara, T.; Inukai, K.; Sakoda, H.; Fujishiro, M.; Fukushima, Y.; Anai, M.; Ono, H.; Horike, N.; et al. Resistin-like molecule beta activates MAPKs, suppresses insulin signaling in hepatocytes, and induces diabetes, hyperlipidemia, and fatty liver in transgenic mice on a high fat diet. *J. Biol. Chem.* **2005**, *280*, 42016–42025. [CrossRef] [PubMed]

56. Rao, X.; Zhong, J.; Xu, X.; Jordan, B.; Maurya, S.; Braunstein, Z.; Wang, T.Y.; Huang, W.; Aggarwal, S.; Periasamy, M.; et al. Exercise protects against diet-induced insulin resistance through downregulation of protein kinase Cbeta in mice. *PLoS ONE* **2013**, *8*, e81364. [CrossRef] [PubMed]

57. Li, M.; Vienberg, S.G.; Bezy, O.; O'Neill, B.T.; Kahn, C.R. Role of PKCdelta in Insulin Sensitivity and Skeletal Muscle Metabolism. *Diabetes* **2015**, *64*, 4023–4032. [CrossRef] [PubMed]

58. Reagan-Shaw, S.; Nihal, M.; Ahmad, N. Dose translation from animal to human studies revisited. *FASEB J.* **2008**, *22*, 659–661. [CrossRef] [PubMed]

59. Efsa Panel on Dietetic Products, Nutrients and Allergies. Scientific Opinion on the substantiation of health claims related to eicosapentaenoic acid (EPA), docosahexaenoic acid (DHA), docosapentaenoic acid (DPA) and maintenance of normal cardiac function (ID 504, 506, 516, 527, 538, 703, 1128, *1317*, 1324, 1325), maintenance of normal blood glucose concentrations (ID 566), maintenance of normal blood pressure (ID 506, 516, 703, 1317, 1324), maintenance of normal blood HDL-cholesterol concentrations (ID 506), maintenance of normal (fasting) blood concentrations of triglycerides (ID 506, 527, 538, 1317, *1324*, 1325), maintenance of normal blood LDL-cholesterol concentrations (ID 527, 538, 1317, *1325*, 4689), protection of the skin from photo-oxidative (UV-induced) damage (ID 530), improved absorption of EPA and DHA (ID 522, 523), contribution to the normal function of the immune system by decreasing the levels of eicosanoids, arachidonic acid-derived mediators and pro-inflammatory cytokines (ID 520, 2914), and "immunomodulating agent" (4690) pursuant to Article 13(1) of Regulation (EC) No 1924/2006. *EFSA J.* **2010**, *8*, 1796–1828.

60. Efsa Panel on Dietetic Products, Nutrients and Allergies. Scientific Opinion on the Tolerable Upper Intake Level of eicosapentaenoic acid (EPA), docosahexaenoic acid (DHA) and docosapentaenoic acid (DPA). *EFSA J.* **2012**, *10*, 2815.

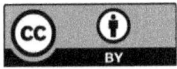

nutrients

MDPI

Article

Lipidomic and Antioxidant Response to Grape Seed, Corn and Coconut Oils in Healthy Wistar Rats

Abraham Wall-Medrano [1,*], Laura A. de la Rosa [1,*], Alma A. Vázquez-Flores [1], Gilberto Mercado-Mercado [1], Rogelio González-Arellanes [1], José A. López-Díaz [1], Aarón F. González-Córdova [2], Gustavo A. González-Aguilar [3], Belinda Vallejo-Cordoba [2] and Francisco J. Molina-Corral [4]

[1] Instituto de Ciencias Biomédicas, Universidad Autónoma de Ciudad Juárez, Anillo Envolvente del PRONAF y Estocolmo s/n, Ciudad Juárez 32310, Chihuahua, Mexico; alma.vazquez@uacj.mx (A.A.V.-F.); gil_4783@yahoo.com.mx (G.M.-M.); rga.nut@gmail.com (R.G.-A.); joslopez@uacj.mx (J.A.L.-D.)

[2] Centro de Investigación en Alimentación y Desarrollo, AC (Unidad Hermosillo), Coordinación de Tecnología de Alimentos de Origen Animal (DTAOA), Carretera a la Victoria km. 0.6, AP 1735, Hermosillo 83000, Sonora, Mexico; aaronglz@ciad.mx (A.F.G.-C.); vallejo@ciad.mx (B.V.-C.)

[3] Centro de Investigación en Alimentación y Desarrollo, AC (Unidad Hermosillo), Tecnología de Alimentos de Origen Vegetal (DTAOV), Carretera a la Victoria km. 0.6, AP 1735, Hermosillo 83000, Sonora, Mexico; gustavo@ciad.mx

[4] Centro de Investigación en Alimentación y Desarrollo, AC. (Unidad Cuauhtémoc), Laboratorio de Tecnología de Alimentos de Origen Vegetal y Toxicología, Ave. Río Conchos s/n, Parque Industrial, AP 781, Cuauhtémoc 31570, Chihuahua, Mexico; javiermolina@ciad.mx

[*] Correspondence: awall@uacj.mx (A.W.-M.); ldelaros@uacj.mx (L.A.d.l.R.);
Tel.: +52-656-688-1821 (A.W.-M. & L.A.d.l.R.); Fax: +52-656-688-1800 (A.W.-M. & L.A.d.l.R.)

Received: 5 November 2016; Accepted: 11 January 2017; Published: 20 January 2017

Abstract: Specialty oils differ in fatty acid, phytosterol and antioxidant content, impacting their benefits for cardiovascular health. The lipid (fatty acid, phytosterol) and antioxidant (total phenolics, radical scavenging capacity) profiles of grapeseed (GSO), corn (CO) and coconut (CNO) oils and their physiological (triacylglycerides, total and HDL-cholesterol and antioxidant capacity (FRAP) in serum and fatty acid and phytosterol hepatic deposition) and genomic (HL, LCAT, ApoA-1 and SR-BP1 mRNA hepatic levels) responses after their sub-chronic intake (10% diet for 28 days) was examined in healthy albino rats. Fatty acid, phytosterol and antioxidant profiles differed between oils ($p \leq 0.01$). Serum and hepatic triacylglycerides and total cholesterol increased ($p \leq 0.01$); serum HDL-Cholesterol decreased ($p < 0.05$); but serum FRAP did not differ ($p > 0.05$) in CNO-fed rats as compared to CO or GSO groups. Hepatic phytosterol deposition was higher (+2.2 mg/g; $p \leq 0.001$) in CO- than GSO-fed rats, but their fatty acid deposition was similar. All but ApoA-1 mRNA level increased in GSO-fed rats as compared to other groups ($p \leq 0.01$). Hepatic fatty acid handling, but not antioxidant response, nor hepatic phytosterol deposition, could be related to a more efficient reverse-cholesterol transport in GSO-fed rats as compared to CO or CNO.

Keywords: specialty oil; fatty acids; grapeseed oil; antioxidant; HDL; coconut oil; corn oil; lipoproteins; phytosterols

1. Introduction

Cardiovascular disease (CVD) continues to be the leading cause of mortality worldwide. It accounts for 17.3 million deaths per year, and it is expected to grow steadily by 2030 [1,2]. The World Health Organization estimates that failure to implement prevention and therapy strategies for CVD could result in an expense of $47 trillion dollars in the next 25 years, a cost that will be borne more heavily by low and middle income countries in which atherosclerotic CVD is the reason for about 50%

of all deaths [1]. CVD includes several illnesses, such as coronary heart disease, atherosclerosis and stroke, in which many environmental and genetic factors concur [3,4]. Fortunately, small dietary and behavioral changes may result in a significant reduction of several CVD risk factors [5].

The association of specific rather than total lipid intake on the risk for CVD has been documented for many years. It is well known that the intake of saturated fatty acids (SFA) increases blood triacylglycerides (TAG), total (TC), very low (VLDL-C) and low density lipoprotein (LDL-C) cholesterol, leading to a higher risk for atherosclerosis and coronary heart disease [6,7]. Despite the latter, in silico and wet lab studies have revealed that lauric acid ($C_{12:0}$) from coconut oil (CNO) may exert a TC-lowering effect [8]. However, a low SFA intake without any other dietary modification reduces not only the atherogenic (LDL-C), but also the cardio-protective (HDL-C) cholesterol [9]; the partial replacement of SFA with either mono- (MUFA) or poly- (PUFA) unsaturated fatty acids (FA) reduces the risk for myocardial infarctions and stroke among high-risk persons [10,11]; and the cardio protective effects of omega 3 (*n*-3) PUFA, particularly α-linolenic acid ($C_{18:3}$), have been extensively documented [12–14].

More recently, phytosterols (PST) and antioxidants (AOX), commonly found in substantial amounts in specialty oils, such as grape seed (GSO) [15], corn (CO) [16] and pecan nut (PNO) [17] oils, have been associated with a lower risk for oxidative stress, inflammation and dyslipidemia that in concerted action affect the endothelial integrity [18,19]; in fact, synergistic effects between these molecules may result in an even better lipidomic effect [20]. However, the aforementioned edible oils and others differ in their FA, PST and AOX profile, which may impact differently their benefits for cardiovascular health [21]. Therefore, the aim of this study was to evaluate the lipid and AOX profile of corn oil (CO), GSO and CNO and their physiological and genomic effect (reverse-cholesterol transport) after a sub-chronic intake (28 days) in healthy Wistar rats.

2. Materials and Methods

2.1. Edible Oils and Chemicals

Commercial grapeseed oil (GSO; Olitalia, Italy) and coconut oil (CNO; Everland Natural Foods, Burnaby, BC, Canada) were imported from Canada, and corn oil (CO; Mazola, ACH Food Companies Inc., Cordoba, TN. USA) was obtained from the local market, wrapped in dark plastic bags and transported to the laboratory under refrigeration (4 °C). Casein (ANRC, 95% protein), AIN-93-vitamin mix, AIN-93G-mineral mix, cellulose and DL-methionine were purchased from Bioserv, Inc. (Frenchtown, NJ, USA).

All other food-grade ingredients used to prepare the experimental diets were purchased in the local market. Folin–Ciocalteu reagent (FCR), trolox (6-hydroxy-2,5,7,8-tetramethylchroman-2-carboxylic acid), DPPH (2,2-diphenyl-1-picrylhydrazyl), $ABTS^{2-}$ (2,2′-azinobis-(3-ethylbenzothiazoline-6-sulphonate), gallic acid, quercetin and choline chloride (99% pure, 74.6% choline) were purchased from Sigma Chemical Co. (St. Louis, MO, USA), while standards of fatty acid methyl esters (Supelco® 37 Component FAME Mix) and sterols (campesterol, ergosterol, stigmasterol and β-Sitosterol) were from Supelco, USA (St. Louis, MO, USA). Kits for lipid determination were from Stanbio Laboratory (Boerne, TX, USA). Unless otherwise specified, all ACS-grade solvents were purchased from JT Baker (Mexico City, Mexico) or Fisher Scientific (Houston, TX, USA). All reagents and chemicals used in gene expression analyses were from Sigma-Aldrich (St. Luis, MO, USA) or Promega (Madison, WI, USA).

2.2. Fatty Acid and Phytosterol Profile of Edible Oils

The fatty acid (FA) composition of GSO, CO or CNO was analyzed by GC-MS as fatty acid methyl esters (FAMEs) [22], following the method proposed by Villa-Rodríguez et al. [23] in a GC-MS (VARIAN Saturn 2100D) equipped with a CP7420 column (100 m, 0.25 mm i.d.) using helium ultra-high purity grade (1 mL/min) as the carrier gas. Operating conditions were: oven (T (°C)/time (min)/rate

(°C/min)): 160/4/20 and 198/42/1, injector (EFC Type 1) and detector temperatures were 250 °C and 180 °C, respectively. The mass spectrometer was operated in the electron impact (EI) mode at 70 eV in the scan range of 40–500 m/z. FAMEs were identified by comparing the peak's retention against commercial standards (Supelco 37 FAME Mix; Sigma Chemical Co., St. Louis, MO, USA) and by comparing the respective ion chromatograms with those reported in the NIST 2008 library (NIST/EPA/NIH Mass Spectral Library, Version 2.0). Phytosterol (PST) composition in all three oils was evaluated by direct saponification (KOH 0.5 M) and capillary gas chromatography following the method proposed by Fleteouris et al. [24] in a 6890 GC System Gas Chromatograph (Hewlett-Packard Development Company, L.P., Houston, TX, USA) equipped with a SP™-2560 Capillary GC Column (L × I.D. 100 m × 0.25 mm, d_f 0.20 µm;) using helium Ultra High Purity grade (1 mL/min) as the carrier gas.

2.3. Total Phenolic Compounds and Antioxidant Capacity

Total phenolic compounds (TP) in edible oils were quantified with the FCR [25] at 665 nm, and results were expressed as milligrams of gallic acid equivalents (GAE) per 100 g of edible oil (mg GAE/100 g). The radical scavenging capacity (RSC) of edible oils was tested against DPPH (518 nm) and $ABTS^{2-}$ (734 nm) radicals, as suggested by Brand-Williams et al. [26] and Re et al. [27], respectively; values were expressed as millimoles of trolox equivalents per liter (mM TE). Lastly, serum (1:1000 dilution) total antioxidant capacity (TAC) was assayed by the ferric reducing/antioxidant power (FRAP) assay at 595 nm using $FeSO_4$ (in water) as the standard as previously reported [28]; values are expressed as mM TE.

2.4. Bioassay Protocol

The experiment was conducted in pathogen-free male Wistar rats (300 g) obtained from the Universidad Autónoma de Ciudad Juárez (UACJ) animal care facility. Rats were randomly assigned to three groups ($n = 6$ each) and fed ad libitum with one of three iso-energetic diets (399 kcal/100 g diet: 23%, 20% and 57% energy from fat, protein and carbohydrates, respectively) (Table 1).

Table 1. Experimental diets (g/100 g).

Ingredient	GSO	CO	CNO	Ingredient	GSO	CO	CNO
GSO [1]	10.0			DL-methionine [2,4]	0.2	0.2	0.2
CO [1]		10.0		Cellulose [2]	5.0	5.0	5.0
CNO [1]			10.0	AIN-93G-Mineral mix [2]	3.5	3.5	3.5
SFA	1.1	1.4	9.2	AIN-93-Vitamin mix [2]	1.0	1.0	1.0
MUFA	3.2	3.2	0.7	Choline chloride [5]	0.02	0.02	0.02
PUFA	5.7	5.4	0.1	Sucrose + maltodextrins [1]	17.6	17.7	17.7
Casein [2,3]	21.0	21.0	21.0	Corn starch [1]	38.7	38.8	38.8

[1] Food-grade (several trademarks); grapeseed oil (GSO), corn oil (CO), coconut oil (CNO); [2] food-grade from Bioserv, Inc. (Frenchtown, NJ, USA); [3] ANRC (American National Research Council) grade: 95% protein, vitamin-free, 2.5 of total sulfur amino acids (TSA)/100 g protein; [4] to reach >0.98 g/100 g diet of TSA [29]; [5] 99% pure (74.6% choline); saturated (SFA), mono- (MUFA) and poly-unsaturated fatty acids (PUFA). All diets were isocaloric (4 kcal/g).

This formulation was initially based on the nutrient requirements to sustain an adequate growth in young rats [29], mimicking the AIN-93G rodent diet, but differing on the amount (10 g instead of 5 g/100 g), caloric contribution (23% instead of 17%) and lipid source (GSO, CO and CNO instead of soybean oil). After 1 week of acclimatization and during the 4 weeks of experimental treatment, rats were housed individually in metabolic cages under controlled environmental conditions (22 ± 2 °C, relative humidity 45%–60%, 12-h light to dark cycles). Animals and residual diets were weighed every other day, and the feed efficiency ratio (FER = weight gain (g)/diet consumed (g)) was calculated. At the end of the study, animals were sacrificed under anesthesia (tiletamine-zolazepam (Zoletil®, 1 mL/kg; Virbac, Barcelona, Spain)) by cervical dislocation after overnight fast.

All experimental procedures were approved by the UACJ-Biomedical Science Institute Ethics Committee (approval date: 24 October 2012), according to the National legislation on the use of animals for (NOM-062-ZOO-1999) [30] and the National Institutes of Health (NIH) Guide for Care and Use of Laboratory Animals.

2.5. Biological Samples

Blood samples were obtained by cardiac puncture during anesthesia, collected in anticoagulant-free tubes and centrifuged at 2000× g for 10 min at 4 °C to obtain serum, which was stored at −80 °C until use. Livers were carefully removed, rinsed with sterile PBS, blotted on a filter paper to remove the excess of water, weighed and the hepatosomatic index calculated (HIS = liver weight × 100 × body weight^{-1}). Livers were frozen in liquid nitrogen and stored at −80 °C until use.

2.6. Serum and Hepatic Lipids

Serum samples were analyzed for TAG, TC and HDL-C as-collected, while hepatic lipids (total fat, TAG and TC) from all 18 samples (6 rats/3 diets) were extracted by the Folch method [31] using ice-cold chloroform: methanol (2:1 v/v) for 20 min. The Folch method is the most effective method for extracting fatty acids, sterols and steroids from biological samples as compared to other lipid extraction methods [32]. The content of total lipids in hepatic samples was expressed as a percentage (%), while the FA and PST profile of liver fat extracts was performed as for edible oils (Section 2.2), and values were expressed as g (FA) or mg (PST) per 100 g of liver fat. TAG were assayed by the glycerol-phosphate oxidase colorimetric method (TAG liquiColor® GPO-PAP; Stanbio Laboratory, USA), while TC and HDL-C by the cholesterol esterase/oxidase method (liquiColor®; Stanbio Laboratory, Boerne, USA) following the manufacturer's protocol. Lipid values are expressed as mM (serum) and mmol/g (hepatic). All assays were performed in quadruplicates in 96-well microplates.

2.7. Gene Expression Analysis

Total RNA was isolated from 100 to 150 mg of each liver sample (n = 18; 6 rats/3 diets) using TRI reagent (T9424; Sigma-Aldrich, St. Louis, MO, USA) according to the manufacturer's instructions. The recovered RNA was treated with RNase-free DNase (Promega, 6PIM610, Madison, WI, USA); its integrity (18S and 28S bands) was evaluated by electrophoresis in 1.0% agarose gels stained with ethidium bromide, and its concentration and purity (260/280 nm ratio >1.8) was evaluated in a Quawell Q3000 UV spectrophotometer (Quawell Technology, Inc., San Jose, CA, USA). Each DNase-treated RNA (2 µg; triplicates) was reverse transcribed (RT) to complementary DNA (cDNA) using the GoScript™ reverse transcription system (A5001; Promega) in a MultiGene™ OptiMax Thermal Cycler (Lab Net International, Inc., Edison, NJ, USA).

One hundred nanograms of each cDNA were further amplified by PCR using the GoTaq® green master mix (M7122; Promega). Reaction mixtures were incubated for 5 min at 25 °C, 60 min at 42 °C and 15 min at 70 °C for enzyme inactivation. End point-PCR amplifications proceeded as follows: Cycle 1 (94 °C/120 s), Cycles 2–35 (denaturing (94 °C/30 s)), annealing (Tm °C/30 s) and extension (72 °C/40 s). PCR products were stored at −80 °C until analysis. All PCR amplifications, from which the semi-quantitative (relative) gene expression (sqRT-PCR) level was estimated, were always performed under the same analytical conditions, the same cDNA stock and the same Taq DNA polymerase dilution. Gene-specific primers pairs were designed (Tm = 57–60 °C) using primer BLAST software from reference sequences deposited in the National Center for Biotechnology Information website (Table 2). Lastly, end point RT-PCR products were separated on 2% agarose gels under 1× TAE buffer, stained with ethidium bromide (0.5 µg/mL in 1× TAE) and visualized using the Protein Simple Red Imager (Protein Simple, Santa Clara, CA, USA). Images were processed and semi-quantified using the ImageJ software (1.47v, WS Rasband-US National Institutes of Health: Bethesda, MD, USA), using 45S pre-rRNA, precursors of 18S, 5.8S and 28S rRNA, as the house-keeping gene (Rn45S; NR_046239.1).

Table 2. PCR primers.

Gene	NCBI-RS	Protein	Primer Pair (5'-3')	*Tm* °C
Rn45s	NR_046239.1		Fw: GTTCCGCTCACACCTCAGAT Rv: CAAGTGCGTTCGAAGTGTCG	58
Lcat	NM_017024.2	LCAT	Fw: ACACAGGCCAAGACTTCGAG Rv: GGTTGGGGACTTAGGAGTGC	56
ApoA1	NM_012738.1	ApoA-1	Fw: CCTGGACAACTGGGACACTC Rv: GCCCAGAACTCCTGAGTCAC	57
Lipc	NM_012597.2	HL	Fw: GCACTATGCTATTGCCGTGC Rv: TTGATGCCCACACTCAGACC	60
Srb1	NM_031541.1	SR-B1	Fw: CCCCATGAACTGTTCCGTGA Rv: GATCTTCCCTGTTTGCCCGA	57

National Center for Biotechnology Information (NCBI) reference sequence (RS); genes: *Rattus norvegicus* 45S pre-ribosomal RNA (Rn45s), lecithin cholesterol acyltransferase (Lcat), apolipoprotein A1 (Apoa1), lipase C hepatic type (Lipc) and scavenger receptor class B, member 1 (Scarb1) mRNA. Primer forward (Fw) and reverse (Rv).

2.8. Statistical Analysis

Normally-distributed data (means ± SD) were analyzed by one-way analysis of variance (ANOVA) and the Tukey–Kramer post hoc test to assess differences between groups' (GSO, CO, CNO) means. Nonparametric variables were evaluated by the Mann–Whitney U test, using the SPSS statistics software 15.0 (SPSS Inc., Chicago, IL, USA). Statistical significance was confirmed as $p < 0.05$.

3. Results

3.1. Lipid and Antioxidant Profile of Edible Oils

The FA, PST and AOX profiles significantly differ between oils. CNO differ ($p \leq 0.01$) from CO and GSO in all thirteen FA reported in Table 3 and ratios in Figure 1.

Table 3. Fatty acid profile in edible oils [1].

Fatty Acid	GSO	CO	CNO
SFA	10.24 ± 0.32 [a]	14.38 ± 0.65 [c]	92.13 ± 2.02 [b]
$C_{6:0}$	≤0.001 [a]	≤0.001 [a]	0.56 ± 0.04 [b]
$C_{8:0}$	≤0.001 [a]	≤0.001 [a]	6.23 ± 0.10 [b]
$C_{10:0}$	≤0.001 [a]	≤0.001 [a]	5.82 ± 0.02 [b]
$C_{12:0}$	≤0.001 [a]	≤0.001 [a]	42.67 ± 1.42 [b]
$C_{14:0}$	0.07 ± 0.03 [a]	0.04 ± 0.02 [a]	21.12 ± 0.97 [b]
$C_{16:0}$	6.63 ± 0.11 [a]	12.47 ± 0.50 [c]	11.69 ± 0.09 [b]
$C_{17:0}$ *	0.03 ± 0.02 [ab]	0.05 ± 0.02 [a]	≤0.001 [b]
$C_{18:0}$	3.49 ± 0.22 [a]	1.79 ± 0.12 [c]	4.03 ± 0.06 [b]
MUFA	32.09 ± 0.99 [a]	31.60 ± 0.52 [a]	6.63 ± 0.10 [b]
$C_{14:1}$	0.03 ± 0.02 [a]	0.02 ± 0.01 [a]	0.13 ± 0.06 [b]
$C_{16:1}$ **	0.09 ± 0.02 [a]	0.10 ± 0.05 [a]	≤0.001 [b]
$C_{18:1}$	32.00 ± 1.00 [a]	31.50 ± 0.53 [a]	6.63 ± 0.10 [b]
PUFA	57.21 ± 1.06 [a]	53.65 ± 0.32 [c]	0.76 ± 0.06 [b]
$C_{18:2}$	57.20 ± 1.06 [a]	53.33 ± 0.32 [c]	0.75 ± 0.05 [b]
$C_{18:3}$	≤0.001 [a]	0.32 ± 0.02 [c]	≤0.001 [a]

[1] Values are expressed as the mean ± SD (g/100 g); different superscript letters within the same line mean statistical differences at $p \leq 0.001$, otherwise specified ($p < 0.05$ *, $p < 0.01$ **).

Individual differences between GSO (higher $C_{16:0}$, $C_{18:2}$) and CO (higher $C_{18:0}$, $C_{18:3}$) were very few (Table 3), but MUFA/SFA, PUFA/SFA and the deterioration index ($C_{18:2}/C_{16:0}$) were higher in GSO ($p \leq 0.01$). Conversely, stigmasterol, β-sitosterol and total PST content was in the order

CO > GSO > CNO ($p \leq 0.001$), and campesterol and ergosterol were only detected in CO (Table 4). Lastly, TP content and radical scavenging capacity (RSC) with the DPPH radical were CO > CNO > GSO and CO > GSO > CNO with the $ABTS^{2-}$ radical ($p \leq 0.001$; Table 4).

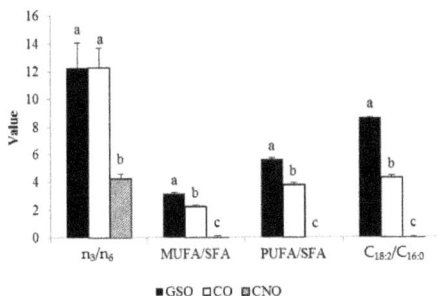

Figure 1. Fatty acid ratios in edible oils. Values are expressed as the mean ± SD ; Different superscripts within the same fatty acid ratio mean statistical differences at $p \leq 0.001$; saturated (SFA), monounsaturated (MUFA), polyunsaturated (PUFA) fatty acids, fat deterioration index ($C_{18:2}/C_{16:0}$).

Table 4. Phytosterol and antioxidant profile of edible oils [1,2]. TE, trolox equivalents.

Variable	GSO	CO	CNO
Phytosterols (mg/g)			
Campesterol	$\leq$0.001 [a]	0.14 ± 0.00 [b]	$\leq$0.001 [a]
Ergosterol	$\leq$0.001 [a]	0.97 ± 0.01 [b]	$\leq$0.001 [a]
Stigmasterol	1.20 ± 0.02 [a]	0.52 ± 0.01 [b]	$\leq$0.001 [c]
β-Sitosterol	1.52 ± 0.01 [a]	8.37 ± 0.04 [b]	$\leq$0.001 [c]
Total	1.72 ± 0.01 [a]	10.0 ± 0.02 [b]	$\leq$0.001 [c]
Antioxidant capacity			
TP (mgGAE/100 g)	2.36 ± 0.12 [a]	2.96 ± 0.12 [b]	2.58 ± 0.14 [c]
ABTS (mM TE)	0.38 ± 0.01 [a]	4.58 ± 0.48 [b]	0.02 ± 0.01 [c]
DPPH (mM TE)	0.55 ± 0.01 [a]	24.68 ± 0.94 [b]	1.95 ± 0.39 [c]

[1] Values are expressed as the mean ± standard deviation from six rats per dietary treatment at the end of the experiment; [2] Different superscript letters within the same line mean statistical differences ($p \leq 0.001$); total phenolic compounds (TP), radical scavenging capacity (ABTS or DPPH).

3.2. Bioassay Parameters

According to Table 5, cumulative (in 28 days) weight gain (~56 g), food (~257 g) and fat (~25.7 g) intake, FER (~0.22), liver weight (~11 g) and water content (~67.3%) and HSI (~3.6) were not different among feeding groups ($p \geq 0.21$). However, CNO-fed rats ate 4.9–5.6-times more SFA, but 0.8- and 0.1-times less MUFA and PUFA than GSO or CO fed-rats ($p \leq 0.001$), leading to a higher deposition of total fats in the liver in CNO-fed rats (~7.0) vs. the other two groups (~5%; $p < 0.01$).

3.3. Serum and Hepatic Lipidomic and Antioxidant Response

Serum (mM) and hepatic (mmol/g) TAG (~2.0 and 0.47) and TC (~2.5 and 0.18) responses to GSO and CO were not different (Figure 2), but lower ($p < 0.01$) than those observed in CNO-fed rats (TC = 3.2 and 0.35; TAG = 3.5 and 0.75). Serum HDL-C (mM) was lower (1.0) in the CNO-fed group ($p < 0.05$) as compared to GSO or CO-fed rats (~1.3).

Except for a slightly higher accumulation of margaric acid ($C_{17:0}$, +0.04 g/100 g liver fat) and total SFA (+1.97 g/100 g liver fat) in CO-fed rats, the liver accumulation of all other FA was quite similar to

GSO-fed rats (Table 6), consistent with the same total liver fat accumulation (Table 5). Furthermore, CNO-fed rats accumulated more SFA (+10 g/100 g liver fat) and MUFA (+8.5 g/100 g liver fat), but less PUFA (−18 g/100 g liver fat) than CO- and GSO-fed rats. Nevertheless, all groups did not differ on hepatic accumulation of the following FA (Appendix A): SFA ($C_{8:0}$, $C_{10:0}$, $C_{15:0}$, $C_{18:0}$, $C_{20:0}$; $p \geq 0.11$), MUFA ($C_{15:1}$, $C_{17:1}$, $C_{20:1}$; $p \geq 0.57$) and PUFA ($C_{18:2n3}$, $C_{22:5n3}$; $p \geq 0.19$). Lastly, with a few exceptions, PST accumulation was CO > GSO or CNO (Table 7), but serum TAC (FRAP) did not differ (~0.47 mM TE; $p = 0.08$) between diets (Appendix A).

Table 5. Bioassay parameters [1,2,3].

Variable	GSO	CO	CNO
Initial body weight	303.8 ± 26.8	298.2 ± 30.0	309.7 ± 24.7
Final body weight	365.8 ± 20.1	358.5 ± 29.1	356.3 ± 27.8
Weight gain	62.0 ± 21.0	60.0 ± 7.2	46.0 ± 11.0
Total food intake	287.2 ± 52.5	254.4 ± 34.3	229.8 ± 37.4
Total fat intake	28.7 ± 5.3	25.4 ± 3.4	23.0 ± 3.7
SFA intake ***	3.2 ± 0.6 [a]	3.6 ± 0.5 [a]	21.1 ± 3.4 [b]
MUFA intake ***	9.2 ± 1.7 [a]	8.1 ± 1.1 [a]	1.6 ± 0.3 [b]
PUFA intake ***	16.4 ± 3.0 [a]	13.7 ± 1.9 [a]	0.2 ± 0.0 [b]
FER	0.22 ± 0.08	0.24 ± 0.03	0.20 ± 0.05
Liver weight	11.7 ± 1.0	11.4 ± 0.8	10.2 ± 2.1
HSI (%)	3.9 ± 0.4	3.8 ± 0.2	3.3 ± 0.7
Liver water (%)	66.7 ± 1.8	67.9 ± 1.2	67.4 ± 0.3
Liver fat (%) **	4.9 ± 1.0 [a]	5.0 ± 0.7 [a]	6.9 ± 1.0 [b]

[1] Values are expressed as the mean (g) ± standard deviation from six rats per dietary treatment accumulated at the 28th day, otherwise specified; [2] Different superscript letter in the same line mean statistical differences (*** $p \leq 0.001$, ** $p \leq 0.01$); [3] food efficiency ratio (FER = weight gain (g)/diet consumed (g)), hepatosomatic index (HSI = liver weight × 100 × body weight^{-1}), saturated (SFA), monounsaturated (MUFA), polyunsaturated (PUFA) fatty acids.

Table 6. Fatty acid deposition in liver [1].

Fatty Acid	GSO	CO	CNO
SFA	31.28 ± 3.67 [a]	33.25 ± 2.08 [b]	42.29 ± 1.87 [c]
$C_{12:0}$	0.11 ± 0.03 [a]	0.08 ± 0.04 [a]	1.20 ± 0.42 [b]
$C_{14:0}$	0.38 ± 0.05 [a]	0.46 ± 0.10 [a]	2.81 ± 0.33 [b]
$C_{16:0}$	16.36 ± 0.80 [a]	18.35 ± 0.57 [a]	23.19 ± 1.08 [b]
$C_{17:0}$	0.34 ± 0.06 [a]	0.38 ± 0.04 [b]	0.21 ± 0.05 [c]
$C_{22:0}$	0.17 ± 0.05 [a,c]	0.16 ± 0.03 [a]	0.26 ± 0.02 [b]
MUFA	13.91 ± 2.73 [a]	15.55 ± 1.93 [a]	23.31 ± 2.65 [b]
$C_{16:1}$	0.88 ± 0.41 [a]	0.88 ± 0.18 [a]	4.03 ± 1.30 [b]
$C_{18:1cis}$	11.82 ± 2.29 [a]	13.63 ± 1.81 [a]	18.12 ± 1.48 [b]
PUFA	53.16 ± 1.37 [a]	51.27 ± 0.75 [a]	34.41 ± 2.52 [b]
$C_{18:2cis}$	25.08 ± 1.11 [a]	23.35 ± 2.16 [a]	10.38 ± 1.37 [b]
$C_{18:3n6}$ **	0.30 ± 0.11 [a]	0.34 ± 0.11 [a]	0.16 ± 0.03 [a]
$C_{20:2}$ **	0.85 ± 0.12 [a]	0.78 ± 0.05 [ab]	0.57 ± 0.23 [b]
$C_{20:3n6}$	0.56 ± 0.09 [a]	0.83 ± 0.25 [a]	1.39 ± 0.16 [b]
$C_{20:4n6}$	22.13 ± 2.09 [a]	21.29 ± 1.91 [a]	15.20 ± 1.33 [b]
$C_{22:4n6}$	0.61 ± 0.14 [a]	0.69 ± 0.09 [a]	0.27 ± 0.06 [b]
$C_{22:6n3}$	2.77 ± 0.39 [a]	2.94 ± 0.47 [a]	5.54 ± 0.28 [b]

[1] Fatty acids were expressed as the mean (g/100 g liver fat) ± standard deviation from six rats per dietary treatment at the end of the experiment (28th day). Different superscript letters within the same line mean statistical differences at $p \leq 0.001$, otherwise specified ($p < 0.01$ **); saturated (SFA), monounsaturated (MUFA), polyunsaturated (PUFA) fatty acids.

Table 7. Phytosterol deposition in liver [1].

Phytosterol	GSO	CO	CNO
Campesterol	0.03 ± 0.02 [a]	0.34 ± 0.05 [b]	0.13 ± 0.04 [c]
Ergosterol	0.32 ± 0.18 [a]	0.75 ± 0.28 [b]	0.07 ± 0.02 [a]
Stigmasterol **	0.09 ± 0.05 [ab]	0.13 ± 0.03 [a]	0.05 ± 0.03 [b]
β-Sitosterol	0.52 ± 0.23 [a]	1.95 ± 0.56 [b]	0.26 ± 0.09 [a]
Total	0.96 ± 0.45 [a]	3.16 ± 0.62 [b]	0.50 ± 0.18 [a]

[1] Values are expressed as the mean (mg/g) $\pm$ standard deviation ($n = 4$); Different superscript letters within the same line means statistical differences at $p \leq 0.001$, otherwise specified ($p < 0.01$ **).

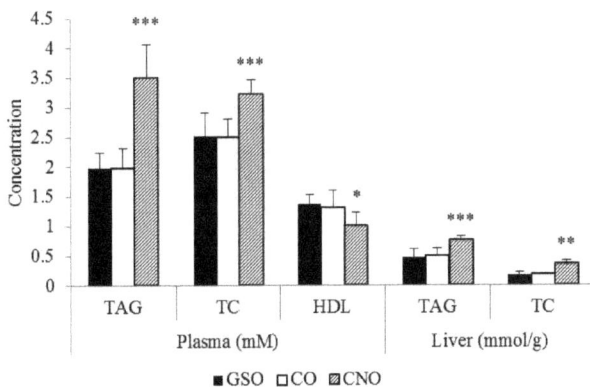

Figure 2. Serum and hepatic lipids. Values are expressed as the mean $\pm$ SD ($n = 6$/group) at the 28th day; [2] $p < 0.05$ *, $p < 0.01$ **, $p \leq 0.001$ ***; triacylglycerides (TAG) and total (TC) and high density lipoprotein-cholesterol (HDL).

3.4. Expression of HDL-Metabolism Related Genes

The sqRT-PCR evaluation revealed that mRNA levels (normalized to Rn45s) of lecithin-cholesterol acyltransferase (LCAT), hepatic lipase (HL) and scavenger receptor class B type 1 (SR-B1), but not that of apolipoprotein A1 (ApoA-1), were upregulated to a higher extent in GSO-fed rats as compared to CO- or CNO-fed rats (Figure 3). Furthermore, the HL lipase mRNA level was higher in CO than CNO-fed rats.

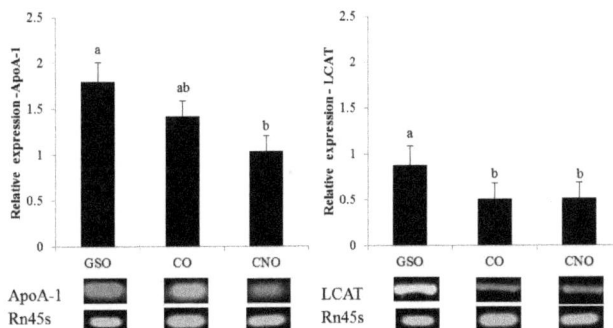

Figure 3. *Cont.*

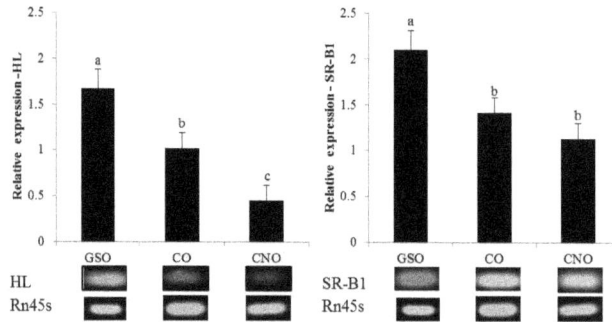

Figure 3. Relative mRNA level of four participants in HDL metabolism. Relative expression normalized to *Rattus norvegicus* 45S pre-ribosomal RNA (Rn45s); data are expressed as the mean ± SD (*n* = 6 rats/group) at the 28th day; Different superscript letters for a same gene means tatistical differences at ≤0.01; lecithin-cholesterol acyltransferase (LCAT), apolipoprotein A1 (ApoA-1), hepatic lipase (HL) and scavenger receptor class B, type 1 (SR-B1).

4. Discussion

The health benefits of unsaturated FA (MUFA, PUFA) have prompted the new market of specialty and functional oils. This niche market has emerged from the fact that nutrition conscious consumers are seeking novel food products to preserve their health and to prevent severe illness, such as CVD. In this regard, several public organizations such as the American Heart Association recommend replacing SFA for MUFA or PUFA in the daily diet [5]. However, more recently, recommendations have been focused on improving the functionality of circulating HDL particles (e.g., improving reverse-cholesterol transport (RCT) and or anti-inflammatory actions) through pharmacological and dietary strategies [33], since HDL is a potent AOX, anti-inflammatory, antithrombotic and vasodilator agent, besides its well-known role in RCT [34]. From a primary prevention standpoint, non-pharmacological strategies, including small dietary changes, may reduce the cost of treatment (secondary prevention) while promoting a healthy lifestyle in at-risk populations [1,3–5]. In this study, three specialty oils differing in their FA, PST and AOX profile were tested for their ability to improve the physiological and genomic response associated with certain aspects of TAG, TC and HDL metabolism, trying to disentangle their overall lipidomic effect in healthy rats.

In countries with a well-established regulation for functional foods, in-market differentiation of specialty oils is based on their specific FA, PST and AOX profile when compared to conventional edible oils, in order to sustain ingredient-based claims. In this sense, all edible oils evaluated in this study (GSO, CO and CNO) qualify as functional oils [8,15,16]. GSO is rich (>85%) in oleic ($C_{18:1}$) + linoleic ($C_{18:2}$) FA (arranged mostly as trilinoleil (43%) and dilinoleil-oleil (23%) TAG), PST (~2.6 mg/g, mainly β-sitosterol), but a moderate source of TP (2.9–36.0 mgGAE/100 g) [15,35–37] and RSC (0.33–0.49 mM against $ABTS^{2-}$) [38], and our results are consistent with this evidence ($C_{18:1}$ + $C_{18:2}$ (89.2%), total PST (1.72 mg/g), β-sitosterol (1.52 mg/g), TP (2.4 mgGAE/100 g) and RSC (0.38 mM against $ABTS^{2-}$)). GSO is also a good source of lipophilic antioxidants, such as α, γ-tocopherols and α, γ-tocotrienols [15,36], although they were not evaluated in this study. The CO profile was very similar to other CO previously reported, at least in its $C_{16:0}$ + $C_{18:1}$ + $C_{18:2}$ (>85 g/100 g) and PST (11 mg/g) content [39,40]. The FA profile of CNO was almost identical to other CNO [15,40], although its TP and PST content was lower than previously reported [40,41]. Nevertheless, lauric acid ($C_{12:0}$) from coconut oil (CNO) may exert a TC-lowering effect [8]; α-linolenic acid ($C_{18:3}$) + PST + TP in CO may reduce several risk factors for atherosclerosis [20], inflammation [18] and dyslipidemia [42]; and the PUFA/SFA ratio in GSO may reduce many risk factors for CVD [12–15].

It is noteworthy that CO showed a higher content of stearic acid ($C_{18:0}$), α-linolenic acid ($C_{18:3}$), total/specific PST, TP and RSC, a similar $n3/n6$ ratio, but a lower PUFA/SFA ratio than GSO, while CNO had the highest SFA content (92%, 73.8% from $C_{12:0}$ and $C_{14:0}$) and a negligible content of PST and TP as compared to GSO and CO. The higher deteriorating index in GSO (8.6) as compared to CO (4.3) indicates that the former is more susceptible to oxidation, and so, it is not suitable for frying [36,43]. However, the quantity (CO > GSO > CNO) and chemical nature of AOX species (TP, tocols and PST) in these specialty oils may confer them a higher shelf life, although this was not evaluated in this study.

Health claims related to CVD prevention require a rigorous scientific sustentation of all (negative and positive) physiological effects after the intake of functional edible oils. These evaluations should be performed in convenient rodent models and/or human intervention trials in order to stablish significant associations between their daily intake and certain physiological outcomes, such as a lower risk for oxidative stress, inflammation, hypertension or dyslipidemia [18–20,42]. In this study, the lipidomic and antioxidant response to GSO, CO and CNO after a sub-chronic ad libitum intake (28 days) of moderate fat diets (10% w/w; 23% energy) in healthy young Wistar rats was studied. This protocol was used with the intention to develop a low degree of metabolic disturbances due to a +5% (w/w) fat intake above the recommendation for Wistar rats [29,39], but not a marked steatosis [44], a higher body fat, dyslipidemia and leptinemia [17] or a higher visceral fat and hyperinsulinemia [39], which are commonly observed in young Wistar rats fed high fat ($\geq$20% w/w; $\geq$50% energy from fat) diets. Furthermore, GSO and CO were selected intentionally due their similar FA profile [15,38,40] and possibly different PST and AOX content; also, a high SFA- and cholesterol-free oil (CNO) with negligible PST or AOX content served as control diet, since isoenergetic SFA-rich diets are more obesogenic than PUFA-rich diets [39,45].

In this study, most bioassay parameters did not change among experimental diets at the 28th day, including weight gain (46–62 g), food intake (230–287 g), FER (0.20–0.24) and HSI (3.3%–3.9%). Alsaif et al. [39] fed male Wistar rats (150–160 g) with 10% fat diets (prepared with CO, olive oil or low fat butter oil) for 35 days observing weight gains between 76 and 80 g and HSI ~3.0% with no apparent differences between edible oils. Dominguez-Avila et al. [17] fed male rats (~148 g) with a 10% fat diet (5% lard/5.0% corn oils) for 63 days observing a weight gain of 271.3 g and an FER of 0.20, while Fakhoury-Sayegh et al. [44] fed male rats (150–180 g) with a 15.2% fat-diet (7% soya/8.2% butter oils; 407.5 kcal/100 g; 31.5% energy from fat) for 112 days observing a weight gain of 229 g and an HSI of 2.1%. Together, all of these studies suggest a time + fat quantity effect on weight gain, but not in FER or HIS, not necessarily associated with a certain type of edible oil at least for protocols with sub-chronic fat consumption such as these; it is noteworthy that the authors did not observed steatohepatitis in their moderate fat-fed rat model.

Furthermore, Hurtado de Catalfo et al. [21] fed male Wistar pups (48 $\pm$ 3 g) for 60 days with normal-fat diets (7% w/w; 17% energy from fat) prepared with CNO (high SFA), olive oil (high MUFA), soybean oil and GSO (different PUFA/SFA), demonstrating a higher rate of body weight gain and FER in CNO-fed rats as compared to all other diets, so an age-related effect on bioassay parameters can be also assumed. Lastly, significant differences ($p \leq 0.001$) on SFA, MUFA and PUFA intakes were observed between diets, which in turn may cause other metabolic derangements, such as dyslipidemia, endothelial dysfunction or higher adiposity (total body, abdominal and hepatic) as those seen with a sub-chronic intake of high fat [17,39,44] or oil-fried (12.3% w/w, 28% energy canola oil (MUFA/SFA = 1.5, PUFA/SFA = 3.9) + peroxynitrites) diets [46].

The effect of reducing and/or changing dietary fat sources instead of modifying other macronutrients in the daily diet (e.g., dietary fiber and protein) seems to be a more promising way to prevent CVD [4,9]. Particularly, dietary fats are well known to affect TAG and cholesterol homeostasis. A lesser SFA intake with no other dietary modification reduces LDL-C, HDL-C and TC simultaneously [3,7,9], while human and animal studies have shown that consuming PUFA (particularly, n3) and MUFA, to a lower extent, reduces blood LDL-C, but increases HDL-C levels when compared to SFA [12,40,47]. Here, serum TAG and TC increased, while HDL-C decreased in CNO-fed rats as compared to CO- or GSO-fed rats whose serum lipid response was quite similar; the latter effect may be related to the nature and sn-2 position of FA in TAGs [48] from these edible oils. Moreover, data from Table 5 indicate that CNO-fed rats had a higher intake of SFA and accumulated more fat in liver (new data in this new version of the manuscript) as total cholesterol, triacylglycerides (Figure 2) and SFA (mainly as palmitic acid ($C_{16:0}$); Table 6), which in turn modified the mRNA levels of certain enzymes and proteins involved in reverse-cholesterol transport. The hypercholesterolemic (high TC and LDL-C, low HDL-C) and hypertriglyceridemic effect of CNO has been previously reported in rats [49] and humans [50], despite the fact that its lauric acid ($C_{12:0}$) alone is efficient to lower TC [8]. Thus, our study provides a further argument as to the null effect of coconut oil as a superfood.

However, the effect of GSO vs. other PUFA-rich edible oils on the murine serum lipidome has generated controversial results. Chang et al. [51] postulated that a higher (PUFA + MFA)/SFA ratio increases serum TC, TAG and VLDL-C levels, and so, GSO (ratio 8.72) should behave worse than CO (ratio 5.93) on this matter. Asadi et al. [52] fed young Wistar rats (~225 g) with CO and GSO, besides water and a chow diet, ad libitum for 10 weeks observing the same feed and oil intake, serum TC and HDL-C, but a lower serum LDL-C level in CO-fed rats. Kim et al. [53] observed significant reductions in TC, LDL-C and the atherogenic index, but a higher HDL-C/TC ratio in GSO-fed rats as compared to those fed with lard or soybean oil. De la Torre-Carbot et al. [54] evaluated the serum lipid profile of male Wistar rats fed with different commercial oils, including GSO (10% *w/w*; 14.4% energy as added oil) for two weeks, showing that GSO promoted a lower liver weight than soybean oil and higher HDL-C and LDL-C levels as compared to other PUFA-rich edible oils. However, Al-Attar [55] showed higher TC and HDL-C levels in CO- vs. GSO-fed (orally administered 2 g/kg BW) Wistar rats (85–93 g BW), both conferring protection against diazinon-induced hepatotoxicity. Discrepancies between all of these studies, including ours, may rely on the duration and dose used, the rat's physiological condition and the source of GSO (e.g., commercial vs. fresh cold-pressed).

This study also showed that the hepatic deposition of FA, but mostly PST, was different between specialty oils. CNO-fed rats accumulated more SFA and MUFA, but less PUFA as compared to CO- and GSO-fed rats, but the FA deposition in CO and GSO was quite similar; in fact, $C_{18:0}$ (higher in GSO) and $C_{18:1cis}$ (higher in CO) were equally deposited, while $C_{17:0}$ (same in CO and GSO) and total SFA (higher in CO) were deposited differently. Moreover, the hepatic deposition of PST was higher in CO- than in GSO-fed rats ($p \leq 0.001$). To our knowledge, the specific hepatic deposition of PST from GSO (1.72 mg/g, mostly β-sitosterol) is reported here for the first time.

The effect of GSO's lipids, other than PST, on serum, hepatic and extrahepatic lipidomes has been studied by others. Hurtado de Catalfo et al. [21] reported that at the end of the feeding period (60 days), CNO, olive and soybean oil and GSO differently modified the hepatic lipid composition; Lastly, Shinagawa et al. [56] evaluated the effect of intra-gastric administration (3 and 6 mL/kg) of a cold-pressed GSO or a soybean oil in male Wistar rats (~54 g BW) for 65 days observing a dose-response effect on the weight of retroperitoneal fat and liver, independently of the administered oil; despite the fact that both edible oils deposited their total SFA and MUFA in liver similarly, differences in PUFA deposition in adipose tissue (retroperitoneal) were observed, particularly a higher $C_{18:3n3}$ deposition in soybean oil-fed rats as compared to GSO. Since liver weight (11.7 g vs. 11.4 g) and water content (66.7% vs. 67.9%; 7.8 g and 7.4 g) were similar between GSO- and CO-fed rats, our results suggest that hepatic FA handling instead of their total deposition as TAG (~3.9 g) could be different. This in turn may affect several metabolic routes, including the regulatory mechanisms related to hepatic FA and cholesterol homeostasis [17,57,58], while a different hepatic deposition of PST may have affected different signaling pathways involved in liver inflammation [18,20] and lipoprotein trafficking [42].

The liver plays a critical role in controlling FA and cholesterol homeostasis [17,34,58] in full integration with peripheral tissues, such as small bowel [34,42,58], muscle [52] and adipose tissue [46,56]. The epigenetic role of FA on the hepatic metabolism of TAG and of PST on cholesterol metabolism has been the traditional approach, although few studies address the communication between these two metabolic pathways. A failure to handle FA may result in hepatic steatosis as that seen with high fat (particularly SFA) and hypercholesterolemic diets, increasing the risk for vascular degeneration, hypertension and insulin resistance [17,39,44] and lowering serum HDL-C levels while increasing LDL-C. This explains the inverse relationship between HDL-C serum levels and the risk for CVD, since HDL-C reflects the body's capacity to return cholesterol from peripheral organs to the liver (also known as RCT) [58] and an efficient enzymatic machinery to convert SFA into MUFA or PUFA under normal conditions [9]. Moreover, because this lipoprotein is also involved in AOX mechanisms [34], pharmaceutical interventions aimed to raise HDL-C levels and/or to increase its functionality (e.g., improving RCT and or anti-inflammatory actions) rather than reducing LDL-C, seems to be the best approach to prevent and/or treat CVD [33].

However, HDL-C metabolism is more complex than that of LDL-C, since many proteins, mostly regulated at the transcriptional level, participate in HDL remodeling, its hepatic clearance and RCT [57,58]. TAG (from dietary FA) and other lipids (including PST and dietary cholesterol) are packed into chylomicrons by intestinal cells, which travel up to the liver [34]. Free cholesterol within cells generates oxysterols, which act as ligands for nuclear liver receptors (LXR) and retinoid receptors (RXR), an action that could be reversed by MUFA + PUFA [17] and PST. HDL particles are packed in plasma, in the extravascular space, the liver and small bowel are involved in nascent HDL synthesis providing ApoA-1 (both) or ApoA-2 (just liver), but also in RCT [58]. RCT is mediated by a basic interaction between the ATP-binding cassette (ABC) transporter-A1 (in intestine and peripheral tissues) and ApoA-1 (in HDL) [59]. TAG-rich remnant lipoproteins are converted to LDL-C, which may interact with its receptor (LDLr) in liver and peripheral tissues and/or interchange its TAG content for cholesteryl esters from HDL particles and vice versa by means of cholesteryl ester transfer protein (CETP), whose expression is regulated by LXR/RXR. HDL_3 (dense, rich in esterified cholesterol) is further metabolized into HDL_2 (less dense, rich in phospholipids) by LCAT and phospholipid transfer protein (PLTP) in a concerted action with HL (synthesized and secreted by hepatocytes and macrophages), which performs the same reaction in the opposite direction. Lastly, HDL_2 (marker of acute myocardial infarction) is hydrolyzed by HL, and its components enter the liver via SR-B1, which removes esterified cholesterol from the liver, which is excreted in bile.

Lastly, our sqRT-PCR assay indicates that HL, LCAT and SR-B1, but not ApoA-1 mRNA levels increased in GSO-fed rats as compared to CO or CNO groups ($p \leq 0.01$). Kim et al. [53] found a lower epididymal, but not hepatic fat in GSO-fed rats as compared to soybean oil or lard, attributing this effect to a concerted action of $C_{18:2}$ (58%–78%), tocotrienols (4.5–5.3 mg/g oil) and TP (0.10–0.34 mg/g) contents in GSO. GSO and CO assayed in this study promoted the same HDL-C serum level, but their TP and PST content differ (higher in CO); so, a more efficient hepatic FA handling, but not serum AOX response, nor PST hepatic deposition, seemed to drive the effects on the expression of these hepatic genes. This hypothesis is based on the fact that a concurrent ApoA-1 (same in CO and GSO) and ABCA1 expression prevents hepatic steatosis by stimulating a lower deposition of FA (as TAG) and TC, while suppressing FA synthesis by reducing 27-hydroxyesterol levels [59]; this effect plus a higher expression of RCT-involved enzymes/proteins in (SR-B1) and out (LCAT/HL) the liver may stimulate a more efficient FA and TC mobilization.

5. Conclusions

Novel insights into the study of HDL metabolism indicate that we are at the beginning of a new line of research on dysfunctional HDL-C (dysHDL-C), although many issues need to be considered before confirming its predictive role of CVD [33,34]. For instance, the RCT-improving and anti-inflammatory effects of HDL-C are emerging subjects of research [57–60]. In this sense, our study attempts to show that the hepatic fatty acid handling, but not antioxidant response, nor hepatic phytosterol deposition, could be related to a more efficient reverse-cholesterol transport in GSO-fed rats as compared to CO or CNO.

The authors recognize that this study has several limitations. Major drawbacks are the lack of HPLC sub-fractionation of serum lipoproteins (VLDL/LDL/IDL/HDL) at the end of the study, the fact that we only measured total and HDL-cholesterol, not considering more efficient and standardized ways to evaluate HDL functionality [57–60], and the failure to specifically link the mRNA expression of four genes related to RCT with the fatty acid and phytosterol deposition and related antioxidant microenvironment in the liver. Particularly, measuring the in vivo function of HDL could be of significant importance to test the effectiveness of different RCT-enhancing diet therapies [60]. The lipidomic approach used in this study (circulating lipids, lipid deposition in liver and gene expression) just provide a little bit of evidence as to the possibility of a more efficient reverse-cholesterol transport (RCT); however, in order to support this evidence, fatty acid and phytosterol tracer studies and/or sub-chronic feeding studies using knockout rodent models should be performed in the near future to get a better understanding of the health benefits of consuming GSO over other specialty oils.

Acknowledgments: The authors are thankful to Abraham Dominguez-Avila (Universidad Autonoma de Ciudad Juarez) and Maria del Carmen Estrada-Montoya (Centro de Investigacion y Alimentacion y Desarrollo, AC; Hermosillo) for their technical assistance in AOX and GC-MS assays and to the Mexico's Faculty Improvement Program for supporting the publication cost of this work. This research did not receive any additional grants from the funding agencies in the public, commercial or not-for-profit sectors.

Author Contributions: All authors substantially contributed to the design of the study, the production, analysis or interpretation of the results and/or preparation of the manuscript. A.W.-M. and G.A.G.-A. conceived of the experimental design, supervised all experiments, drafted the manuscript and performed data handling and statistical analyses. A.W.-M. and J.A.L.-D. performed raw lipid analysis (serum and liver) and formulated experimental diets. A.F.G.-C., B.V.-C. and F.J.M.-C. performed and supervised the GC-MS analysis of fatty acids and phytosterols in edible oils and liver samples. A.A.V.-F. and G.M.-M. performed the bioassay and collected all biological samples. L.A.d.l.R. and R.G.-A. performed and supervised all gene expression analyses. All authors read and approved the final manuscript.

Conflicts of Interest: The authors declare no conflict of interest.

Appendix A

Table A1. Non-modified physiological parameters after GSO, CO and CNO intake [1,2].

Variable	GSO	CO	CNO	*p*
Hepatic FA (mg/g)				
$C_{8:0}$	0.25 ± 0.04	0.18 ± 0.10	0.16 ± 0.05	0.11
$C_{10:0}$	0.08 ± 0.04	0.06 ± 0.03	0.09 ± 0.01	0.36
$C_{15:0}$	0.22 ± 0.03	0.20 ± 0.02	0.20 ± 0.03	0.49
$C_{18:0}$	14.96 ± 2.37	13.25 ± 1.48	14.14 ± 0.58	0.29
$C_{20:0}$	0.07 ± 0.02	0.11 ± 0.02	0.07 ± 0.07	0.16
$C_{15:1}$	0.13 ± 0.03	0.11 ± 0.02	0.13 ± 0.03	0.57
$C_{17:1}$	0.45 ± 0.16	0.50 ± 0.09	0.44 ± 0.05	0.68
$C_{20:1}$	0.24 ± 0.02	0.27 ± 0.03	0.24 ± 0.12	0.75
$C_{18:2n3}$	0.43 ± 0.12	0.49 ± 0.15	0.34 ± 0.12	0.19
$C_{22:5n3}$	0.39 ± 0.10	0.41 ± 0.10	0.50 ± 0.17	0.32
Serum TAC				
FRAP (mM TE)	0.47 ± 0.01	0.48 ± 0.02	0.46 ± 0.01	0.08

[1] Values are expressed as the mean ± standard deviation, 28-day consumption; [2] grapeseed oil (GSO), corn oil (CO), coconut oil (CNO), ferric reducing ability (FRAP), total antioxidant capacity (TAC).

References

1. Zyriax, B.-C.; Windler, E. Dietary fat in the prevention of cardiovascular disease—A review. *Eur. J. Lipid Sci. Technol.* **2000**, *102*, 355–365. [CrossRef]

2.   Laslett, L.J.; Alagona, P.; Clark, B.A.; Drozda, J.P.; Saldivar, F.; Wilson, S.R.; Poe, C.; Har, M. The worldwide environmental of cardiovascular disease: Prevalence, diagnosis, therapy, and policy issues: A report from the American College of Cardiology. *J. Am. Coll. Cardiol.* **2012**, *60* (Suppl. 25), S1–S49. [CrossRef] [PubMed]

3.   Astrup, A.; Dyerberg, J.; Elwood, P.; Hermansen, K.; Hu, F.B.; Jakobsen, M.U.; Kok, F.J.; Krauss, R.M.; Lecerf, J.M.; LeGrand, P.; et al. The role of reducing intakes of saturated fat in the prevention of cardiovascular disease: Where does the evidence stand in 2010? *Am. J. Clin. Nutr.* **2011**, *93*, 684–688. [CrossRef] [PubMed]

4.   Torres, N.; Guevara-Cruz, M.; Granados, J.; Vargas-Alarcón, G.; González-Palacios, B.; Ramos-Barragan, V.E.; Quiroz-Olguín, G.; Flores-Islas, I.M.; Tovar, A.R. Reduction of serum lipids by soy protein and soluble fiber is not associated with the ABCG5/G8, apolipoprotein E, and apolipoprotein A1 polymorphisms in a group of hyperlipidemic Mexican subjects. *Nutr. Res.* **2009**, *29*, 728–735. [CrossRef] [PubMed]

5.   Pearson, T.A.; Palaniappan, L.P.; Artinian, N.T.; Carnethon, M.R.; Criqui, M.H.; Daniels, S.R.; Goldstein, L.B.; Hong, Y.; Mensah, G.A.; Sallis, J.F.; et al. American Heart Association guide for improving cardiovascular health at the community level, 2013 update a scientific statement for public health practitioners, healthcare providers, and health policy makers. *Circulation* **2013**, *127*, 1730–1753. [CrossRef] [PubMed]

6.   Yamagishi, K.; Iso, H.; Yatsuya, H.; Tanabe, N.; Date, C.; Kikuchi, S.; Yamamoto, A.; Inaba, Y.; Tamakoshi, A. JACC Study Group Dietary intake of saturated fatty acids and mortality from cardiovascular disease in Japanese: The Japan collaborative cohort study for evaluation of cancer risk (JACC) study. *Am. J. Clin. Nutr.* **2012**, *92*, 759–765. [CrossRef] [PubMed]

7.   Manson, P.; Porter, S.C.; Berry, S.E.; Stillman, P.; Steele, C.; Kirby, A.; Griffin, B.A.; Minihane, A.M. Saturated fatty acid consumption: Outlining the scale of the problem and assessing the solutions. *Nutr. Bull.* **2009**, *34*, 74–84. [CrossRef]

8.   Sheela, D.L.; Nazeem, P.A.; Narayanankutty, A.; Manalil, J.J.; Raghavamenon, A.C. In silico and wet lab studies reveal the cholesterol lowering efficacy of lauric acid, a medium chain fat of coconut oil. *Plant Foods Hum. Nutr.* **2016**. [CrossRef]

9.   Grundy, S.M.; Denke, M.A. Dietary influences on serum lipids and lipoproteins. *J. Lipid Res.* **1990**, *31*, 1149–1172. [PubMed]

10.   Estruch, R.; Ros, E.; Salas-Salvado, J.; Covas, M.I.; Corella, D.; Aros, F.; Gómez-Gracia, E.; Ruiz-Gutiérrez, V.; Fiol, M.; Lapetra, J.; et al. Primary prevention of cardiovascular disease with a Mediterranean diet. *N. Engl. J. Med.* **2013**, *368*, 1279–1290. [CrossRef] [PubMed]

11.   Oh, K.; Hu, F.B.; Manson, J.E.; Stampfer, M.J.; Willet, W.C. Expand+Dietary fat intake and risk of coronary heart disease in women: 20 Years of follow-up of the nurses' health study. *Am. J. Epidemiol.* **2005**, *161*, 672–679. [CrossRef] [PubMed]

12.   Larsson, S.C.; Orsini, N.; Wolk, A. Long-chain omega-3 polyunsaturated fatty acids and risk of stroke: A meta-analysis. *Eur. J. Epidemiol.* **2012**, *27*, 895–901. [CrossRef] [PubMed]

13.   Kotwal, S.; Jun, M.; Sullivan, D.; Perkovic, V.; Neal, B. Omega 3 fatty acids and cardiovascular outcomes: Systematic review and meta-analysis. *Circ. Cardiovasc. Qual. Outcomes* **2012**, *5*, 808–818. [CrossRef] [PubMed]

14.   Pan, A.; Chen, M.; Chowdhury, R.; Wu, J.H.; Sun, Q.; Campos, H.; Mozaffarian, D.; Hu, F.B. α-linolenic acid and risk of cardiovascular disease: A systematic review and meta-analysis. *Am. J. Clin. Nutr.* **2012**, *96*, 1262–1273. [CrossRef] [PubMed]

15.   Garavaglia, J.; Markoski, M.M.; Oliveira, A.; Marcadenti, A. Grape seed oil compounds: Biological and chemical actions for health. *Nutr. Metab. Insights* **2016**, *9*, 59–64. [PubMed]

16.   Hassanien, M.F.R. Tocol and phytosterol composition of edible oils in the Egyptian market. *J. Food Process. Preserv.* **2012**, *36*, 531–538. [CrossRef]

17.   Domínguez-Ávila, J.A.; Álvarez-Parrilla, E.; López-Díaz, J.A.; Maldonado-Mendoza, I.E.; Gómez-García, M.C.; de la Rosa, L.A. The pecan nut (*Carya illinoinensis*) and its oil and polyphenolic fractions differentially modulate lipid metabolism and the antioxidant enzyme activities in rats fed high-fat diets. *Food Chem.* **2015**, *168*, 529–537. [CrossRef] [PubMed]

18.   Rocha, V.A.; Ras, R.T.; Gagliardi, A.C.; Mangili, L.C.; Trautwein, E.A.; Santos, R.D. Effects of phytosterols on markers of inflammation: A systematic review and meta-analysis. *Atheroesclerosis* **2016**, *248*, 76–83. [CrossRef] [PubMed]

19.   Wang, Y.; Chun, O.K.; Song, W.O. Plasma and dietary antioxidant status as cardiovascular disease risk factors: A review of human studies. *Nutrients* **2013**, *5*, 2969–3004. [CrossRef] [PubMed]

20. Deng, Q.; Yu, X.; Xu, J.; Kou, X.; Zheng, M.; Huang, F.; Huang, Q.; Wang, L. Single frequency intake of α-linolenic acid rich phytosterol esters attenuates atherosclerosis risk factors in hamsters fed a high fat diet. *Lipids Health. Dis.* **2016**, *15*, 23. [CrossRef] [PubMed]

21. De Catalfo, G.E.H.; de Alaniz, M.J.; Marra, C.A. Dietary lipid-induced changes in enzymes of hepatic lipid metabolism. *Nutrition* **2013**, *28*, 462–469. [CrossRef] [PubMed]

22. Park, P.W.; Goins, R.E. In situ preparation of fatty acid methyl esters for analysis of fatty acid composition of foods. *J. Food Sci.* **1994**, *59*, 1262–1266. [CrossRef]

23. Villa-Rodríguez, J.A.; Molina-Corral, F.J.; Ayala-Zavala, J.F.; Olivas, G.I.; González-Aguilar, G.A. Effect of maturity stage on the content of fatty acids and antioxidant activity of 'Hass' avocado. *Food Res. Int.* **2011**, *44*, 1231–1237. [CrossRef]

24. Fletouris, D.J.; Botsoglou, N.A.; Psomas, I.E.; Mantis, A.I. Rapid determination of cholesterol in milk and milk products by direct saponification and capillary gas chromatography. *J. Dairy Sci.* **1998**, *81*, 2833–2840. [CrossRef]

25. Berker, K.I.; Ozdemir, O.F.A.; Ozyurt, D.; Demirata, B.; Apak, R. Modified Folic-Ciocalteu antioxidant capacity assay for measuring lipophilic antioxidants. *J. Agric. Food Chem.* **2013**, *61*, 4783–4791. [CrossRef] [PubMed]

26. Brand-Williams, W.; Cuvelier, M.E.; Berset, C.L.W.T. Use of a free radical method to evaluate antioxidant activity. *LWT Food Sci. Technol.* **1995**, *28*, 25–30. [CrossRef]

27. Re, R.; Pellegrini, N.; Proteggente, A.; Pannala, A.; Yang, M.; Rice-Evans, C. Antioxidant activity applying an improved ABTS radical cation decolorization assay. *Free Rad. Biol. Med.* **1999**, *26*, 1231–1237. [CrossRef]

28. Álvarez-Parrilla, E.; de la Rosa, L.A.; Legarreta, P.; Sáenz, L.; Rodrigo-García, J.; González-Aguilar, G.A. Daily consumption of apple, pear and orange juice differently affects plasma lipids and antioxidant capacity of smoking and non-smoking adults. *Int. J. Food Sci. Nutr.* **2010**, *61*, 369–380. [CrossRef] [PubMed]

29. National Research Council (NRC). Nutrient requirements of the laboratory rat. In *Nutrient Requirements of Laboratory Animals*, 4th ed.National Academy Press: Washington, DC, USA, 1995; pp. 11–16. Available online: https://www.nap.edu/catalog/4758/nutrient-requirements-of-laboratory-animals-fourth-revised-edition-1995 (accessed on 5 November 2016).

30. NOM-062-ZOO-1999. Especificaciones Técnicas para la Producción, Cuidado y uso de Los Animales de Laboratorio. Available online: http://www.fmvz.unam.mx/fmvz/principal/archivos/062ZOO.PDF (accessed on 5 November 2016).

31. Folch, J.; Lees, M.; Sloane Stanley, G.H. A simple method for the isolation and purification of total lipids from animal tissues. *J. Biol. Chem.* **1957**, *226*, 497–509. [PubMed]

32. Reis, A.; Rudnitskaya, A.; Blackburn, G.J.; Fauzi, N.M.; Pitt, A.R.; Spickett, C.M. A comparison of five lipid extraction solvent systems for lipidomic studies of human LDL. *J. Lipid Res.* **2013**, *54*, 1812–1824. [CrossRef] [PubMed]

33. Agouridis, A.P.; Banach, M.; Mikhailidis, D.P. Dysfunctional high-density lipoprotein: Not only quantity but first of all quality. *Arch. Med. Sci.* **2015**, *11*, 230–231. [CrossRef] [PubMed]

34. Santos-Gallego, C.G.; Badimon, J.J.; Rosenson, S.S. Beginning to understand high-density lipoproteins. *Endocrinol. Metab. Clin. N. Am.* **2014**, *43*, 913–947. [CrossRef] [PubMed]

35. Sabir, A.; Unver, A.; Kara, Z. The fatty acid and tocopherol constituents of the seed oil extracted from 21 grape varieties (*Vitis* spp.). *J. Sci. Food Agric.* **2012**, *92*, 1982–1987. [CrossRef] [PubMed]

36. Madawala, S.R.P.; Kochhar, S.P.; Dutta, P.C. Lipid components and oxidative status of selected specialty oils. *Grasas y Aceites* **2012**, *63*, 143–151. [CrossRef]

37. De Marchi, F.; Seraglia, R.; Molin, L.; Traldi, P.; De Rosso, M.; Panighel, A.; Dalla Vedova, A.; Gardiman, M.; Giust, M.; Flamini, R. Seed oil triglyceride profiling of thirty-two hybrid grape varieties. *J. Mass Spectrom.* **2012**, *47*, 1113–1119. [CrossRef] [PubMed]

38. Fernandes, L.; Casal, S.; Cruz, R.; Pereira, J.A.; Ramalhosa, E. Seed oils of ten traditional Portuguese grape varieties with interesting chemical and antioxidant properties. *Food Res. Int.* **2013**, *50*, 161–166. [CrossRef]

39. Alsaif, M.A.; Duwaihy, M.M.S. Influence of dietary fat quantity and composition on glucose tolerance and insulin sensitivity in rats. *Nutr. Res.* **2004**, *24*, 417–425. [CrossRef]

40. Gunstone, F. *Vegetable Oils in Food Technology: Composition, Properties and Uses*, 2nd ed.; John Wiley & Sons: Oxford, UK, 2011; pp. 169–174, 273–286. Available online: http://197.14.51.10: 81/pmb/AGROALIMENTAIRE/Vegetable%20Oils%20in%20Food%20Technology%20Composition% 20Properties%20and%20Uses.pdf (accessed on 5 November 2016).

41. Wagner, K.H.; Wotruba, F.; Elmadfa, I. Antioxidative potential of tocotrienols and tocopherols in coconut fat at different oxidation temperatures. *Eur. J. Lipid Sci. Technol.* **2001**, *103*, 746–751. [CrossRef]

42. Gylling, E.; Simonen, P. Phytosterols, phytostanols, and lipoprotein metabolism. *Nutrients* **2015**, *7*, 7965–7977. [CrossRef] [PubMed]

43. Tekin, L.; Aday, M.S.; Yilmaz, E. Physicochemical changes in hazelnut, olive pomace, grapeseed and sunflower oils heated at frying temperatures. *Food Sci. Technol. Res.* **2009**, *15*, 519–524. [CrossRef]

44. Fakhoury-Sayegh, N.; Trak-Smayra, V.; Khazzaka, A.; Esseily, F.; Obeid, O.; Lahoud-Zouein, M.; Younes, H. Characteristics of nonalcoholic fatty liver disease induced in wistar rats following four different diets. *Nutr. Res. Pract.* **2015**, *9*, 350–357. [CrossRef] [PubMed]

45. Legrand, P.; Rioux, V. Specific roles of saturated fatty acids: Beyond epidemiological data. *Eur. J. Lipid Sci. Technol.* **2015**, *127*, 1489–1499. [CrossRef]

46. Bautista, R.; Carreón-Torres, E.; Luna-Luna, M.; Komera-Arenas, Y.; Franco, M.; Fragoso, J.M.; López-Olmos, V.; Cruz-Robles, D.; Vargas-Barrón, J.; Vargas-Alarcón, G.; et al. Early endothelial nitrosylation and increased abdominal adiposity in Wistar rats after long-term consumption of food fried in canola oil. *Nutrition* **2014**, *30*, 1055–1060. [CrossRef] [PubMed]

47. Mensink, R.P.; Zock, P.L.; Kester, A.D.; Katan, M.B. Effects of dietary fatty acids and carbohydrates on the ratio of serum total to HDL cholesterol and on serum lipids and apolipoproteins: A meta-analysis of 60 controlled trials. *Am. J. Clin. Nutr.* **2003**, *77*, 1146–1155. [PubMed]

48. The, S.S.; Voon, P.T.; Ng, Y.T.; Ong, S.H.; Ong, A.S.H.; Choo, Y.M. Effects of fatty acids at different positions in the triglycerides on cholesterol levels. *J. Oil Palm. Res.* **2016**, *28*, 211–221.

49. Dauqan, E.; Sani, H.; Abdullah, A.; Kasim, Z. Effect of different vegetable oils (red palm olein, palm olein, corn oil and coconut oil) on lipid profile in rat. *Food Nutr. Sci.* **2011**, *2*, 253–258. [CrossRef]

50. Eyres, L.; Eyres, M.F.; Chisholm, A.; Brown, R.C. Coconut oil consumption and cardiovascular risk factors in humans. *Nutr. Rev.* **2016**, *74*, 267–280. [CrossRef] [PubMed]

51. Chang, N.-W.; Wu, C.-T.; Chen, F.-N.; Huang, P.-C. Effect of dietary ratios of fatty acids on cholesterol metabolism in rats and on low density lipoprotein uptake in hepatocytes. *Nutr. Res.* **2005**, *25*, 781–790. [CrossRef]

52. Asadi, F.; Shahriari, A.; Chahardah-Cheric, M. Effect of long-term optional ingestion of canola oil, grape seed oil, corn oil and yogurt butter on plasma, muscle and liver cholesterol status in rats. *Food Chem. Toxicol.* **2010**, *48*, 2454–2457. [CrossRef] [PubMed]

53. Kim, D.-J.; Jeon, G.; Sung, J.; Oh, S.-K.; Hong, H.-C.; Lee, J. Effect of grape seed oil supplementation on serum lipid profiles in rats. *Food Sci. Biotechnol.* **2010**, *19*, 249–252. [CrossRef]

54. De la Torre-Carbot, K.; Chávez-Servín, J.L.; Reyes, P.; Ferriz, R.A.; Gutiérrez, E.; Escobar, K.; Aguilera, A.; Anaya, M.A.; García, T.; García, O.P.; et al. Changes in lipid profile of Wistar rats after sustained consumption of different types of commercial vegetable oil: A preliminary study. *Universal J. Food Nutr. Sci.* **2015**, *3*, 10–18. [CrossRef]

55. Al-Attar, A.M. Effect of grapeseed oil on diazinon-induced physiological and histopathological alterations in rats. *Saudi J. Biol. Sci.* **2015**, *22*, 284–292. [CrossRef] [PubMed]

56. Shinagawa, F.B.; Santana, F.C.D.; Mancini-Filho, J. Effect of cold pressed grape seed oil on rats' biochemical markers and inflammatory profile. *Rev. Nutr.* **2015**, *28*, 65–76. [CrossRef]

57. Rohatgi, A.; Khera, A.; Berry, J.D.; Givens, E.G.; Ayers, C.R.; Wedin, K.E.; Neeland, I.J.; Yuhanna, I.S.; Rader, D.R.; de Lemos, J.A.; et al. HDL cholesterol efflux capacity and incident cardiovascular events. *N. Engl. J. Med.* **2014**, *371*, 2383–2393. [CrossRef] [PubMed]

58. Khera, A.V.; Cuchel, M.; de la Llera-Moya, M.; Rodrigues, A.; Burke, M.F.; Jafri, K.; French, B.C.; Phillips, J.A.; Mucksavage, M.L.; Wilensky, R.L.; et al. Cholesterol efflux capacity, high-density lipoprotein function, and atherosclerosis. *N. Engl. J. Med.* **2011**, *364*, 127–135. [CrossRef] [PubMed]

59. Ma, D.; Liu, W.; Wang, Y. ApoA-I or ABCA1 expression suppresses fatty acid synthesis by reducing 27-hydroxycholesterol levels. *Biochimie* **2014**, *103*, 101–108. [CrossRef] [PubMed]
60. Santos-Gallego, C.G.; Giannarelli, C.; Badimón, J.J. Experimental models for the investigation of high density lipoprotein-mediated cholesterol efflux. *Curr. Atheroescler. Rep.* **2011**, *13*, 266–276. [CrossRef] [PubMed]

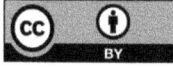

nutrients

MDPI

Review

Genetic Variations as Modifying Factors to Dietary Zinc Requirements—A Systematic Review

Kaitlin J. Day [†,‡], Melissa M. Adamski [‡], Aimee L. Dordevic and Chiara Murgia *

Department of Nutrition, Dietetics and Food, Monash University, Notting Hill VIC 3168, Australia; kjday1@student.monash.edu (K.J.D.); melissa.adamski@monash.edu (M.M.A.); aimee.dordevic@monash.edu (A.L.D.)

* Correspondence: chiara.murgia@monash.edu; Tel.: +61-03-9902-4264
† Current address: School of Biomedical Sciences, University of Surrey, Guilford, Surrey, UK.
‡ These authors contribute equally to this work.

Received: 11 January 2017; Accepted: 13 February 2017; Published: 17 February 2017

Abstract: Due to reduced cost and accessibility, the use of genetic testing has appealed to health professionals for personalising nutrition advice. However, translation of the evidence linking polymorphisms, dietary requirements, and pathology risk proves to be challenging for nutrition and dietetic practitioners. Zinc status and polymorphisms of genes coding for zinc-transporters have been associated with chronic diseases. The present study aimed to systematically review the literature to assess whether recommendations for zinc intake could be made according to genotype. Eighteen studies investigating 31 Single Nucleotide Polymorphisms (SNPs) in relation to zinc intake and/or status were identified. Five studies examined type 2 diabetes; zinc intake was found to interact independently with two polymorphisms in the zinc-transporter gene *SLC30A8* to affect glucose metabolism indicators. While the outcomes were statistically significant, the small size of the effect and lack of replication raises issues regarding translation into nutrition and dietetic practice. Two studies assessed the relationship of polymorphisms and cognitive performance; seven studies assessed the association between a range of outcomes linked to chronic conditions in aging population; two papers described the analysis of the genetic contribution in determining zinc concentration in human milk; and two papers assessed zinc concentration in plasma without linking to clinical outcomes. The data extracted confirmed a connection between genetics and zinc requirements, although the direction and magnitude of the dietary modification for carriers of specific genotypes could not be defined. This study highlights the need to summarise nutrigenetics studies to enable health professionals to translate scientific evidence into dietary recommendations.

Keywords: zinc requirements; SNPs; nutrigenetics; nutritional genomics

1. Introduction

Genetic background can affect a person's nutritional status. This may have the potential to modify an individual's optimal nutrient requirements and risk of developing specific pathologic conditions [1]. Zinc (Zn) is an essential micronutrient that plays fundamental roles in several aspects of physiology, cellular metabolism, and gene expression [2]. In Australia, the current Recommended Dietary Intake (RDI) for Zn is 14 mg/day for men and 8 mg/day for women (19+ years), with an upper limit of 40 mg/day [3]. Similarly, in the US, the current Recommended Dietary Allowance for Zn is 11 mg/day for men and 8 mg/day for women (19+ years) [4]. Zn deficiency is the cause of a complex syndrome [5], more subtle and difficult to assess is marginal Zn deficiency; while currently not well-understood, it may be a contributing factor in chronic disease development [6]. Zn deficiency can arise from several causes including specific genetic background [7]. For example, mutations in the gene coding for the intestinal transporter *SLC39A4* cause the inherited disorder Acrodermatitis Enteropathica (AE), a condition caused by the inability to absorb Zn and resulting in systemic deficiency that is resolved with lifelong Zn supplementation (1 mg/kg/day body weight) [8].

Zn crosses biological membranes with the aid of specialized trans-membrane proteins. More than 20 proteins coordinate their activity to maintain systemic and cellular Zn homeostasis; in mammals, ZnT (coded by *SLC30A* genes) and ZIP (coded by *SLC39A* genes) were identified for this role. Intracellular Zn concentration is buffered by Metallothioneins (MTs), a class of proteins with high affinity for metals [9]. With the completion of the human genome sequence, all Zn transporter genes were identified and several common polymorphisms and rare mutations were found to be associated with human pathologies [6,10].

Insulin metabolism in the pancreatic β-cells requires Zn [11], and intracellular Zn directly acts on insulin receptors' intracellular pathways. A Single Nucleotide Polymorphism (SNP) in the gene coding for the Zn transporter *SLC30A8* (rs13266634) has been identified as being associated with increasing the risk of developing type 2 diabetes (T2D); as such, modification of Zn requirements was hypothesized as a potential method to reduce the risk of T2D for rs13266634 carriers [12,13]. Another condition that is impacted by genetic polymorphisms in Zn transporters is mammary gland secretion of Zn in milk. Null mutations in genes coding for transporters expressed in mammary epithelium result in milk Zn concentrations that are insufficient to support the growth of babies, ultimately leading to poor infant health outcomes [8,14,15]. Zn status has been also associated with cognitive performance [16]. Genetic variations have been explored in cognitive studies and may also play a role in conditions such as Alzheimer's Disease (AD) [17], a concept that is yet to be investigated in human studies [18]. Many studies have investigated genetic polymorphisms in regards to gene-nutrient interactions and nutrient status in the onset and progression of specific diseases. However, the question remains; is there sufficient evidence to make specific dietary and nutrition recommendations based on genotype? [19]. The aim of this paper was to systematically review the evidence to answer whether specific polymorphisms modify individual dietary Zn requirements and whether current evidence can inform clinical dietetic practice.

2. Materials and Methods

2.1. Search Methods

A literature search was conducted in October, 2015. The following search strategy was used to search Medline, Embase, and CENTRAL. This strategy was then adapted to search Web of Science, CINAHL and Scopus databases (S1). (See PRISMA checklist (S2)).

1. Zinc.ti,ab.
2. Zn.ti,ab.
3. Zinc/
4. Zinc compounds/
5. Finger*.ti,ab.
6. 1 OR 2 OR 3 OR 4
7. 6 NOT 5
8. (Polymorph* OR Allel* OR Genet* OR Geno* OR Gene OR Genes).ti,ab.
9. Exp Polymorphism, Genetic/
10. 8 OR 9
11. Exp Cation Transport Proteins/
12. (Zinc adj2 deficienc*).ti,ab.
13. (Zn adj2 deficienc*).ti,ab.
14. (Zinc adj2 transporter*).ti,ab.
15. (Zn adj2 transporter*).ti,ab.
16. 11 OR 12 OR 13 OR 14 OR 15
17. 7 AND 10 AND 16

2.2. Inclusion Criteria

Studies were included if they were conducted in mammals, in particular humans, mice, and rats, if they investigated polymorphisms within the population, if they modulated plasma Zn concentrations or investigated whether this interaction was modulated by Zn status. Study designs that were observational, case-control, and clinical trials were eligible for inclusion in this review.

2.3. Exclusion Criteria

Studies were excluded that were not written in English. Studies were also excluded that were examining type 1 diabetes, conducted before 1995 (when the first gene coding for a Zn transporter was identified [20]), single case studies, book chapters, editorial letters, conference proceedings, and reviews.

2.4. Data Collection and Analysis

2.4.1. Selection of Studies

Three reviewers (KD, MA, and CM) independently screened the titles and abstracts of the studies retrieved by the above search strategy. Full articles were then retrieved and were independently assessed by the same three reviewers for inclusion using the criteria outlined above. Conflicts were discussed and decided upon as a group. Reference lists of relevant studies and reviews were also manually searched.

2.4.2. Data Extraction

An extraction table was developed to include information about study design, association of genetic variants with phenotypic traits, and other relevant outcomes. Three review authors (KD, MA, and CM) independently extracted the data into an extraction table which included zinc status method, genotyping method, polymorphisms identified, association between SNP, zinc status and biomarkers, association between SNP, zinc status, and disease state. The data were then cross-verified by another author (AD). Any discrepancies were resolved through group discussion. Corresponding authors for the papers [21–24] were contacted with requests for more information; unfortunately, we were unable to obtain answers to the questions we sought.

2.5. Quality Assessment

A suitable, validated quality assessment (QA) tool was not available for the types of studies and outcomes reviewed in this study. Therefore, an original quality assessment tool was created by merging and adapting the American Dietetic Association (ADA) quality criteria checklist for Randomized Control Trials (RCTs) and cohorts [25], the Cochrane risk of bias [26], and the STROBE statement checklist for observational studies [27] (Figure 1). The key domain that was included and considered particularly pertinent for this review was "polymorphisms are with the Hardy-Weinberg equilibrium" [28] and whether the association of the genetic variants with specific phenotypic traits was properly reported. The final checklist included 13 "yes" or "no" statements. Similar to the ADA quality criteria checklist and Cochrane risk of bias tool, each study was assigned as positive, neutral, or negative based on the number of "yes", "no", or "not applicable" answers. A study was assigned positive if the majority of statements received "yes", or were assigned negative if the majority of statements received "no". If a study had the same number of yes and no statements it was assigned neutral (Figure 1). Two reviewers (KD, MA, and AD) independently performed the quality assessment and any discrepancies were discussed as a group.

	Breast Milk		Insulin and Glucose Regulation					Memory Impairment		Chronic Disease and Aging							Zn Homeostasis	
	Alam 2015	Qian 2012	Billings 2014	Jansen 2012	Kanoni 2011	Maruthur 2015	Shan 2014	Da Rocha 2013	Flinn 2014	Giacconi 2005	Giacconi 2006	Giacconi 2007	Giacconi 2010	Kanoni 2010	Mariani 2007	Mocchegiani 2008	Da Rocha 2014	Whitfield 2010
Q1																		
Q2																		
Q3																		
Q4																		
Q5																		
Q6																		
Q7																		
Q8																		
Q9																		
Q10																		
Q11																		
Q12																		
Q13																		
Overall	+	+	+	−	+	+	+	+	+	−	−	−	⊕	−	−	−	+	+

− = negative + = positive ⊕ = neutral ☐ = Yes ☐ = No ■ = Not Applicable to study design

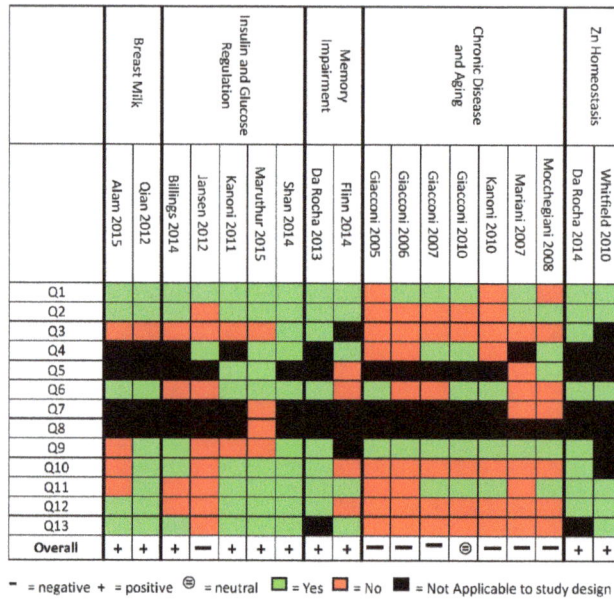

Figure 1. Quality Assessment (QA) results for each included study. Q1. Research question; Q2. Study Design; Q3. Subjects/patients bias; Q4. Group comparisons; Q5. Intervention/therapeutic description; Q6. Outcomes; Q7. Withdrawals; Q8. Blinding; Q9. Hardy-Weinberg equilibrium; Q10. Association between Zn intake or Zn status and Single Nucleotide Polymorphisms (SNPs); Q11. Appropriateness of statistics; Q12. Supported conclusions; Q13. Funding bias [29].

3. Results

3.1. Description of Included Studies

The result of the systematic search of the databases is shown in the PRISMA flowchart (Figure 2); eighteen studies matched the inclusion and exclusion criteria. Of these 18 studies, eight were observational cross-sectional [21,30–35], six were case control studies [23,36–41], three were non-randomised clinical control trials ([24,42,43], and one was a cross-sectional meta-analysis [22]. Nine separate genes with 31 SNPs (Table 1), and one study that looked at twins [34] were identified across the 18 studies. The studies selected were grouped according to the association between one or more polymorphisms with a phenotypic trait. Using this criterion, the studies were classified into the following five groups: polymorphisms in genes relating to Zn transporters for breastmilk, insulin and glucose regulation, cognitive performance, chronic disease in the ageing population, and Zn homeostasis (Table 1).

The 18 studies were scored for their quality against a list of 13 items; a summary of the results of the quality assessment is summarised in Figure 1. Overall, the studies scored positively on the identification of the research questions and validation of methods; the studies identified as scoring negatively did so mainly in the selection of study participants, or providing conclusions that did not take into consideration the limitations of the study or study bias. Due to the lack of consistency across grouped studies, identification of outcomes, and methods of determining associations, conclusions on how to translate the information into recommendations in practice could not be drawn.

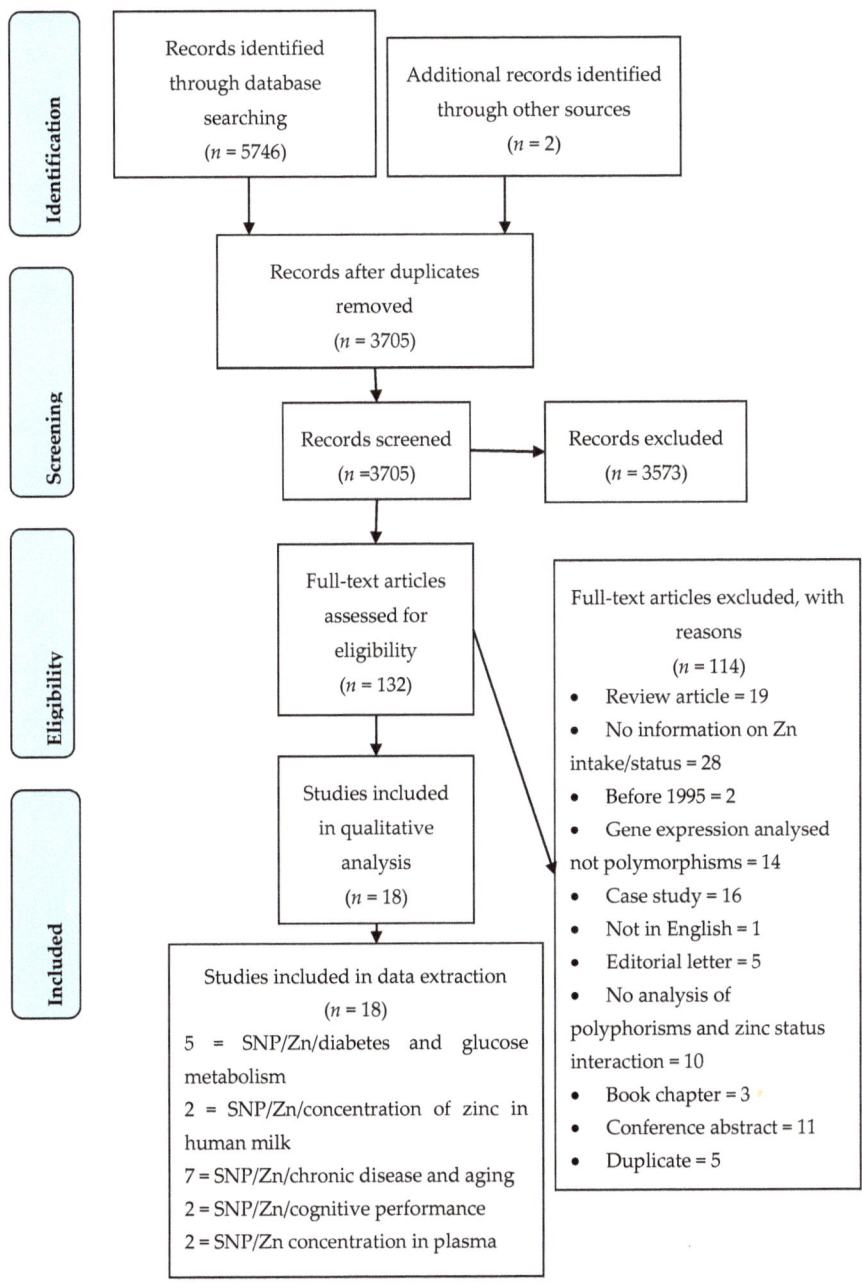

Figure 2. PRISMA 2009 Flow Diagram adapted from [44].

Table 1. Data extraction of each study identified. T1D, type 1 diabetes; T2D, type 2 diabetes.

Study Reference	Study Design	Sample Description	SNPs Associated with a Phenotype (Gene, rs# and Nucleotide Change)	Description of the SNPs Association with Phenotypic Trait	SNPs Association with Plasma Zn Concentration ^	SNPs Association with Zn Intake or Zn Supplementation	Outcomes
Polymorphisms in Zn transporters for Breast milk							
Alam et al. 2015 [30]	Cross-sectional	54 F, healthy American. Inclusion: 18–40 years who were breastfeeding one healthy infant at ≈4 months post-partum. Exclusion: Pre-term births (<37 week gestation), multiple births, smokers	12 novel SNPs identified as missense by sequencing. $SLC30A2$ gene: $A^{28}D$, $K^{66}N$, $Q^{71}H$, $D^{108}E$, $A^{105}P$ $Q^{117}H$, $T^{288}S$, $A^{310}T$, $L^{311}V$, $T^{312}K$, $V^{313}G$, $Q^{315}R$.	$D^{108}E$ found associated with low [Zn] breastmilk.	N/A	N/A	Variability in the concentration of Zn in human milk was associated with $SLC30A2$ SNPs. Possibly because of the small sample size, the other association did not reach significance.
Qian et al. 2012 [31]	Cross-sectional	750 F, healthy Chinese. Inclusion: 18–36 years breastfeeding day 42 postpartum. Exclusion: multiple gestations, multiparity, pre-existing maternal diseases, foetal malformation and lactation failure, complicated pregnancy	1 SNP in the promoter region and 1 in the coding region of the coding sequence of $SLC30A2$ gene (rs117153535 (G/T); No rs-$SLC30A2$/1031A > G)	Association between genetic polymorphisms and milk Zn concentration: rs117153535 T allele associated with lower [Zn]; $SLC30A2$/1031A > G allele associated with lower [Zn].	N/A	N/A	Variability in the concentration of Zn in human milk was associated with $SLC30A2$ SNPs.
Polymorphisms in genes relating to Insulin and Glucose Regulation							
Billings et al. 2014 [21]	Cross-sectional from RCT	2997 male and female participants in the Diabetes Prevention Program (US). Inclusion: high risk of developing T2D (overweight with elevated fasting glucose and IGT) randomised to placebo, metformin 850 mg twice daily, or lifestyle intervention and consented to genetic testing	44 novel SNPs including: $SLC30A8$: rs2464591 (C/T), rs2466296 (C/T), rs2466297 (A/G), rs2466299 (C/T). $SLC30A8$: rs2466293 (C/T)	Associated with improvement in β-cell function. Decrease in β-cell function.	No association between Zn intake and SNPs on diabetes incidence	N/A	$SLC30A8$ variants influence T2D risk, insulin secretion traits and β-cell function. Zn intake did not modify the genetic risk. None of the SNPs had a large effect.
Shan et al. 2014 [41]	Cross-sectional Case-control study	1796 male and female Chinese Han ethnicity. Inclusion: newly diagnosed IGR and T2D. ≥30 years, BMI ≥ 40 kg/m², no history of diabetes diagnosis or pharmacological treatment for hyperlipidaemia. Exclusion: clinically significant neurological, endocrine, or other systemic diseases, as well as acute illness, chronic inflammatory, or infectious diseases.	$SLC30A8$, rs13266634 (C/T)	C allele was associated with increased odds of T2D.	Decreased risk of T2D in carriers of risk (C) allele with high plasma Zn concentration.	N/A	$SLC30A8$ rs13266634 is associated with T2D. CC genotype and low plasma Zn increase T2D risk and Impaired Glucose Regulation. High plasma Zn concentration (third highest tertile ≥197.58 ug/dL) decreased risk of T2D in carriers of risk C allele.

Table 1. *Cont.*

Study Reference	Study Design	Sample Description	SNPs Associated with a Phenotype (Gene, rs# and Nucleotide Change)	Description of the SNPs Association with Phenotypic Trait	SNPs Association with Plasma Zn Concentration ^	SNPs Association with Zn Intake or Zn Supplementation	Outcomes
Polymorphisms in genes relating to Insulin and Glucose Regulation							
Kanoni et al. 2011 [22]	Cross-sectional Meta-analysis	Meta-analysis from 14 cohort studies, 46,021 participants. **Inclusion:** no diabetes (fasting glucose ≥ 7 mmol/L or use of antidiabetic medications). Sample size for interaction analysis between dietary Zn intake and SNPs ranged from 27,010 to 45,821.	20 SNPs analysed including: SLC30A8, rs11558471 (A/G)	N/A	Zn intake of 14 mg/day associated with 0.024 mmol/L decrease in fasting glucose concentration in A carriers in comparison to GG (0.048 mmol/L reduction for AA homozygotes)	Interaction only significant with zinc diet and supplementation	Increased Zn intake improves diabetes risk dependent for A allele carriers of SNP rs11558471.S
Jansen et al. 2012 [36]	Case-control study	150 male and female (22 T1D; 53 T2D; 7 matched controls). **Inclusion:** ≥18 years, patients with type 1 or 2 diabetes; **Exclusion:** acute infection, recent, cancer, liver or renal disease.	SLC30A8 rs13266634 (C/T) MT1A rs11640851 (A/C), rs8052394 (A/G)	No significance in SNP association T1D or T2D	N/A	N/A	Serum Zn decreased in patients with diabetes, no association with any SNPs and disease biomarkers. Small sample size.
Maruthur et al. 2015 [43]	Non-randomised supplement clinical trial	55 male and female Old Order Amish from Lancaster, PA, USA. **Inclusion:** 21–70 years no diagnosis of diabetes and random glucose less than 11.10 mmol/L [200 mg/dL].	SLC30A8, rs13266634 (C/T) (R325W). The (C) allele encodes the arginine (R), and the (T) allele encodes the tryptophan (W)	Carriers of allele T showed increased insulin response after supplementation	Serum Zn concentration increased by 23% for CC genotypes and 33% for CT/TT genotypes after supplementation	Oral Zn acetate 50 mg, twice daily × 14 days	Carriers of risk T allele showed increased insulin response after supplementation with Zn; these participants may benefit most from Zn supplementation
Polymorphisms in genes relating to Memory Impairment							
Da Rocha et al. 2014a [32]	Cross-sectional study	240 male and female mature, elderly adults **Inclusion:** ≥50 years, absence of dementia, owning intellect enough to continue production, present complaint of progressive memory loss, show objective evidence of memory deficits. **Exclusion:** symptoms of depression, anxiety, or stress, JQ < 70, use of vitamin supplements containing micronutrients of interest	SLC30A3, rs73924411 (C/T) rs11126936 (G/T)	Increased frequency of rs11126936 TT carriers in people with memory deficits.	When serum Zn was below recommended concentration: rs11126936 T carriers had better memory scores, whereas CC carriers' performance decreased.	N/A	Recommended Zn concentration may be neurotoxic for T carriers suffering from memory deficit. CC genotype may benefit from increased Zn intake when Zn serum is low
Flinn et al. 2014 [37]	Case-control on mouse-model	22 Mouse strain CRND8 with human ApoE ε4; 23 Mouse strain CRND8; 24 WT controls	ApoE ε4 (Apoliprotein E isoform SNP in NCBI rs7412)	Carriers of human ApoE ε4 showed impaired spatial memory	N/A	10 ppm of ZnCO₃ in water	Increased dietary Zn significantly impaired spatial memory of mice carrying ApoE ε4 human compared with WT and CRND8. The amount of Zn consumed daily was not reported

Table 1. *Cont.*

Study Reference	Study Design	Sample Description	SNPs Associated with a Phenotype (Gene, rs# and Nucleotide Change)	Description of the SNPs Association with Phenotypic Trait	SNPs Association with Plasma Zn Concentration ^	SNPs Association with Zn Intake or Zn Supplementation	Outcomes
Polymorphisms in genes relating to chronic disease in the aging population							
Giacconi et al. 2007 [40]	Case-control study	506 male and female elderly adults (288 with coronary artery stenosis; 218 healthy, age and sex matched controls living at home) **Inclusion:** older individuals born and living in Central Italy admitted to INRCA Geriatric Hospital, Ancona, Italy, for endarterectomy	MT2A rs10636 (C/G)	C allele more frequent amongst patients with carotid stenosis	Low plasma [Zn] associated with C allele	N/A	MT2A rs10636 C allele is associated with low plasma Zn and independently with carotid stenosis. No conclusive evidence that modifying Zn intake is beneficial for C allele carriers
Kanoni et al. 2010 [35]	Cross-sectional study	819 male and female elderly adults (272 from Italy, 163 from Greece, 137 from Germany, 128 from France, and 119 from Poland). **Inclusion:** (ZINCAGE Project: www.zincage.org). ≥ 60 years old, non-institutionalised, free of medication and supplements. **Exclusion:** autoimmune, neurodegenerative, cardiovascular, kidney, or liver disease, diabetes, infections, cancer, sickle cell, skin ulcerations, and endocrine disorders.	−174 IL-6 G/C (inNational Center for Biotechnology Information (NCBI)rs1800795 C/G)	GG genotype had greater increase in IL-6 levels with increased 'Zn diet score' than CG and CC genotypes	Significant interaction of 'Zn diet score' and GG genotype of rs1800795	N/A	Method developed to calculate Zn dietary intake and correlate it with plasma Zn "Zn score". Association observed between Zn score, G allele and IL-6 levels
Giacconi et al. 2005 [38]	Case-control study	279 male and female born and living in Central Italy, (91 T2D; 188 age and sex-matched controls living at home). **Inclusion:** (ZINCAGE Project: www.zincage.org) older adults, diagnosis of T2D with carotid stenosis, control individuals living at home, no hypertension, diabetes or carotid stenosis, no history of Coronary Heart Disease (CHD), normal electrocardiography and no sign of myocardial ischemia	MT2A rs1610216 A/G (in NCBI database C/T)	AA genotype associated with carotid stenosis and T2D, inflammation markers. A allele more frequent in patients than controls	Plasma Zn concentration decreased in AA genotype compared with AG genotypes	N/A	MT2A rs1610216, AA genotype associated with disease biomarkers and low serum Zn concentration. No evidence supporting that increased serum Zn would be beneficial
Giacconi et al. 2010 [39]	Case-control study	459 male and female elderly Italian adults (215 Cardio-Vascular Diseases (CVD) 244 age and sex-matched healthy controls); 374 male and female elderly Greek adults (154 CVD 220 age and sex-matched healthy controls). **Inclusion:** (ZINCAGE Project: www.zincage.org) Italian: diagnosis of ischemic heart disease and/or carotid heart disease; Greek: diagnoses history of angina, heart failure, coronary heart disease, stroke, myocardial infarction, or heart surgery. **Exclusion:** Italian controls: diabetes diagnosis	MT1A rs8052394 (A/C), rs11640851 (A/G)	Increased frequency of rs11640851 G allele carriers in Greek patients with ischemic heart and/or carotid heart disease in comparison to Greek controls. No difference between Italian patients and controls.	Intracellular zinc of peripheral blood cells decreased in CVD patients MT1A haplotype CG+ compared with MT1A CG−/CG− haplotype	N/A	No evidence of association between genotype, Zn, and biomarkers of disease, including inflammation and circulating lipids

Table 1. *Cont.*

Study Reference	Study Design	Sample Description	SNPs Associated with a Phenotype (Gene, rs# and Nucleotide Change)	Description of the SNPs Association with Phenotypic Trait	SNPs Association with Plasma Zn Concentration ^	SNPs Association with Zn Intake or Zn Supplementation	Outcomes
Polymorphisms in genes relating to chronic disease in the aging population							
Giacconi et al. 2006 [23]	Case-control study	406 male and female older adults born and living in central Italy (105 with carotid stenosis and CVD (C); 111 with cardioischaemia (D); 190 age and sex-matched controls). **Inclusion:** ≥70 years, older individuals born and living in Central Italy admitted to INRCA Geriatric Hospital, Ancona, Italy, for endarterectomy	1267 *Hsp70-2* (A/G); (in NCBI database rs780016316 C/T) -308 *TNFα* G/A (in NCBI rs1800629 A/G)	1267 *Hsp70-2* G allele more frequent in (C) group than (D)	Plasma Zn similar across genotypic groups	N/A	No evidence of association between genotype, Zn, and biomarkers of disease, including hypertension and circulating lipids.
Mocchegiani et al. 2008 [42]	Non-randomised supplement clinical trial	110 male and female healthy, non-institutionalised older adults from Italy, France, Germany, Poland, and Greece. **Inclusion:** (ZINCAGE Project: www.zincage.org). 60–84 years old, free of medication, plasma zinc ≤ 10.5 μM. **Exclusion:** autoimmune, neurodegenerative, cardiovascular, kidney or liver diseases, diabetes, infections, cancer, chronic inflammatory bowel disease or acrodermatitis enteropathica, sickle cell anaemia, chronic skin ulcerations, and endocrine disorders	−174 *IL-6* G/C (in NCBI rs1800795 C/G)	No significant difference between carriers of alleles for immune parameters	GG genotype had significantly lower plasma Zn than C carriers. GG genotypes with normal plasma Zn still presented with impaired Zn status	10 mg/day Zn-aspartate for 48 ± 2 days	Low plasma Zn associated with impaired immune response and psychological function independent of genotype GG genotype carriers are more predisposed to Zn deficiency and suggested as better candidates for supplementation
Mariani et al. 2008 [24]	Non-randomised supplement clinical trial	39 male and female healthy older adults **Inclusion:** (ZINCAGE Project: www.zincage.org). 60–83 years old, healthy old people, still living independently, plasma Zn < 11 μmol/L. **Exclusion:** taking medication, nutritional integrators, or vitamin complexes.	+647 A/C *MT1A* −174 *IL-6* (in NCBI rs1800795 (C/G)	+647 *MT1A* genotype associated with increased inflammatory biomarkers	+647 *MT1A* C− allele associated with lower plasma Zn than C+ at basal and after supplementation.	10 mg/day Zn-aspartate for 48 ± 2 days. Plasma Zn concentration significantly increased after supplementation in C+ carriers of −174 *IL6*.	Carriers of C− genotype of *MT1A* had lowest concentration of plasma zinc. Increment after supplementation was more pronounced in subjects carrying C- allele of *MT1A* /C+ −174 *IL-6*. Carriers of C− *MT1A*/C −174 *IL-6* did not respond to zinc supplementation.
Polymorphisms relating to Zn homeostasis							
Whitfield et al. 2010 [34]	Cross-sectional study	2926 male and female adult twins living in Australia **Inclusion:** Born between 1903 and 1964 (30–92 years old), enrolled in the Australian Twin Registry	N/A	N/A	20% of the variation in plasma Zn concentration is due to genetic factors.	N/A	Genetic variability is contributing factor to Zn plasma variability. Specific genotypes not reported
Da Rocha et al. 2014b [33]	Cross-sectional study	110 male and female older adults **Inclusion:** ≥50 years old adults **Exclusion:** use of vitamin supplements containing micronutrients	*SLC30A3* rs11126936 (A/C)	N/A	CC genotypes had lower plasma Zn concentration than A carriers. CC genotype more frequent in participants with low plasma Zn	N/A	*SLC30A3* polymorphism rs11126936 was associated with differences in plasma Zn concentration

3.2. Does Dietary Zn Modulate the Effect of SLC30A2 Polymorphisms on Human Milk Zinc Content?

Two cross-sectional studies examined the association of polymorphisms within *SLC30A2* gene and Zn content variability in human milk from a total of 794 healthy, breastfeeding mothers with children from single births, without complications. Zn concentrations in breastmilk were examined at 42 days and 4 months postpartum [28]. *SLC30A2* SNPs found to be associated with variability in milk Zn concentrations are listed in Table 1. SNP rs-numbers were only reported in Qian et al. [30], whereas SNPs were identified as "novel" without associated rs-numbers in Alam et al. [28], which makes identifying common SNPs between the studies difficult. Qian et al. identified five SNPs in the Chinese mothers, with two associated with decreased concentrations and three with no association with Zn in breastmilk. In the US, Alam et al. identified 12 polymorphisms in mothers, of which two variants were associated with decreased concentrations of Zn in breastmilk. Low concentration of Zn in breastmilk were defined as 21.5 μmol/L [30], and less than 1 mg per L (15.3 μmol/L) [28]. Neither study reported whether maternal dietary Zn intake or plasma Zn modulated Zn concentrations of milk in mothers carrying polymorphisms associated with low breastmilk Zn concentrations [28,30]. Both of these studies were assessed by QA rating P (Figure 1).

3.3. Does Dietary Zn Modulate the Association between Gene Variants and Glucose Metabolism Traits in Relation to Type-2 Diabetes?

Five independent studies examined the association between SNPs for the *SLC30A8* gene, Zn intake, the risk of T2D diabetes, and glucose metabolism biomarkers (Table 1). Three out of five studies examined the SNP rs13266634 [36,41,43]; of these studies, all but Jansen et al. [36] confirmed the increased risk of T2D associated with the T allele of this SNP (Table 1). While Jansen and colleagues showed contradicting results, the small sample size may have not allowed the association to be significant, and this was discussed by the authors. When the effect of dietary Zn intake was investigated in carriers of the T allele for the SNP rs13266634, Shan et al. [41] reported a reversed risk for T2D with high plasma Zn concentration (third highest tertile $\geq$ 197.58 μg/dL). Maruthur et al. also reported that after Zn supplementation for 14 days carriers of the T allele experienced increased insulin response to glucose by 15% and 14% at 5 and 10 minutes, respectively, compared with individuals carrying the CC genotype [43].

The hypothesis that more variants of SLC30A8 are associated with impaired glucose metabolism was explored by Billings and co-workers in a study that sequenced the exome of the gene in 380 subjects classified as possessing an increased risk of developing T2D [21]. This study identified 44 novel *SLC30A8* variants; four of which demonstrated a positive association, and one that showed a negative association with pancreatic β-cell function biomarkers (Table 1). The authors concluded that dietary Zn intake did not modify the genetic predisposition to T2D, suggesting a limited role for dietary manipulation in affecting risk in relation to the SNPs identified. The study's main limitation was a lack of description of a method to measure dietary intake which prevented the results from properly supporting the conclusion (Table 1 and Figure 1). The authors were contacted on this matter, however, we did not obtain a response.

The fifth study was a cross-sectional meta-analysis on 14 cohorts including a total of 46,021 individuals of European ancestry with fasting glucose <6 mmol/L [22]. The association of dietary zinc intake with fasting glucose, and the interaction with 20 genetic variants known to be related to glucose metabolism traits was examined. This study identified the *SLC30A8* SNP rs11558471, where carriers of the A allele have increased fasting glucose. An association was observed with the SNP rs11558471, fasting glucose, and total Zn intake, suggesting that Zn intake has an inverse association with fasting glucose plasma concentration in carriers of the A allele for that SNP. Fasting glucose of individuals carrying the A allele of rs11558471 responded to increased Zn intake compared with GG genotype carriers; for each milligram of Zn intake per day, a reduction of -0.0017 mmol/L fasting glucose was reported (Table 1) [22]. Quality of the meta-analysis was assessed as positive, however, the rationale for examining the specific SNP was not reported.

3.4. Does Dietary Zn Modulate the Effect of Gene Variants on Cognitive Performance?

Two studies, one in humans and one in mice, were identified that examined Zn, genes, and cognition. The human study examined the interaction between SNPs for the *SLC30A3* gene, cognitive performance, and Zn dietary intake in 240 healthy people over 50 years of age, but with memory deficit [32]. The authors reported a gene-nutrient interaction for SLC30A3 rs73924411 and serum Zn concentration (Table 1). Carriers of the T allele displayed higher memory score than the CC genotype carriers when serum Zn concentration was below the recommended concentration (<0.70 mg/L = 0.01 mmol/L). This suggests a possible neurotoxicity effect of Zn for T allele carriers with serum Zn > 0.70 mg/L = 0.01 mmol/L.

The mouse model study examined late-onset AD, and analysed the interaction between Zn dietary intake and the isoform ε4 of the apolipoprotein E (ApoE) human gene [37] corresponding to SNP rs7412 in the NCBI database. The authors tested whether high Zn intake worsened the spatial memory of mice in which the endogen APOE gene was replaced with the isoform ε4 of human ApoE. The ApoE isoform ε4 is over-represented in AD patients and promotes the binding of Zn to amyloid plaques [45]. Although in a mouse model, Flinn's group showed that high Zn intake was associated with worse performance in tests aimed at evaluating spatial memory in carriers of the ApoE isoform ε4 [37]. However, the authors did not report actual Zn intake, as the mice were allowed to drink Zn-spiked water ad-libitum.

Both these studies reported that high Zn intake, in association with specific gene variants, significantly impaired the memory scores of older adults and spatial memory in an AD mouse model, respectively. Flinn's study scored negative in the QA assessment mainly because the lack of reporting of Zn intake. Da Rocha et al., although with some limitations, was assessed as positive in the QA (Figure 1) [32,37].

3.5. Does Dietary Zn Modulate the Association between Gene Variants and the Development of Chronic Diseases in the Aging Population?

Seven studies aimed to identify carriers of genetic polymorphisms that would benefit from Zn supplementation to support healthy ageing [23,24,35,38–40,46]. Unlike the other studies reported in this review, Zn and healthy ageing have not been associated with Zn transporter genes, but rather genes that are associated with inflammation and oxidative stress. Three papers investigated the association between Interleukin-6 (IL-6) SNP rs1800795 and serum Zn in a group of older adults, but did not show any conclusive relationship (Table 1) [24,35,46]. All papers in this group reported on SNPs in relation to separate outcomes, often in small sample sizes. Differing targets and the lack of consistency in reporting across the group prevents reaching a clinically relevant conclusion (Table 1) [23,35,38–40,42]. These studies were all assessed negative or neutral in the QA score (Figure 1).

3.6. Do Polymorphisms in Genes Involved in Zn Transport and Metabolism Affect Plasma Zn Concentration?

Two of the 18 papers identified did not explore the interaction between polymorphisms in Zn metabolism and dietary Zn in relation to a clinical biomarker/disease state, but they investigated the influence of polymorphisms only on plasma Zn concentrations and whether this is affected by dietary Zn intake [33,34]. Da Rocha et al. looked at the influence of SNPs rs11126936 and rs73924411 in the gene *SLC20A3* and found that Zn serum concentrations were significantly lower in carriers of C allele of rs11126936 compared to T carriers ($p = 0.014$). When subjects were grouped by serum Zn concentrations the CC genotype was more frequently observed in subjects with low Zn serum. Da Rocha and colleagues did not find any association between serum Zn concentration and rs73924411. This finding needs to be evaluated against another study from the same group that found a significant association between rs73924411 and Zn concentrations in relation to cognitive impairment scores [32]. This suggests the interaction is only observed in relation to cognitive impairment. Finally, Whitfield et al. [34] investigated to what extent Zn concentrations in erythrocytes are influenced by genetic effects by obtaining samples from twins. The group used model-fitting and grouped twins according to zygosity in order to establish to what extent the Zn concentration variation was due to genetic or environmental factors including diet. They concluded that 20% of the variation in Zn concentration is due to genetic factors [34].

4. Discussion

The completion of the Human Genome Project held the promise of resolving the complexity of individual response to diet and one-size fits all public health guidelines, and to reveal the role of genetics in shaping nutritional requirements [1,19]. Zn exemplifies this paradigm; this essential micronutrient is distributed throughout all organs, Zn absorption and metabolism involves numerous gene products, and it is expected that genetic variability is capable of affecting requirements [6].

The Zn transporter *SLC30A8* is a gene expressed in insulin secreting pancreas β-cells; *SLC30A8* SNP rs13266634 has been associated with increased risk of T2D [31,47–50]. The discovery of a relationship between Zn transporter gene variants and T2D led to the hypothesis that Zn intake may affect insulin and/or glucose metabolism [51], thus making *SLC30A8* polymorphisms good candidates to modify Zn requirements. This systematic review highlighted the role of Zn intake and its interaction with *SLC30A8* SNPs. In the meta-analysis performed by Kanoni et al. 2011, the gene dependent nutrient interaction with glucose metabolism markers was confirmed. Kanoni et al. demonstrated that total Zn intake has a stronger inverse association with fasting glucose concentration in individuals carrying the glucose-raising A allele of rs11558471. The interaction resulted in a reduction of 0.024 mmol/L in blood sugar concentration per 1 mg of Zn. The normal range for blood glucose concentration is considered 4–8 mmol/L; this finding, while interesting, may not be easily utilised in clinical practice due to the relatively small effects [22]. *SLC30A8* has been linked to pancreatic islets function [12], but this was the first time that rs11558471 was investigated in the context of glucose metabolism outcomes. rs11558471 was reported to be in strong linkage disequilibrium with rs13266634, although no further explanation was offered on why this SNP was selected. Different SNPs on *SLC30A8* were tested by Shan's group, showing that the risk of T2D and impaired glucose regulation could be attenuated by increasing plasma Zn concentrations in CC carriers of rs13266634. These observations support the concept that Zn intervention could play a role in T2D, and that Zn recommendations may benefit from being personalised according to *SLC30A8* genotypes. This study was assessed positive on quality, however, its use in clinical practice is limited, as it does not provide indications on the magnitude of an intervention (i.e., within or above the RDI) [41]. Jansen and collaborators reported rs13266634 in the same gene and presented conflicting results, reporting a lack of association with glucose metabolism biomarkers, possibly due to the small sample analysed [36]. This highlights the importance of further larger scale research projects that seek to clarify any gene-nutrient interactions and provide clear understanding of any intervention requirements.

The potential associations of genetic polymorphisms with cognitive performance in relation to Zn intake were investigated in two of the selected studies [32,37]. The *SLC30A3* gene was identified in 1996 and raised major interest, as the corresponding protein was shown to transport Zn into pre-synaptic vesicles of glutamatergic neurones of the cerebral cortex and hippocampus, key regions for the memory formation and with a role in the development of amyloid β plaques in AD [52,53]. Da Rocha and colleagues analysed the role of *SLC30A3* rs73924411 in memory [32]. Another study analysed another genetic variation associated with AD, the ApoE isoform ε4 [54]. Both reports suggested that carriers of T allele of *SLC30A3* rs73924411 and ApoE isoform ε4 (rs7412 in NCBI), respectively, could benefit from Zn plasma concentration on the lower side of the recommended cut-off and suggested that what is considered the optimal concentration could have a neurotoxic effect for the carriers of these polymorphisms. Those observations can lead to the conclusion that individuals with these genotypes would be better off in terms of cognitive performance with Zn intakes lower than the recommended amounts. Although one of these reports analysed a small sample [32] and the other did not report Zn intake correctly [54], they are examples of where one size fits all nutrient recommendations may not be appropriate. The quest to slow down the inevitable process of aging and the development of

Nutrients **2017**, *9*, 148

diseases associated with it has included the attempt to optimise diet to support the metabolic needs of elderly people. Seven papers indicated that there may be a potential interaction between markers of chronic disease in the elderly and the variation of Zn intake, with outcomes being dependent on genetic variations. However, these findings should be treated with caution until further research that explicitly quantifies the association of Zn intake and genotype, not just Zn status, is conducted. Therefore, no conclusions can be drawn at this time in relation to clinical practice.

5. Perspectives

Healthcare professionals need to be able to translate genetic information in the context of the health priorities of patients, to take into consideration the scenario of a patient carrying one or more SNPs in genes affecting Zn metabolism in different organs and the possibility of the results of these different genotypes modifying the risk of two pathologies in opposite/different ways. This would ideally require bioinformatics tools to evaluate the function and effect size of each relevant variant, along with clinical information. To develop dietary recommendations that incorporate information of common polymorphisms, more studies need to be conducted looking at the association of genetic variants, disease biomarkers, and dietary intake. The majority of the studies included in this report analysed the association of only two out of three of these factors, making it difficult to draw a conclusion about personalised dietary recommendations based on genotypes. Moreover, a reliable biomarker to assess Zn status is still an open debate; serum concentration is generally used, but this measure is affected by several transient factors, such as infections and acute inflammation [55].

A number of studies identified in this review confirmed the concept of genetic makeup modifying the response to Zn and possibly Zn requirements; however, we are still left with a number of questions such as what is the optimal Zn intake for specific genetic variations? Should the advice on Zn intake change in relation to a reduction in disease risk or to be used as a therapeutic tool to make treatments more effective? Most studies did not assess dietary Zn intake, so while associations between Zn status and SNPs may have been identified, there is no mention of whether current dietary recommendations are appropriate for different genotypes for general good health or in relation to disease outcomes. Another point of reflection is that most studies were performed on small cohorts, in specific sub groups of the population, not representing the variability present in the human species. These questions are important for research in the current environment, where more nutrigenetic tests are being developed and advertised as tools to tailor dietary advice; the public have increasing access to these tests through both a range of healthcare professionals and the internet. While tests may correctly report on the associations between genetics and health effects, they do not take into consideration the effect size and the direction of the intervention. The limited clear evidence on how variations affect dietary requirements for general good health, therapeutic treatments, and disease reduction, raises the question of deciding when it is useful to use the results to modify nutrient intake advice. Healthcare professionals with appropriate knowledge in both genetics and nutrition are required to help individuals understand whether and how information within nutrigenetic tests should be used to inform dietary intake. Limitations of this systematic study include the lack of homogeneity between the studies selected, which prevented the possibility of performing a meta-analysis, thereby making it difficult to reach a decisive conclusion that provides clear directions for application.

Supplementary Materials: The following are available online at http://www.mdpi.com/2072-6643/9/2/148/s1, Figure S1: Databases' search strategy, Figure S2: PRISMA checklist.

Acknowledgments: We thank Anne Yung for assisting with the initial database searches.

Author Contributions: C.M. and M.M.A. conceived the study. K.J.D., M.M.A. and C.M. performed the database searches and wrote the first draft of the manuscript; A.L.D., M.M.A. and K.J.D. assessed the quality of the selected studies. A.L.D. assisted with the final editing of the manuscript.

Conflicts of Interest: The authors declare no conflict of interest.

References

1. Ferguson, L.R.; De Caterina, R.; Görman, U.; Allayee, H.; Kohlmeier, M.; Prasad, C.; Kang, J.X. Guide and Position of the International Society of Nutrigenetics/Nutrigenomics on Personalised Nutrition: Part 1—Fields of Precision Nutrition. *J. Nutrigenet. Nutrigenom.* **2016**, *9*, 12–27. [CrossRef] [PubMed]
2. Lonnerdal, B. Dietary factors affecting trace element absorption in infants. *Acta Paediatr. Scand. Suppl.* **1989**, *351*, 109–113. [CrossRef] [PubMed]
3. National Health and Medical Research Council. Nutrient Reference Values. 2006. Available online: http://www.nrv.gov.au (accessed on 24 May 2016).
4. Maret, W.; Sandstead, H.H. Zinc requirements and the risks and benefits of zinc supplementation. *J. Trace Elem. Med. Biol.* **2006**, *20*, 3–18. [CrossRef] [PubMed]
5. Prasad, A.S.; Miale, A., Jr.; Farid, Z.; Sandstead, H.H.; Schulert, A.R. Zinc metabolism in patients with the syndrome of iron deficiency anemia, hepatosplenomegaly, dwarfism, and hypognadism. *J. Lab. Clin. Med.* **1963**, *61*, 537–549. [PubMed]
6. Devirgiliis, C.; Zalewski, P.D.; Perozzi, G.; Murgia, C. Zinc fluxes and zinc transporter genes in chronic diseases. *Mutat. Res.* **2007**, *622*, 84–93. [CrossRef] [PubMed]
7. Hambidge, K.M.; Krebs, N.F. Zinc deficiency: A special challenge. *J. Nutr.* **2007**, *137*, 1101–1105. [PubMed]
8. Ackland, M.L.; Michalczyk, A. Zinc deficiency and its inherited disorders—A review. *Genes Nutr.* **2006**, *1*, 41–49. [CrossRef] [PubMed]
9. Kimura, T.; Kambe, T. The Functions of Metallothionein and ZIP and ZnT Transporters: An Overview and Perspective. *Int. J. Mol. Sci.* **2016**, *17*, 336. [CrossRef] [PubMed]
10. Kambe, T.; Tsuji, T.; Hashimoto, A.; Itsumura, N. The Physiological, Biochemical, and Molecular Roles of Zinc Transporters in Zinc Homeostasis and Metabolism. *Physiol. Rev.* **2015**, *95*, 749–784. [CrossRef] [PubMed]
11. Huang, L. Zinc and its transporters, pancreatic beta-cells, and insulin metabolism. *Vitam. Horm.* **2014**, *95*, 365–390. [PubMed]
12. Rutter, G.A.; Chimienti, F. *SLC30A8* mutations in type 2 diabetes. *Diabetologia* **2015**, *58*, 31–36. [CrossRef] [PubMed]
13. Fan, M.; Li, W.; Wang, L.; Gu, S.; Dong, S.; Chen, M.; Jiang, X. Association of *SLC30A8* gene polymorphism with type 2 diabetes, evidence from 46 studies: A meta-analysis. *Endocrine* **2016**, *53*, 381–394. [CrossRef] [PubMed]
14. Lee, S.; Hennigar, S.R.; Alam, S.; Nishida, K.; Kelleher, S.L. Essential Role for Zinc Transporter 2 (ZnT2)-mediated Zinc Transport in Mammary Gland Development and Function during Lactation. *J. Biol. Chem.* **2015**, *290*, 13064–13078. [CrossRef] [PubMed]
15. Murgia, C.; Vespignani, I.; Rami, R.; Perozzi, G. The Znt4 mutation inlethal milk mice affects intestinal zinc homeostasis through the expression of other Zn transporters. *Genes Nutr.* **2006**, *1*, 61–70. [CrossRef] [PubMed]
16. Adlard, P.A.; Parncutt, J.; Lal, V.; James, S.; Hare, D.; Doble, P.; Bush, A.I. Metal chaperones prevent zinc-mediated cognitive decline. *Neurobiol. Dis.* **2015**, *81*, 196–202. [CrossRef] [PubMed]
17. Adlard, P.A.; Parncutt, J.M.; Finkelstein, D.I.; Bush, A.I. Cognitive loss in zinc transporter-3 knock-out mice: A phenocopy for the synaptic and memory deficits of Alzheimer's disease? *J. Neurosci.* **2010**, *30*, 1631–1636. [CrossRef] [PubMed]
18. Greenough, M.A.; Camakaris, J.; Bush, A.I. Metal dyshomeostasis and oxidative stress in Alzheimer's disease. *Neurochem. Int.* **2013**, *62*, 540–555. [CrossRef] [PubMed]
19. Hesketh, J. Personalised nutrition: How far has nutrigenomics progressed? *Eur. J. Clin. Nutr.* **2013**, *67*, 430–435. [CrossRef] [PubMed]
20. Palmiter, R.D.; Findley, S.D. Cloning and functional characterization of a mammalian zinc transporter that confers resistance to zinc. *EMBO J.* **1995**, *14*, 639–649. [PubMed]
21. Billings, L.K.; Jablonski, K.A.; Ackerman, R.J.; Taylor, A.; Fanelli, R.R.; McAteer, J.B.; Franks, P.W. The Influence of Rare Genetic Variation in *SLC30A8* on Diabetes Incidence and beta-Cell Function. *J. Clin. Endocrinol. Metab.* **2014**, *99*, E926–E930. [CrossRef] [PubMed]
22. Kanoni, S.; Nettleton, J.A.; Hivert, M.F.; Ye, Z.; Van Rooij, F.J.; Shungin, D.; Gustafsson, S. Total zinc intake may modify the glucose-raising effect of a zinc transporter (*SLC30A8*) variant: A 14-cohort meta-analysis. *Diabetes* **2011**, *60*, 2407–2416. [CrossRef] [PubMed]

23. Giacconi, R.; Cipriano, C.; Muti, E.; Costarelli, L.; Malavolta, M.; Caruso, C.; Mocchegiani, E. Involvement of-308 TNF-α and 1267 Hsp70-2 polymorphisms and zinc status in the susceptibility of coronary artery disease (CAD) in old patients. *Biogerontology* **2006**, *7*, 347–356. [CrossRef] [PubMed]

24. Mariani, E.; Neri, S.; Cattini, L.; Mocchegiani, E.; Malavolta, M.; Dedoussis, G.V.; Facchini, A. Effect of zinc supplementation on plasma IL-6 and MCP-1 production and NK cell function in healthy elderly: Interactive influence of +647 MT1a and -174 IL-6 polymorphic alleles. *Exp. Gerontol.* **2008**, *43*, 462–471. [CrossRef] [PubMed]

25. Association, A.D. *Evidence Analysis Manual: Steps in the ADA Evidence Analysis Process*; American Dietetic Association: Chicago, IL, USA, 2008.

26. Higgins, J.P.; Altman, D.G.; Gøtzsche, P.C.; Jüni, P.; Moher, D.; Oxman, A.D.; Sterne, J.A. The Cochrane Collaboration's tool for assessing risk of bias in randomised trials. *Br. Med. J.* **2011**, *343*, d5928. [CrossRef] [PubMed]

27. STROBE Statement. Checklist of items that should be included in reports of observational studies (STROBE initiative). *Int. J. Public Health* **2008**, *53*, 3–4.

28. Salanti, G.; Amountza, G.; Ntzani, E.E.; Ioannidis, J.P. Hardy-Weinberg equilibrium in genetic association studies: An empirical evaluation of reporting, deviations, and power. *Eur. J. Hum. Genet.* **2005**, *13*, 840–848. [CrossRef] [PubMed]

29. A Logo for Human Rights. ONE WORLD EQUAL RIGHTS. Available online: http://www.humanrightslogo.net/en/submission/one-world-%E2%80%93-equal-rights (accessed on 15 February 2017).

30. Alam, S.; Hennigar, S.R.; Gallagher, C.; Soybel, D.I.; Kelleher, S.L. Exome Sequencing of *SLC30A2* Identifies Novel Loss- and Gain-of-Function Variants Associated with Breast Cell Dysfunction. *J. Mammary Gland Biol. Neoplasia* **2015**, *20*, 159–172. [CrossRef] [PubMed]

31. Qian, L.; Wang, B.; Tang, N.; Zhang, W.; Cai, W. Polymorphisms of *SLC30A2* and selected perinatal factors associated with low milk zinc in Chinese breastfeeding women. *Early Hum. Dev.* **2012**, *88*, 663–668. [CrossRef] [PubMed]

32. Da Rocha, T.J.; Blehm, C.J.; Bamberg, D.P.; Fonseca, T.L.R.; Tisser, L.A.; de Oliveira Junior, A.A.; Fiegenbaum, M. The effects of interactions between selenium and zinc serum concentration and *SEP15* and *SLC30A3* gene polymorphisms on memory scores in a population of mature and elderly adults. *Genes Nutr.* **2014**, *9*, 377. [CrossRef] [PubMed]

33. Da Rocha, T.J.; Korb, C.; Schuch, J.B.; Bamberg, D.P.; de Andrade, F.M.; Fiegenbaum, M. *SLC30A3* and *SEP15* gene polymorphisms influence the serum concentrations of zinc and selenium in mature adults. *Nutr. Res.* **2014**, *34*, 742–748. [CrossRef] [PubMed]

34. Whitfield, J.B.; Dy, V.; McQuilty, R.; Zhu, G.; Heath, A.C.; Montgomery, G.W.; Martin, N.G. Genetic Effects on Toxic and Essential Elements in Humans: Arsenic, Cadmium, Copper, Lead, Mercury, Selenium, and Zinc in Erythrocytes. *Environ. Health Perspect.* **2010**, *118*, 776–782. [CrossRef] [PubMed]

35. Kanoni, S.; Dedoussis, G.V.; Herbein, G.; Fulop, T.; Varin, A.; Jajte, J.; Giacconi, R. Assessment of gene-nutrient interactions on inflammatory status of the elderly with the use of a zinc diet score—ZINCAGE study. *J. Nutr. Biochem.* **2010**, *21*, 526–531. [CrossRef] [PubMed]

36. Jansen, J.; Rosenkranz, E.; Overbeck, S.; Warmuth, S.; Mocchegiani, E.; Giacconi, R.; Rink, L. Disturbed zinc homeostasis in diabetic patients by in vitro and in vivo analysis of insulinomimetic activity of zinc. *J. Nutr. Biochem.* **2012**, *23*, 1458–1466. [CrossRef] [PubMed]

37. Flinn, J.M.; Bozzelli, P.L.; Adlard, P.A.; Railey, A.M. Spatial memory deficits in a mouse model of late-onset Alzheimer's disease are caused by zinc supplementation and correlate with amyloid-beta levels. *Front. Aging Neurosci.* **2014**, *6*, 174. [CrossRef] [PubMed]

38. Giacconi, R.; Cipriano, C.; Muti, E.; Costarelli, L.; Maurizio, C.; Saba, V.; Mocchegiani, E. Novel -209A/G MT2A polymorphism in old patients with type 2 diabetes and atherosclerosis: Relationship with inflammation (IL-6) and zinc. *Biogerontology* **2005**, *6*, 407–413. [CrossRef] [PubMed]

39. Giacconi, R.; Kanoni, S.; Mecocci, P.; Malavolta, M.; Richter, D.; Pierpaoli, S.; Piacenza, F. Association of MT1A haplotype with cardiovascular disease and antioxidant enzyme defense in elderly Greek population: Comparison with an Italian cohort. *J. Nutr. Biochem.* **2010**, *21*, 1008–1014. [CrossRef] [PubMed]

40. Giacconi, R.; Muti, E.; Malavolta, M.; Cipriano, C.; Costarelli, L.; Bernardini, G.; Mocchegiani, E. The +838 C/G MT2A polymorphism, metals, and the inflammatory/immune response in carotid artery stenosis in elderly people. *Mol. Med.* **2007**, *13*, 388–395. [CrossRef]

41. Shan, Z.L.; Bao, W.; Zhang, Y.; Rong, Y.; Wang, X.; Jin, Y.; Liu, L. Interactions Between Zinc Transporter-8 Gene (*SLC30A8*) and Plasma Zinc Concentrations for Impaired Glucose Regulation and Type 2 Diabetes. *Diabetes* **2014**, *63*, 1796–1803. [CrossRef] [PubMed]

42. Mocchegiani, E.; Giacconi, R.; Costarelli, L.; Muti, E.; Cipriano, C.; Tesei, S.; Gasparini, N. Zinc deficiency and IL-6−174G/C polymorphism in old people from different European countries: Effect of zinc supplementation. *ZINCAGE study. Exp. Gerontol.* **2008**, *43*, 433–444. [CrossRef] [PubMed]

43. Maruthur, N.M.; Clark, J.M.; Fu, M.; Kao, W.L.; Shuldiner, A.R. Effect of zinc supplementation on insulin secretion: Interaction between zinc and *SLC30A8* genotype in Old Order Amish. *Diabetologia* **2015**, *58*, 295–303. [CrossRef] [PubMed]

44. Moher, D.; Liberati, A.; Tetzlaff, J.; Altman, D.G.; Prisma Group. Preferred reporting items for systematic reviews and meta-analyses: The PRISMA statement. *PLoS Med.* **2009**, *6*, e1000097. [CrossRef] [PubMed]

45. Verghese, P.B.; Castellano, J.M.; Holtzman, D.M. Apolipoprotein E in Alzheimer's disease and other neurological disorders. *Lancet Neurol.* **2011**, *10*, 241–252. [CrossRef]

46. Mocchegiani, E.; Zincage, C. Zinc, metallothioneins, longevity: Effect of zinc supplementation on antioxidant response: A zincage study. *Rejuvenation Res.* **2008**, *11*, 419–423. [CrossRef] [PubMed]

47. Sladek, R.; Rocheleau, G.; Rung, J.; Dina, C.; Shen, L.; Serre, D.; Balkau, B. A genome-wide association study identifies novel risk loci for type 2 diabetes. *Nature* **2007**, *445*, 881–885. [CrossRef] [PubMed]

48. Diabetes Genetics Initiative of Broad Institute of Harvard and MIT, Lund University, and Novartis Institutes of BioMedical Research; Saxena, R.; Voight, B.F.; Lyssenko, V.; Burtt, N.P.; de Bakker, P.I.; Chen, H.; Roix, J.J.; Kathiresan, S.; Hirschhorn, J.N.; et al. Genome-wide association analysis identifies loci for type 2 diabetes and triglyceride levels. *Science* **2007**, *316*, 1331–1336. [PubMed]

49. Zeggini, E.; Weedon, M.N.; Lindgren, C.M.; Frayling, T.M.; Elliott, K.S.; Lango, H.; Barrett, J.C. Replication of genome-wide association signals in UK samples reveals risk loci for type 2 diabetes. *Science* **2007**, *316*, 1336–1341. [CrossRef] [PubMed]

50. Scott, L.J.; Weedon, M.N.; Lindgren, C.M.; Frayling, T.M.; Elliott, K.S.; Lango, H.; Barrett, J.C. A genome-wide association study of type 2 diabetes in Finns detects multiple susceptibility variants. *Science* **2007**, *316*, 1341–1345. [CrossRef] [PubMed]

51. Mocchegiani, E.; Giacconi, R.; Malavolta, M. Zinc signalling and subcellular distribution: Emerging targets in type 2 diabetes. *Trends Mol. Med.* **2008**, *14*, 419–428. [CrossRef] [PubMed]

52. Palmiter, R.D.; Cole, T.B.; Quaife, C.J.; Findley, S.D. ZnT-3, a putative transporter of zinc into synaptic vesicles. *Proc. Natl. Acad. Sci. USA* **1996**, *93*, 14934–14939. [CrossRef] [PubMed]

53. Cole, T.B.; Quaife, C.J.; Findley, S.D. Elimination of zinc from synaptic vesicles in the intact mouse brain by disruption of the *ZnT3* gene. *Proc. Natl. Acad. Sci. USA* **1999**, *96*, 1716–1721. [CrossRef] [PubMed]

54. Tai, L.M.; Ghura, S.; Koster, K.P.; Liakaite, V.; Maienschein-Cline, M.; Kanabar, P.; Green, S.J. APOE-modulated Abeta-induced neuroinflammation in Alzheimer's disease: Current landscape, novel data, and future perspective. *J. Neurochem.* **2015**, *133*, 465–488. [CrossRef] [PubMed]

55. Lowe, N.M.; Fekete, K.; Decsi, T. Methods of assessment of zinc status in humans: A systematic review. *Am. J. Clin. Nutr.* **2009**, *89*, 2040S–2051S. [CrossRef] [PubMed]

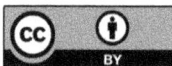

nutrients

MDPI

Article

Evaluating Changes in Omega-3 Fatty Acid Intake after Receiving Personal *FADS1* Genetic Information: A Randomized Nutrigenetic Intervention

Kaitlin Roke [1], Kathryn Walton [2], Shannon L. Klingel [1], Amber Harnett [1], Sanjeena Subedi [3], Jess Haines [2] and David M. Mutch [1,*]

1   Department of Human Health and Nutritional Sciences, University of Guelph, Guelph, ON N1G 2W1, Canada; kroke@uoguelph.ca (K.R.); sklingel@uoguelph.ca (S.L.K.); aharnett@uoguelph.ca (A.H.)
2   Department of Family Relations and Applied Nutrition, University of Guelph, Guelph, ON N1G 2W1, Canada; kwalton@uoguelph.ca (K.W.); jhaines@uoguelph.ca (J.H.)
3   Department of Mathematics and Statistics, University of Guelph, Guelph, ON N1G 2W1, Canada; sdang@binghamton.edu
*   Correspondence: dmutch@uoguelph.ca; Tel.: +1-519-824-4120 (ext. 53322)

Received: 25 January 2017; Accepted: 3 March 2017; Published: 6 March 2017

Abstract: Nutrigenetics research is anticipated to lay the foundation for personalized dietary recommendations; however, it remains unclear if providing individuals with their personal genetic information changes dietary behaviors. Our objective was to evaluate if providing information for a common variant in the fatty acid desaturase 1 (*FADS1*) gene changed omega-3 fatty acid (FA) intake and blood levels in young female adults (18–25 years). Participants were randomized into Genetic (intervention) and Non-Genetic (control) groups, with measurements taken at Baseline and Final (12 weeks). Dietary intake of eicosapentaenoic acid (EPA) and docosahexaenoic acid (DHA) was assessed using an omega-3 food frequency questionnaire. Red blood cell (RBC) FA content was quantified by gas chromatography. Implications of participation in a nutrigenetics study and awareness of omega-3 FAs were assessed with online questionnaires. Upon completion of the study, EPA and DHA intake increased significantly ($p = 1.0 \times 10^{-4}$) in all participants. This change was reflected by small increases in RBC %EPA. Participants in the Genetic group showed increased awareness of omega-3 terminology by the end of the study, reported that the dietary recommendations were more useful, and rated cost as a barrier to omega-3 consumption less often than those in the Non-Genetic group. Providing participants *FADS1* genetic information did not appear to influence omega-3 intake during the 12 weeks, but did change perceptions and behaviors related to omega-3 FAs in this timeframe.

Keywords: omega-3 fats; nutrigenomics; personalized nutrition; eicosapentaenoic acid; EPA; docosahexaenoic acid; DHA; single nucleotide polymorphisms; SNPs; fatty acid desaturase 1

1. Introduction

The field of nutritional genomics, or nutrigenetics, aims to unravel the genetic basis for why individuals respond differently to the same nutrients and/or foods [1–3]. The long-term outcomes of this research are expected to lay the foundation for personalized dietary recommendations to help prevent the development of chronic diseases. A more direct outcome of nutrigenetics research may simply entail the use of personal genetic information as an additional factor to help motivate people to adopt healthier dietary behaviors.

To date, the vast majority of nutrigenetic studies have examined and assessed perceptions of genetic and health information in various populations [3–5]. When individuals were queried, many reported to be interested in undergoing genetic testing for the prevention of chronic diseases [6–9]. However, there are currently a limited number of randomized controlled nutrigenetic trials assessing if providing genetic information actually changes dietary behaviors. The few nutrigenetic intervention studies performed to date suggest that individuals who receive personal genetic information may make more changes to their diet compared to controls [10–13].

Omega-3 fatty acids (FAs) represent an ideal nutrient to examine in the context of a nutrigenetics intervention for several reasons. From a global health perspective, it is widely recognized that increased intake of omega-3 FAs, in particular eicosapentaenoic acid (EPA, 20:5n-3) and docosahexaenoic acid (DHA, 22:6n-3), is beneficial for cardiovascular, metabolic, developmental and cognitive health [14–16]. However, the consumption of EPA- and DHA-rich foods such as fatty fish is low, specifically within the Western diet [17,18]. Therefore, finding new ways to motivate people to increase their consumption of omega-3 FAs are necessary.

From a genetic perspective, EPA and DHA are endogenously produced to a limited extent through a well-characterized pathway that desaturates and elongates the essential omega-3 FA, alpha-linolenic acid (ALA, 18:3n-3). The fatty acid desaturase 1 and 2 genes (*FADS1* and *FADS2*) play critical roles in this pathway [19,20]. It has consistently been demonstrated that single nucleotide polymorphisms (SNPs) in the *FADS* genes influence the degree of endogenous conversion of ALA into EPA and DHA [21,22]. Specifically, individuals who carry the minor allele in one or more SNP(s) in *FADS1* and/or *FADS2* have been reported to have reduced desaturase activity, resulting in lower levels of EPA [21,22]. Gillingham et al. showed that when minor allele carriers were provided dietary ALA, blood EPA levels were increased to a level equivalent to that observed in major allele carriers [23]. This suggests that giving individuals their personal *FADS* genotype information may yield a new approach to encourage increased intake and optimize dietary recommendations for omega-3 FAs.

Providing personal genetic information in relation to omega-3 FAs in the context of a randomized intervention represents a novel area of investigation. Therefore, the objective of this study was to test the impact of providing personal genetic information for *FADS1* on the consumption of omega-3 FAs in a population of female adults over a 12-week period. We examined changes in EPA and DHA intake from foods and supplements, analyzed blood omega-3 FA levels, and assessed perceptions of nutrition and genetics.

2. Materials and Methods

2.1. Participants and Ethics

Female adults (between 18–25 years) were recruited through emails and poster advertisements displayed around the University of Guelph campus. Individuals completed an online screening questionnaire prior to acceptance into the study. Individuals were ineligible to participate in the study if they regularly consumed omega-3 FA supplements and/or fish more than two times per week. Baseline and Final (week 12) study visits were scheduled when participants were menstruating to minimize variability in lipid levels within an individual, as recommended by Mumford et al. [24]. Therefore, participants who reported having a regular menstrual cycle in the online screening questionnaire and would expect their period (approximately) every 28 days were eligible for the study. Study design and participant flow through the study is reported using Consolidated Standards of Reporting Trials (CONSORT) guidelines (Figure 1). Ethical approval for the study was granted by the University of Guelph Human Research Ethics Board (REB#:15AP019). The trial was registered at clinicaltrials.gov (NCT02829138).

2.2. Study Design

Participants attended three in-person study visits. Participants signed the consent form and provided a saliva sample to be used for DNA analysis at visit #1. Once all DNA samples were analyzed, participants were randomized into either a Genetic group (intervention) or Non-Genetic group (control) using a random number generator by two individuals external to the study intervention. The randomization process used also ensured that each group would have an equivalent number of major and minor allele carriers. The lead investigator for the study intervention was blinded to this assignment. Participants were informed of which group they were in at Visit #2.

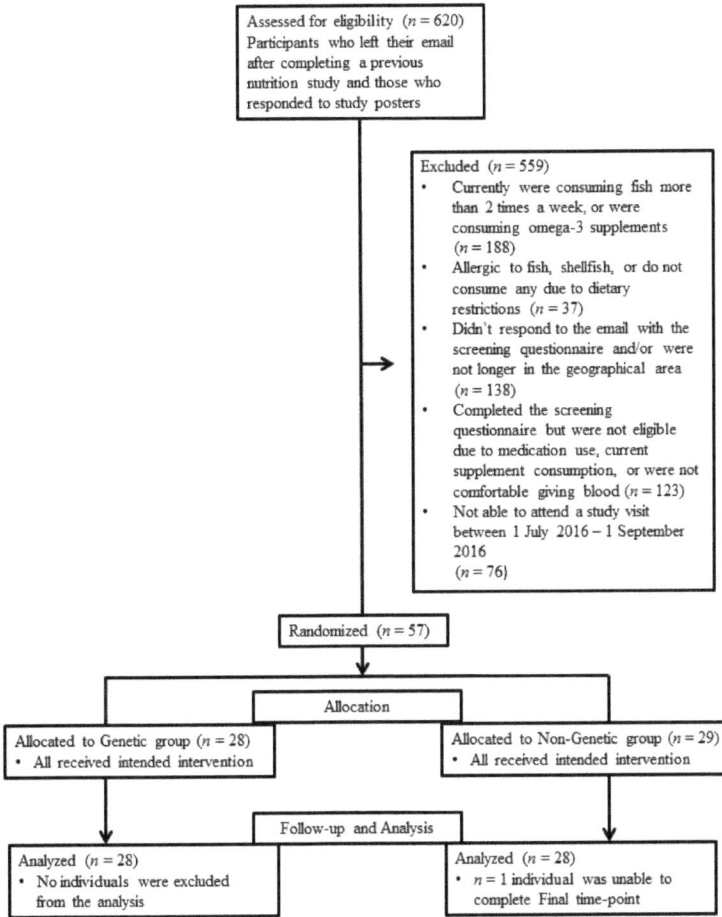

Figure 1. Study flow chart. Consolidated Standards of Reporting Trials (CONSORT) guidelines were used for reporting.

Visit #2 corresponded to the baseline study visit. Participants provided fasted blood samples, had a one-on-one information session, and received a copy of all study intervention materials. At this visit, all participants were also given a generic information document that provided details of omega-3 FAs, and an overview of the association between SNPs in *FADS1* and omega-3 metabolism. Specifically, this document provided information about omega-3 FAs, including general nutritional information, foods and supplements that have these FAs, and possible health effects associated with their consumption; compiled from the Dietitians of Canada fact sheets [25,26]. Furthermore, the document also provided a brief overview of the reported difference in omega-3 FA levels in relation to a common SNP in *FADS1* (rs174537). Specifically, it was indicated that individuals who are homozygote GG allele carriers have been reported to have more EPA in their bodies and an increased ability to convert ALA into EPA and

DHA [27–29], while individuals with at least one copy of the minor allele (GT or TT) were shown to have less EPA in their bodies and a reduced ability to convert ALA into EPA and DHA [21,22]. This generic information document was provided to all study participants to ensure that individuals in both the Genetic and Non-Genetic groups had a similar level of knowledge regarding omega-3 FAs and the influence of genetic variation in *FADS1*.

At the end of Visit #2, each participant was given a security-style sealed envelope to open after their appointment that made them aware if they had been randomly selected to the Genetic Group or the Non-Genetic Group. If participants were assigned to the Genetic group, the letter identified them as either a major (GG) or minor (GT + TT) allele carrier, according to their personal *FADS1* genotype. If the participants were in the Non-Genetic group, the letter indicated that they would receive their genetic information at the end of the study. Importantly, we did not provide any dietary advice in a genotype-specific manner, as the primary goal of the study was to assess if individuals who were given their personal *FADS1* genetic information changed their omega-3 dietary habits or not.

Visit #3 corresponded to the final week 12 study visit. All participants provided a fasted blood sample. Participants in the Non-Genetic group were given their personal *FADS1* genetic information at this point.

Participants were contacted by email throughout the study for survey distribution and appointment scheduling. Participants were not provided with additional omega-3 FA or genetic information throughout the intervention; however, we acknowledge it is possible that participants may have sought out more information independently (not monitored by the research team).

2.3. Online Surveys

Participants completed online food frequency questionnaires (FFQs) at Baseline and Final (week 12) to assess dietary intake of omega-3 FAs. Data on the awareness of omega-3 FAs, perceptions of receiving genetic information, and overall perceptions of the study intervention was also assessed through online questionnaires at Final (week 12). Qualtrics software (V13.28.05, ©2015, Provo, UT, USA) was used to host the online surveys. The online surveys were pilot-tested to ensure ease of completion. Participants could complete the surveys within a week of their distribution, on an electronic device of their choosing. There were questions of various types (multiple choice, select all that apply, Likert-style rating questions, sliding bar scales, and open text boxes). Survey questions are provided in Supplementary File.

2.3.1. Food Frequency Questionnaires

Dietary intake of omega-3 FAs (specifically EPA and DHA) was assessed at Baseline and Final (week 12) using a validated Canadian FFQ [30] that was updated to be reflective of the omega-3 enriched foods currently available on the market (e.g., newer brands of eggs and spreads fortified with EPA and DHA). This FFQ was then translated to an online version for participant completion. For each category of whole food, functional food, or supplement, the FFQ prompted specific product names/brands, frequency of consumption, and portion size consumed during the past week. The Canadian Nutrient File (version 2015) was used to assess the amount of EPA and DHA in whole foods (e.g., fish, eggs, poultry) [31]. Researchers used food labels obtained from Internet searches and conducted visits to local grocery stores to confirm amounts of omega-3 FAs in functional foods and supplements enriched with EPA and DHA. Many food products do not distinguish between the amount of EPA or DHA within a food product, and thus EPA and DHA are represented together as a summation of both FAs. To reflect the current Canadian dietary recommendations for both EPA and DHA, the total daily intake of EPA and DHA was combined and calculated for each participant in this analysis.

2.3.2. Diet and Genetics Questionnaire

This survey was comprised of researcher-generated and literature-generated questions. We examined the participants' awareness of terminology used to describe omega-3 FAs, including the full scientific names (alpha-linolenic acid, eicosapentaenoic acid, docosahexaenoic acid) and their corresponding abbreviations (ALA, EPA, and DHA), at the start and end of the intervention. After the final study visit, participants completed a questionnaire regarding perceived dietary changes and perceptions of the study intervention (questions in Supplementary File). Questions that focused on general perceptions in nutrition and health were incorporated based on the work from the Canadian Behaviour, Attitude and Nutrition Knowledge Survey (BANKS) [32]. Additionally, participants in the Genetic group received questions regarding perceptions of genetic information, which included some questions from a nutrigenomics survey previously developed by Nielsen and El-Sohemy [33].

2.4. Experimental Procedures

2.4.1. Genotyping

DNA was extracted from saliva using the Oragene DNA collection kit, according to manufacturer's instructions (DNA Genotek, Ottawa, ON, Canada). Participants were genotyped for the rs174537 SNP in *FADS1* using a validated TaqMan genotyping assay (Life Technologies, Carlsbad, CA, USA). This SNP was first reported in a large genome wide association study [21], and has been consistently reported by both our lab [34,35] and others [22,27,36–38] to influence blood FAs and estimated desaturase activity. We used a dominant model to group individuals carrying at least one copy of the minor allele (GT or TT) into a single group (GT + TT). The association between *rs174537* and estimated desaturase activity was confirmed in the present study [39].

2.4.2. Gas Chromatography for FA Analysis

Following an overnight fast, venous blood samples were collected from participants at Baseline and Final (week 12) visits. Serum and red blood cells (RBCs) were separated by centrifugation and frozen at -80 °C for subsequent analyses. RBC FAs were extracted with chloroform:methanol (2:1, v/v), using the methodology established by Folch et al. [40]. Gas chromatography was performed as previously described [41], with only minor modifications. Briefly, frozen RBC samples were thawed on ice for approximately 1.5 h prior to extraction. After the addition of 10 μL (0.1 mg/mL stock) of an internal free FA standard (C17:0), total lipids were extracted from 100 μL of RBC. The next day, samples were centrifuged at 1460 rpm for 10 min. The extraction process was repeated once using an equivalent volume of chloroform. Pooled lipids were saponified using 2 mL of 0.5 mol/L KOH in methanol at 100 °C for 1 h. The resulting free FAs were trans-esterified at 100 °C for 1.5 h. The organic phase was extracted, evaporated under nitrogen gas, and reconstituted in 100 μL of hexane for analysis. FA methyl esters were separated by gas chromatography using an Agilent 6890B gas chromatograph (Agilent Technologies, Santa Clara, CA, USA). FAs of interest were reported as percent FA composition: ALA, EPA, DHA, linoleic acid (LA; 18:2*n*-6) and arachidonic acid (AA; 20:4*n*-6). The Omega-3 Index was calculated by summing %EPA and %DHA [42]. FADS pathway activity was estimated by dividing %AA/%LA, as previously reported [27,36,41].

2.4.3. Clinical Measurements

Following an overnight fast, venous blood samples were collected from participants at Baseline and Final (week 12) visits. Fasted serum samples were sent to LifeLabs Medical Laboratory Services (Guelph, ON, Canada) for the analysis of triglycerides (TAG), total cholesterol, LDL-cholesterol (LDL-c), and HDL-cholesterol (HDL-c).

2.5. Statistics

R software (R Core Team, Version 3.3.0, Vienna, Austria) was used to determine a sufficient sample size prior to commencing the study. A minimum sample size of $n = 25$ individuals per group was calculated using changes in RBC %EPA reported in previous omega-3 FA intervention studies, and differences in RBC %EPA based on SNPs in *FADS1*. The %EPA values used to calculate the effect sizes were based on past work from our lab [34,43] and others [28,44]. Sample size was determined using an alpha level of 0.05 and a power level of 0.8. Intention to treat analysis was implemented (CONSORT), where participants remained in their original intervention groups throughout data analysis.

All survey data including FFQs, and diet and genetics questionnaires were analyzed using SPSS (IBM Corporation, Version 23, Armonk, North Castle, NY, USA). Descriptive statistics were completed for all questions to determine trends and potential issues before individual question analysis. A repeated measures two-way analysis of variance (ANOVA) assuming unequal variance was used to analyze dietary intakes of EPA and DHA using Group (Genetic vs. Non-Genetic), Time (Baseline vs. Final), and the Group × Time interaction. As a secondary outcome, major (GG) and minor (GT + TT) allele carriers within the Genetic group were also compared to determine any differences related to genotype. A repeated measures two-way ANOVA was also used to analyze awareness of omega-3 terminology, using Group and Time effects as described above. Pearson's χ^2 tests were used for questions requiring a determination of difference in proportions between the Genetic and Non-Genetic groups. An independent samples *t*-test was used to determine differences in the means between the Genetic and Non-Genetic groups when analyzing Likert-style questions (scale from 1–7).

GraphPad Prism (GraphPad Software, Version 6, La Jolla, CA, USA) was used to assess normality of the data, and to evaluate differences in anthropometric, clinical, and FA data at Baseline and Final with a repeated measures two-way ANOVA, using Group, Time and Group × Time effects, as described above. A $p \leq 0.05$ was considered statistically significant. R software (R Core Team, Version 3.3.0, Vienna, Austria) was used for correction of multiple comparisons using the Benjamini Hochberg approach [45,46].

3. Results

3.1. Participant Characteristics

The age of participants ranged from 19–25 years (mean = 22.0 ± 1.5 years). On average, participants rated interest in their personal health as 8.5 ± 1.3, out of a possible score of 10. Self-selected ethnicity, school or employment status, field of study/area of work, and contraceptive use were not different between the Genetic and Non-Genetic groups (Table 1).

All participants were genotyped for *rs174537* in *FADS1*. Our population consisted of 26 homozygous major (GG), 23 heterozygous (GT), and 8 homozygous minor allele (TT) carriers (Table 1). The SNP was confirmed to be in Hardy-Weinberg equilibrium. Hereon, we refer to individuals with the GG genotype as "major allele carriers" and individuals with either GT or TT genotypes as "minor allele carriers". Genotypes were evenly and randomly divided between the intervention and control groups.

3.2. FFQ Analysis

At baseline, participants were consuming an average of 200 ± 29 mg EPA and DHA/day. There were no significant differences in EPA and DHA intake between Genetic and Non-Genetic groups at Baseline (Table 2). As indicated by the Group × Time interaction, the nutrigenetic intervention did not differentially influence dietary intake of EPA and DHA ($p = 0.27$) (Table 2); however, both groups significantly increased their intake of EPA and DHA during the intervention ($p = 1.0 \times 10^{-4}$).

Table 1. Demographics of the Genetic and Non-Genetic groups at Baseline.

	Genetic (*n* = 28)	Non-Genetic (*n* = 29)	χ^2 *p*-Value
FADS1 (rs174537) Genotype Frequency			
Major (GG)	13/28 (46.4%)	13/29 (44.8%)	0.79
Minor (GT + TT)	15/28 (53.6%)	16/29 (55.2%)	
Field of study/area of work			
Life Science	19/28 (67.9%)	21/29 (72.4%)	
Social Science	7/28 (25.0%)	4/29 (13.8%)	0.46
Other	2/28 (7.1%)	4/29 (13.8%)	
Current Position			
Undergraduate student	20/28 (71.4%)	19/29 (65.5%)	
Graduate student	7/28 (25.0%)	8/29 (27.6%)	0.36
Working full-time	1/28 (3.6%)	2/29 (6.9%)	
Self-Reported Ethnicity			
White/Caucasian	18/28 (64.3%)	22/29 (75.9%)	
Asian	4/28 (14.3%)	3/29 (10.3%)	0.47
European	4/28 (14.3%)	1/29 (3.5%)	
Other	2/28 (7.1%)	3/29 (10.3%)	
Contraceptive use			
Not taking contraceptives	8/28 (28.6%)	9/29 (31.0%)	
Oral contraceptive	17/28 (60.7%)	18/29 (62.1%)	0.89
IUD contraceptive	3/28 (10.7%)	2/29 (6.9%)	

n = 57 participants completed Baseline measurements and questionnaires. This data is reported as proportions (n/n total) and percentages (%). Percentages are provided in parentheses and are reported as a percentage of either the Genetic or the Non-Genetic group. Pearson's χ^2 analysis were conducted to determine a difference in the proportions between the Genetic and Non-Genetic groups for each parameter. $p \leq 0.05$ was considered statistically significant. IUD, intra-uterine device.

The Genetic group was further investigated to determine if there were any differences in EPA and DHA consumption when stratified according to *FADS1* genotype. Dietary intake of EPA and DHA tended to be higher in GT + TT individuals (272 ± 71 mg/day) than GG individuals (141 ± 38 mg/day) at Baseline (*p* = 0.06). The same trend was seen at final (week 12), where dietary intake of EPA and DHA was higher in GT + TT individuals (432 ± 112 mg/day; ~59% higher than Baseline) than GG individuals (198 ± 34 mg/day; ~40% higher than Baseline) (*p* = 0.08). However, the Group × Time interaction revealed there was no significant difference in EPA and DHA intake between GG and GT + TT individuals at Final (week 12) (*p* = 0.29).

There were 10/56 (~18%) participants (four in the Genetic Group and six in the Non-Genetic Group) who reported initiating supplement use after the first study visit and who continued taking these supplements up to week 12. Out of these 10 participants, nine participants took fish oil supplements and one participant took an algae oil supplement. These participants were amongst those with the highest EPA and DHA intakes measured with the FFQ at Final (week 12).

3.3. FA Analysis

There were no differences between the Genetic and Non-Genetic groups at Baseline for %ALA, %DHA or the Omega-3 Index (Table 2). %EPA was higher in the Non-Genetic group compared to the Genetic group at Baseline. At the end of the study intervention, %EPA increased similarly in both groups (*p* = 0.02) (Table 2). The Omega-3 Index also showed a significant Time effect. The Group × Time interaction analysis revealed the nutrigenetic intervention had no differential effect on these FAs (Table 2).

Table 2. Characteristics of the Genetic and Non-Genetic groups at Baseline and Final.

	Genetic (n = 28)		Non-Genetic (n = 28)		Group	Time	Group × Time Interaction
	Baseline	Final	Baseline	Final	p-Value	p-Value	p-Value
Omega-3 Dietary Intake (FFQ)							
EPA and DHA (mg/day)	211.50 ± 43.16	323.23 ± 65.27	190.16 ± 39.21	395.82 ± 70.60	0.70	1.0×10^{-4}	0.27
RBC FA levels							
ALA (%)	0.43 ± 0.02	0.44 ± 0.02	0.41 ± 0.02	0.42 ± 0.02	0.66	0.14	0.79
EPA (%)	0.45 ± 0.02	0.51 ± 0.03	0.55 ± 0.02	0.61 ± 0.04	3.9×10^{-3} *	0.02	0.89
DHA (%)	3.40 ± 0.11	3.42 ± 0.09	3.42 ± 0.11	3.54 ± 0.11	0.64	0.20	0.36
Omega-3 Index	3.86 ± 0.11	3.97 ± 0.11	3.97 ± 0.12	4.15 ± 0.13	0.34	0.04	0.66
Clinical Data							
BMI (kg/m²)	23.01 ± 0.60	22.87 ± 0.61	23.41 ± 0.50	23.55 ± 0.53	0.50	0.99	0.11
TAG (mmol/L)	0.90 ± 0.07	1.02 ± 0.08	1.02 ± 0.07	1.02 ± 0.06	0.24	0.06	0.06
Cholesterol (mmol/L)	4.40 ± 0.19	4.67 ± 0.20	4.43 ± 0.14	4.72 ± 0.14	0.87	2.0×10^{-4} *	0.85
HDL (mmol/L)	1.76 ± 0.06	1.75 ± 0.07	1.75 ± 0.09	1.78 ± 0.09	0.94	0.66	0.48
Chol/HDL ratio	2.58 ± 0.13	2.70 ± 0.11	2.67 ± 0.12	2.77 ± 0.12	0.60	0.04	0.81
LDL (mmol/L)	2.18 ± 0.15	2.31 ± 0.14	2.22 ± 0.13	2.47 ± 0.12	0.58	2.6×10^{-3} *	0.32
Non-HDL Chol	2.65 ± 0.18	2.88 ± 0.18	2.68 ± 0.13	2.94 ± 0.12	0.83	2.0×10^{-4} *	0.92
Questionnaire Data (Omega-3 terminology)							
Alpha-linolenic acid	16/28 (57.1%)	23/28 (82.1%)	18/29 (62.1%)	20/28 (71.%)	0.73	2.0×10^{-3} *	0.33
Eicosapentaenoic acid	12/28 (42.9%)	22/28 (78.6%)	12/29 (41.4%)	13/28 (46.4%)	0.08	1.0×10^{-3} *	0.07
Docosahexaenoic acid	14/28 (50.0%)	22/28 (78.6%)	12/29 (41.4%)	14/28 (50.0%)	0.04	5.0×10^{-3} *	0.21
ALA	12/28 (42.9%)	23/28 (82.1%)	19/29 (65.5%)	20/28 (71.4%)	0.71	0.01 *	0.04
EPA	15/28 (53.6%)	23/28 (82.1%)	20/29 (69.0%)	20/28 (71.4%)	0.86	0.01 *	0.05
DHA	19/28 (67.9%)	25/28 (89.3%)	19/29 (65.5%)	22/28 (78.6%)	0.46	0.01 *	0.49

n = 56 participants completed Baseline and Final questionnaires (omega-3 dietary intake, questionnaire data), and blood draws for clinical data analysis. n = 55 participants completed Baseline and Final blood draws for RBC fatty acid (FA) data. Using a ROUT outlier analysis, 4 individuals were removed from the TAG data, and 1 individual was removed from the Cholesterol, %EPA, and %ALA data. For the omega-3 dietary intake, clinical and RBC FA data, values represent mean ± SEM. The questionnaire data is represented as the proportion of participants who answered "yes". Percentages are provided in parentheses. A repeated measures 2-way ANOVA was used to evaluate the effects of Group (Genetic vs. Non-Genetic) and Time (Baseline vs. Final), as well as the Group × Time interaction. p-values < 0.05 are shown in bold. RBC FA, clinical and questionnaire data were adjusted for multiple comparisons using a Benjamini Hochberg approach. Values significant after correction for multiple testing are indicated with a *. The question associated with omega-3 terminology data can be found in Supplementary File: Q1. ALA, alpha-linolenic acid; ANOVA, analysis of variance; BMI, body mass index; DHA, docosahexaenoic acid; EPA, eicosapentaenoic acid; FA, fatty acid; FFQ, food frequency questionnaire; HDL, high density lipoprotein cholesterol; LDL, low density lipoprotein cholesterol; ROUT, robust regression and outlier removal; SEM, standard error of mean; TAG, triglycerides.

3.4. Clinical Blood Lipid Analysis

There were no differences between the Genetic and Non-Genetic groups at Baseline for any of the clinical parameters measured (Table 2). As indicated by the Group × Time interaction, the nutrigenetic intervention did not differentially affect any of the parameters between the two groups (Table 2). However, both groups experienced small increases in Total cholesterol, the Chol/HDL ratio, LDL and Non-HDL from Baseline to Final (Table 2). The change in the Chol/HDL ratio was not significant after correction for multiple comparisons.

3.5. Diet and Genetics Questionnaires

3.5.1. Awareness of Omega-3 FA Terminology

The Genetic and Non-Genetic groups were well matched for their level of awareness of omega-3 terminology at Baseline (Table 2, Supplementary File: Q1). A group effect was observed regarding the awareness of docosahexaenoic acid, where more individuals in the Genetic group said they were familiar with the term at Final (week 12) compared to the Non-Genetic group (Table 2). Awareness of both abbreviations and full scientific names increased in both groups during the intervention and remained significant after correction for multiple testing (Table 2). Lastly, Group × Time interactions were observed for both the ALA and EPA abbreviations, with individuals in the Genetic group reporting greater awareness of these terms compared to the Non-Genetic group.

3.5.2. Perceptions and Use of Generic Omega-3 Nutritional Information

Overall, there was a significant difference in perceptions of the study intervention between the Genetic and Non-Genetic groups at Final (week 12) (Table 3, Supplementary File: Q2). Specifically, the Genetic group reported to agree more strongly that the generic omega-3 FA information document was new to them ($p = 0.05$) and that this information was useful when they considered their diet throughout the study ($p = 0.03$), in comparison to the Non-Genetic group (Table 3).

Table 3. Rating of selected statements regarding the study intervention.

	Genetic ($n = 28$)	Non-Genetic ($n = 28$)	p-Value
	Average	Average	
I understood the nutrition information about omega-3 fats provided at the start of the study	6.21 ± 0.26	6.21 ± 0.23	1.0
The recommendations about omega-3 fats that were provided in the document at the start of the study were new to me	4.64 ± 1.75	3.71 ± 0.31	0.05
I enjoyed learning about the dietary recommendations related to omega-3 fats	6.14 ± 1.18	5.89 ± 1.07	0.41
The dietary recommendations were useful when I considered my diet throughout the study	5.68 ± 1.21	4.93 ± 1.25	0.03
When I am in the grocery store or supplement store, I can confidently determine foods that have been fortified, or have added EPA and DHA omega-3 fats	5.43 ± 1.48	5.32 ± 1.19	0.77
I would like to know more about the dietary recommendations related to omega-3 fats	5.64 ± 1.47	5.39 ± 1.47	0.53
I am interested in the relationship between diet and genetics	6.12 ± 1.45	6.61 ± 0.79	0.11

These questions were asked in the Final (week 12) study questionnaire. Participants were asked to indicate on a scale from 1–7, how much they disagreed (strongly disagreed = 1) or agreed (strongly agreed = 7) with the corresponding statements (4 was neutral). The average for each question is represented as mean ± SEM. An independent samples 2-sided *t*-test was used to determine differences between Genetic and Non-Genetic groups. A $p < 0.05$ was considered statistically significant and is indicated in bold font. The question associated with the data can be found in Supplementary File: Q2. SEM, standard error of mean.

3.5.3. Perceived Dietary Changes

At Final (week 12), we asked participants to self-report if they had made changes in their consumption of omega-3 foods, fortified products, or supplements over the course of the study (Supplementary File: Q3–Q6). When asked about consumption of omega-3 foods, there were 8, 5 and 15 individuals in the Genetic Group, and 6, 9, and 13 in the Non-Genetic group who said "*yes*", "*no*" and "*sometimes*" to making changes to overall omega-3 consumption in their diet, respectively. Participants who said "*yes*" or "*sometimes*" were then asked a subsequent question about the factors contributing to their dietary changes.

There were 8/28 (28.6%) in the Genetic Group and 5/28 (17.9%) in the Non-Genetic group who reported that the reason for their dietary changes were related to the generic omega-3 information document provided to them at the start of the study ($p = 0.09$) (Supplementary File: Q7). However, there were 5/28 (17.9%) individuals in the Genetic group who reported that their personal genetic information was the reason they made changes to their diet. We also asked participants to identify obstacles that may have influenced their ability to change their omega-3 dietary habits (Table 4, Supplementary File: Q8). Response rates between the Genetic and Non-Genetic group were not statistically different (Table 4), although there was a trend that fewer individuals in the Genetic Group (32%) reported that "*Omega-3 foods are expensive*" compared to the Non-Genetic group (61%).

Table 4. Obstacles or barriers to change diet and omega-3 FA consumption.

	Genetic (*n* = 28)	Non-Genetic (*n* = 28)	χ^2 *p*-Value
Omega-3 foods are expensive	9/28 (32.1%)	17/28 (60.7%)	
When I get busy I don't make time to eat healthy foods	8/28 (28.6%)	4/28 (14.3%)	
I didn't experience any barriers to change throughout this study	3/28 (10.7%)	1/28 (3.6%)	0.17
Other obstacles/barriers #	8/28 (28.6%)	6/28 (21.4%)	

These questions were asked at the end of the study in the Final questionnaire. The data is represented as the proportion of participants who answered "*yes*" to that answer option. This data is reported as proportions (n/n total) and percentages (%). Percentages are provided in parentheses and are reported as a percentage of either the Genetic or the Non-Genetic group. Pearson's Chi-squared analysis (χ^2) was conducted to determine a difference in the proportions between the Genetic and Non-Genetic groups. $p \leq 0.05$ was considered statistically significant. The question associated with the data can be found in Supplementary File: Q8. # Other obstacles/barriers that could be selected by participants: It is difficult for me to get to a grocery store (Genetic *n* = 1, Non-Genetic *n* = 0); I am not involved in the grocery shopping in my home (Genetic *n* = 1, Non-Genetic *n* = 0); I eat most of my meals away from home (Genetic *n* = 0, Non-Genetic *n* = 1); I have an allergy to an omega-3 containing food (Genetic *n* = 1, Non-Genetic *n* = 1); I do not buy fortified products (Genetic *n* = 1, Non-Genetic n = 1); I do not have time to cook foods high in omega-3 fats (Genetic *n* = 2, Non-Genetic *n* = 1); I do not like fish (Genetic *n* = 1, Non-Genetic *n* = 1); I do not like taking supplements (Genetic *n* = 1, Non-Genetic *n* = 1).

4. Discussion

This study examined the effect of providing individuals with their personal *FADS1* genetic information on the consumption of omega-3 FAs. We found that individuals in both the Genetic and Non-Genetic groups increased their intake of EPA and DHA by the end of the study, and this was reflected by significant increases in RBC %EPA. Both the Genetic and the Non-Genetic groups were meeting the minimum dietary reccomendation of 300 mg EPA and DHA/day (according to the Dietitians of Canada) by the end of the study. Providing individuals with their personal *FADS1* genetic information did not lead to significant differences in dietary intake or blood levels of omega-3 FAs compared to controls. However, the results suggest that providing individuals with genetic information can increase awareness of omega-3 FA terminology, render generic omega-3 nutritional information more useful in the context of their genetic information, and minimize barriers to the consumption of omega-3 FAs. Consequently, providing individuals with their personal *FADS1* genetic information may have an impact on longer-term omega-3 FA intake.

Our FFQ analysis revealed that Baseline intake of EPA and DHA was ~200 mg/day in our study participants, which is slightly higher than recent global reports of EPA and DHA intake (~100 mg DHA/day in developed countries) [17,18,47], although this is still lower than the minimum recommendations by Dietitians of Canada (300 mg EPA and DHA/day) [25,48]. Individuals in both the Genetic and Non-Genetic groups increased their EPA and DHA intake during the study, suggesting that providing generic omega-3 nutritional information was sufficient to motivate increased EPA and DHA consumption in young female adults. This increased dietary intake was reflected by significantly increased %EPA in RBCs. Interestingly, when examining individuals in the Genetic group more closely, minor allele carriers appeared to increase EPA and DHA consumption to a greater extent (59%) than major allele carriers (40%).

Our findings regarding the limited impact of providing personal genetic information on dietary behavior appears to conflict with previous investigations; however, important differences exist between our trial and these previous studies. For example, Hietaranta-Luoma et al. gave adults (n = 107, 20–67 years, 69% female) information about their risk for cardiovascular disease (CVD) in relation to their personal apolipoprotein E (*APOE*) genetic make-up [11]. Individuals with the highest risk for CVD showed the greatest improvements in fat quality in their diets [11]. However, our study focused on benefits to health rather than risk reduction; thus it is plausible that individuals may alter their behavior more substantially if they feel it will reduce the risk for disease instead of potentially improving health. In another study, Arkadianos et al. provided genetic information related to the Mediterranean diet to participants (*n* = 93, 46 ± 12 years, 43% women) enrolled in a weight loss program [12]. After 100 days, there were no differences between the Genetic and Non-Genetic groups; however, after ~300 days, 57% of the Genetic group maintained weight loss compared to 25% who maintained weight loss in the Non-Genetic group [12]. Therefore, it is possible that if we continued our investigation over a longer period of time, the impact of personal *FADS1* genetic information on omega-3 intake may have been more pronounced in the Genetic group compared to the Non-Genetic group.

While we did not see differences in omega-3 FA intake between the Genetic and Non-Genetic groups, it is interesting to note that participants in the Genetic group rated (using a Likert-scale) the generic omega-3 FA information document we provided at the onset of the study as new and useful (5.7/7) more often than those in the Non-Genetic group (4.9/7). This aligns with findings by Nielsen and El-Sohemy, who found that young adults who received personal genetic information related to four dietary components (caffeine, vitamin C, sodium, and sugars) reported to have a greater understanding and utility for the dietary advice provided to them [33]. Additionally, we show that participants in the Genetic group of our study reported greater awareness of omega-3 terminology after the intervention, specifically with regards to the ALA and EPA abbreviations. Similarly, when asked about barriers to omega-3 FA consumption, 61% of the Non-Genetic group rated that *"Omega-3 foods are expensive"* compared to 32% of the Genetic group. Interestingly, this could suggest that having personal genetic information could change attitudes about the value of healthy eating. Thus, greater awareness and a reduced perception of cost as a barrier to omega-3 intake may render these individuals more likely to choose foods with omega-3 FAs in the future.

The present study has some limitations that warrant consideration. First, the current study only included female participants who were primarily of Caucasian/European descent. Gender and ethnicity may influence dietary behavior changes upon receiving personal genetic information; therefore, a more diverse participant population is needed in future studies. Second, our population consisted solely of well-educated young adults. Future studies should examine the role of personal *FADS1* genetic information on dietary behavior changes in different subgroups of the population, such as those outside academia. Third, the FFQ used in this study was validated for EPA and DHA [30], but not ALA. Future studies should create an updated FFQ to add ALA-rich foods, fortified products, and supplements in order to better estimate the consumption of this important omega-3 FA. Since FADS1 is critical for conversion from ALA into EPA and DHA, having an estimation of ALA intake may provide more insight into differences in consumption patterns between individuals stratified according to their *FADS1* genotype. Fourth, increasing the sample size and expanding the analysis to other age groups will provide independent validation of our results. Finally, providing personalized genetic information represents a new area of investigation, therefore future research should focus on thoroughly assessing the qualitative effect of genetic information (i.e., perceptions, reactions, emotions) using focus groups.

5. Conclusions

The present study represents the first of its kind to explore the provision of *FADS1* genetic information and subsequent changes in omega-3 FA intake. We found little evidence that providing personal *FADS1* genetic information affected EPA and DHA intake and circulating blood levels compared to the control group. However, we did find that individuals who received their genetic information had greater awareness of omega-3 terminology, rated cost as a barrier to omega-3 consumption less often, and found their genetic information to be useful in the context of generic nutritional information pertaining to omega-3 FAs compared to the control group. Therefore, providing personal *FADS1* genetic information to young adults may provide an additional factor to help motivate behavior changes to increase the consumption of omega-3 FAs.

Supplementary Materials: The following are available online at http://www.mdpi.com/2072-6643/9/3/240/s1, Supplementary File: Survey Questions and Response Options.

Acknowledgments: We would like to thank the participants for their time and dedication to this study. We would also like to thank the phlebotomists, Jaime-Lee Munroe and James Turgeon. We extend our thanks to Isaac Bell for his assistance with data preparation for the FFQ analysis. Finally, we would like to thank Emily Christofides for her advice for the provision of genetic information to our participants. This work was supported by grant #450115 from the Canadian Institutes of Health Research.

Author Contributions: K.R., K.W., J.H. and D.M.M. designed the study and prepared the intervention materials and questionnaires; K.R., S.K. and D.M.M. ran the clinical trial visits; A.H. created a database for EPA and DHA rich foods; and S.S. aided with statistical analysis. All authors read and approved the final manuscript.

Conflicts of Interest: The authors declare no conflict of interest.

References

1. Mutch, D.M.; Wahli, W.; Williamson, G. Nutrigenomics and nutrigenetics: The emerging faces of nutrition. *FASEB J.* **2005**, *19*, 1602–1616. [CrossRef] [PubMed]
2. Ordovas, J.M.; Mooser, V. Nutrigenomics and nutrigenetics. *Curr. Opin. Lipidol.* **2004**, *15*, 101–108. [CrossRef] [PubMed]
3. McBride, C.M.; Koehly, L.M.; Sanderson, S.C.; Kaphingst, K.A. The behavioral response to personalized genetic information: Will genetic risk profiles motivate individuals and families to choose more healthful behaviors? *Annu. Rev. Public Health* **2010**, *31*, 89–103. [CrossRef] [PubMed]
4. Makeeva, O.A.; Markova, V.V.; Puzyrev, V.P. Public interest and expectations concerning commercial genotyping and genetic risk assessment. *Pers. Med.* **2009**, *6*, 329–341. [CrossRef]
5. Stewart-Knox, B.J.; Bunting, B.P.; Gilpin, S.; Parr, H.J.; Pinhao, S.; Strain, J.; de Almeida, M.D.; Gibney, M. Attitudes toward genetic testing and personalised nutrition in a representative sample of European consumers. *Br. J. Nutr.* **2009**, *101*, 982–989. [CrossRef] [PubMed]
6. Nielsen, D.E.; Shih, S.; El-Sohemy, A. Perceptions of genetic testing for personalized nutrition: A randomized trial of dna-based dietary advice. *J. Nutrigenet. Nutrigenom.* **2014**, *7*, 94–104. [CrossRef] [PubMed]
7. Cormier, H.; Tremblay, B.; Paradis, A.M.; Garneau, V.; Desroches, S.; Robitaille, J.; Vohl, M.C. Nutrigenomics—Perspectives from registered dietitians: A report from the quebec-wide e-consultation on nutrigenomics among registered dietitians. *J. Hum. Nutr. Diet.* **2014**, *27*, 391–400. [CrossRef] [PubMed]
8. Horne, J.; Madill, J.; O'Connor, C. Exploring knowledge and attitudes of personal nutrigenomics testing among dietetic students and its value as a component of dietetic education and practice. *Can. J. Clin. Nutr.* **2016**, *4*, 50–62. [CrossRef]
9. Beery, T.A.; Williams, J.K. Risk reduction and health promotion behaviors following genetic testing for adult-onset disorders. *Genet. Test.* **2007**, *11*, 111–123. [CrossRef] [PubMed]
10. Nielsen, D.E.; El-Sohemy, A. Disclosure of genetic information and change in dietary intake: A randomized controlled trial. *PLoS ONE* **2014**, *9*, e112665. [CrossRef] [PubMed]

11. Hietaranta-Luoma, H.-L.; Tahvonen, R.; Iso-Touru, T.; Puolijoki, H.; Hopia, A. An intervention study of individual, apoe genotype-based dietary and physical-activity advice: Impact on health behavior. *J. Nutrigenet. Nutrigenom.* **2014**, *7*, 161–174. [CrossRef] [PubMed]

12. Arkadianos, I.; Valdes, A.M.; Marinos, E.; Florou, A.; Gill, R.D.; Grimaldi, K.A. Improved weight management using genetic information to personalize a calorie controlled diet. *Nutr. J.* **2007**, *6*, 29. [CrossRef] [PubMed]

13. Livingstone, K.M.; Celis-Morales, C.; Navas-Carretero, S.; San-Cristobal, R.; Macready, A.L.; Fallaize, R.; Forster, H.; Woolhead, C.; O'Donovan, C.B.; Marsaux, C.F. Effect of an internet-based, personalized nutrition randomized trial on dietary changes associated with the Mediterranean diet: The Food4Me study. *Am. J. Clin. Nutr.* **2016**, *104*, 288–297. [CrossRef] [PubMed]

14. Davis, B.C.; Kris-Etherton, P.M. Achieving optimal essential fatty acid status in vegetarians: Current knowledge and practical implications. *Am. J. Clin. Nutr.* **2003**, *78*, S640–S646.

15. Bell, G.A.; Kantor, E.D.; Lampe, J.W.; Kristal, A.R.; Heckbert, S.R.; White, E. Intake of long-chain ω-3 fatty acids from diet and supplements in relation to mortality. *Am. J. Epidemiol.* **2014**, *179*, 710–720. [CrossRef] [PubMed]

16. Kim, Y.-S.; Xun, P.; Iribarren, C.; Van Horn, L.; Steffen, L.; Daviglus, M.L.; Siscovick, D.; Liu, K.; He, K. Intake of fish and long-chain omega-3 polyunsaturated fatty acids and incidence of metabolic syndrome among American young adults: A 25-year follow-up study. *Eur. J. Nutr.* **2016**, 1–10. [CrossRef] [PubMed]

17. Langlois, K.; Ratnayake, W.M. Omega-3 index of Canadian adults. *Health Rep.* **2015**, *26*, 3–11. [PubMed]

18. Forsyth, S.; Gautier, S.; Salem, N., Jr. Global estimates of dietary intake of docosahexaenoic acid and arachidonic acid in developing and developed countries. *Ann. Nutr. Metab.* **2016**, *68*, 258–267. [CrossRef] [PubMed]

19. Merino, D.M.; Ma, D.W.; Mutch, D.M. Genetic variation in lipid desaturases and its impact on the development of human disease. *Lipids Health Dis.* **2010**, *9*, 63. [CrossRef] [PubMed]

20. Nakamura, M.T.; Nara, T.Y. Structure, function, and dietary regulation of δ6, δ5, and δ9 desaturases. *Annu. Rev. Nutr.* **2004**, *24*, 345–376. [CrossRef] [PubMed]

21. Tanaka, T.; Shen, J.; Abecasis, G.R.; Kisialiou, A.; Ordovas, J.M.; Guralnik, J.M.; Singleton, A.; Bandinelli, S.; Cherubini, A.; Arnett, D. Genome-wide association study of plasma polyunsaturated fatty acids in the inchianti study. *PLoS Genet.* **2009**, *5*, e1000338. [CrossRef] [PubMed]

22. Smith, C.E.; Follis, J.L.; Nettleton, J.A.; Foy, M.; Wu, J.H.; Ma, Y.; Tanaka, T.; Manichakul, A.W.; Wu, H.; Chu, A.Y. Dietary fatty acids modulate associations between genetic variants and circulating fatty acids in plasma and erythrocyte membranes: Meta-analysis of nine studies in the charge consortium. *Mol. Nutr. Food Res.* **2015**, *59*, 1373–1383. [CrossRef] [PubMed]

23. Gillingham, L.G.; Harding, S.V.; Rideout, T.C.; Yurkova, N.; Cunnane, S.C.; Eck, P.K.; Jones, P.J. Dietary oils and FADS1-FADS2 genetic variants modulate [13C] α-linolenic acid metabolism and plasma fatty acid composition. *Am. J. Clin. Nutr.* **2013**, *97*, 195–207. [CrossRef] [PubMed]

24. Mumford, S.L.; Dasharathy, S.; Pollack, A.Z.; Schisterman, E.F. Variations in lipid levels according to menstrual cycle phase: Clinical implications. *Clin. Lipidol.* **2011**, *6*, 225–234. [CrossRef] [PubMed]

25. Dietitians of Canada. *Eating Guidelines for Omega-3 Fats*; Dietitians of Canada: Toronto, ON, Canada, 2013.

26. Dietitians of Canada. *Food Sources of Omega-3 Fats*; Dietitians of Canada: Toronto, ON, Canada, 2013.

27. Bokor, S.; Dumont, J.; Spinneker, A.; Gonzalez-Gross, M.; Nova, E.; Widhalm, K.; Moschonis, G.; Stehle, P.; Amouyel, P.; De Henauw, S. Single nucleotide polymorphisms in the FADS gene cluster are associated with delta-5 and delta-6 desaturase activities estimated by serum fatty acid ratios. *J. Lipid Res.* **2010**, *51*, 2325–2333. [CrossRef] [PubMed]

28. Cormier, H.; Rudkowska, I.; Lemieux, S.; Couture, P.; Julien, P.; Vohl, M.-C. Effects of FADS and ELOVL polymorphisms on indexes of desaturase and elongase activities: Results from a pre-post fish oil supplementation. *Genes Nutr.* **2014**, *9*, 1–15. [CrossRef] [PubMed]

29. Malerba, G.; Schaeffer, L.; Xumerle, L.; Klopp, N.; Trabetti, E.; Biscuola, M.; Cavallari, U.; Galavotti, R.; Martinelli, N.; Guarini, P. Snps of the *FADS* gene cluster are associated with polyunsaturated fatty acids in a cohort of patients with cardiovascular disease. *Lipids* **2008**, *43*, 289–299. [CrossRef] [PubMed]

30. Patterson, A.C.; Hogg, R.C.; Kishi, D.M.; Stark, K.D. Biomarker and dietary validation of a Canadian food frequency questionnaire to measure eicosapentaenoic and docosahexaenoic acid intakes from whole food, functional food, and nutraceutical sources. *J. Acad. Nutr. Diet.* **2012**, *112*, 1005–1014. [CrossRef] [PubMed]

31. Canadian Nutrient File. Health Canada: 2015. Available online: http://webprod3.hc-sc.gc.ca/cnf-fce/index-eng.jsp-fce/index-eng.jsp (accessed on 1 February 2016).

32. Lafave, L.M.Z.; Lafave, M.R.; Nordstrom, P. *Development of a Canadian Behaviour, Attitude and Nutrition Knowledge Survey (BANKS)*; The Canadian Council on Learning (CCL): Calgary, AB, Canada, 2009.

33. Nielsen, D.E.; El-Sohemy, A. A randomized trial of genetic information for personalized nutrition. *Genes Nutr.* **2012**, *7*, 559–566. [CrossRef] [PubMed]

34. Roke, K.; Mutch, D.M. The role of FADS1/2 polymorphisms on cardiometabolic markers and fatty acid profiles in young adults consuming fish oil supplements. *Nutrients* **2014**, *6*, 2290–2304. [CrossRef] [PubMed]

35. Roke, K.; Jannas-Vela, S.; Spriet, L.L.; Mutch, D.M. FADS2 genotype influences whole-body resting fat oxidation in young adult men. *Appl. Physiol. Nutr. Metab.* **2016**, *41*, 791–794. [CrossRef] [PubMed]

36. Davidson, E.A.; Pickens, C.A.; Fenton, J. Supplementation with dietary EPA/DHA influences red blood cell fatty acid desaturase estimates and reflects tissue changes in fatty acids in systemic organs. *FASEB J.* **2016**, *30*, 267.1.

37. Martinelli, N.; Girelli, D.; Malerba, G.; Guarini, P.; Illig, T.; Trabetti, E.; Sandri, M.; Friso, S.; Pizzolo, F.; Schaeffer, L. FADS genotypes and desaturase activity estimated by the ratio of arachidonic acid to linoleic acid are associated with inflammation and coronary artery disease. *Am. J. Clin. Nutr.* **2008**, *88*, 941–949. [PubMed]

38. Vessby, B.; Gustafsson, I.-B.; Tengblad, S.; Berglund, L. Indices of fatty acid desaturase activity in healthy human subjects: Effects of different types of dietary fat. *Br. J. Nutr.* **2013**, *110*, 871–879. [CrossRef] [PubMed]

39. Roke, K.; Mutch, David M. Unpublished work. 2017.

40. Folch, J.; Lees, M.; Sloane-Stanley, G. A simple method for the isolation and purification of total lipids from animal tissues. *J. Biol. Chem.* **1957**, *226*, 497–509. [PubMed]

41. Merino, D.M.; Johnston, H.; Clarke, S.; Roke, K.; Nielsen, D.; Badawi, A.; El-Sohemy, A.; Ma, D.W.; Mutch, D.M. Polymorphisms in *FADS1* and *FADS2* alter desaturase activity in young caucasian and asian adults. *Mol. Genet. Metab.* **2011**, *103*, 171–178. [CrossRef] [PubMed]

42. Harris, W.S. The omega-3 index as a risk factor for coronary heart disease. *Am. J. Clin. Nutr.* **2008**, *87*, S1997–S2002.

43. Zulyniak, M.A.; Perreault, M.; Gerling, C.; Spriet, L.L.; Mutch, D.M. Fish oil supplementation alters circulating eicosanoid concentrations in young healthy men. *Metabolism* **2013**, *62*, 1107–1113. [CrossRef] [PubMed]

44. Al-Hilal, M.; AlSaleh, A.; Maniou, Z.; Lewis, F.J.; Hall, W.L.; Sanders, T.A.; O'Dell, S.D. Genetic variation at the *FADS1-FADS2* gene locus influences delta-5 desaturase activity and lc-pufa proportions after fish oil supplement. *J. Lipid Res.* **2013**, *54*, 542–551. [CrossRef] [PubMed]

45. Benjamini, Y.; Hochberg, Y. Controlling the false discovery rate: A practical and powerful approach to multiple testing. *J. R. Stat. Soc. Ser. B Methodol.* **1995**, 289–300.

46. Benjamini, Y.; Drai, D.; Elmer, G.; Kafkafi, N.; Golani, I. Controlling the false discovery rate in behavior genetics research. *Behav. Brain Res.* **2001**, *125*, 279–284. [CrossRef]

47. Stark, K.D.; Van Elswyk, M.E.; Higgins, M.R.; Weatherford, C.A.; Salem, N. Global survey of the omega-3 fatty acids, docosahexaenoic acid and eicosapentaenoic acid in the blood stream of healthy adults. *Prog. Lipid Res.* **2016**, *63*, 132–152. [CrossRef] [PubMed]

48. Global Organization for EPA and DHA Omega-3. *Global Recommendations for EPA and DHA Intake*; Global Organization for EPA and DHA Omega-3: Salt Lake City, UT, USA, 2014.

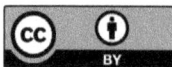

nutrients

MDPI

Review

Genetic Variations Associated with Vitamin A Status and Vitamin A Bioavailability

Patrick Borel and Charles Desmarchelier

NORT, Aix-Marseille Université, INRA, INSERM, 13005 Marseille, France; patrick.borel@univ-amu.fr (P.B.); charles.desmarchelier@univ-amu.fr (C.D.); Tel.: +33-4-9132-4277 (P.B.)

Received: 24 January 2017; Accepted: 6 March 2017; Published: 8 March 2017

Abstract: Blood concentration of vitamin A (VA), which is present as different molecules, i.e., mainly retinol and provitamin A carotenoids, plus retinyl esters in the postprandial period after a VA-containing meal, is affected by numerous factors: dietary VA intake, VA absorption efficiency, efficiency of provitamin A carotenoid conversion to VA, VA tissue uptake, etc. Most of these factors are in turn modulated by genetic variations in genes encoding proteins involved in VA metabolism. Genome-wide association studies (GWAS) and candidate gene association studies have identified single nucleotide polymorphisms (SNPs) associated with blood concentrations of retinol and β-carotene, as well as with β-carotene bioavailability. These genetic variations likely explain, at least in part, interindividual variability in VA status and in VA bioavailability. However, much work remains to be done to identify all of the SNPs involved in VA status and bioavailability and to assess the possible involvement of other kinds of genetic variations, e.g., copy number variants and insertions/deletions, in these phenotypes. Yet, the potential usefulness of this area of research is exciting regarding the proposition of more personalized dietary recommendations in VA, particularly in populations at risk of VA deficiency.

Keywords: genetic polymorphisms; absorption; bioavailability; β-carotene; retinyl palmitate; retinol; nutrigenetics; blood concentration; provitamin A; carotenoids; β-cryptoxanthin; α-carotene; postprandial

1. Introduction

The term vitamin A (VA) is employed generically for all derivatives of β-ionone (other than the carotenoids) that possess the biological activity of all-*trans* retinol (RET) or are closely related to it structurally [1]. This encompasses a group of fat-soluble molecules that are found as preformed VA (mainly RET and its esters, retinal and retinoic acid) in animals and animal products and as provitamin A (proVA) carotenoids in fruit and vegetables. VA is essential to human health and is involved in many metabolic and physiological processes, such as vision [2–5], cell differentiation [6,7], embryonic development [8,9] and immunity [10]. VA deficiency is still a serious public health problem in developing countries, where it still affects about one-third of children [11]. It greatly increases the severity of common childhood infections (e.g., measles, malaria) by compromising the immune system. Symptoms include impaired vision, in extreme cases irreversible blindness, impaired epithelial integrity, exposing the affected individuals to infections and reduced immune response. Night blindness is estimated to affect 250,000–500,000 children each year, of which 50% die within the following year. VA deficiency also contributes to the global burden of growth retardation, which affects 160 million children under five.

The current recommended dietary allowance in France is 600 μg RET activity equivalents (RAE) per day for women and 800 μg RAE/day for men. International committees have established RAE, considering the variability in carotenoid bioavailability depending on the matrix in which they are incorporated, as follows:

- 1 µg RAE = 1 µg RET
- 1 µg RAE = 2 µg all-*trans* β-carotene (βC) from supplements
- 1 µg RAE = 12 µg of all-*trans* βC from food
- 1 µg RAE = 24 µg α-carotene or β-cryptoxanthin from food
- 1 µg RAE = 3.33 IU RET

Although it is well established that there is an insufficient VA intake in developing countries, usually due to an insufficient availability of VA-rich foods (i.e., animal products), leading to VA deficiency, recent data have pointed to intakes below recommendation levels in several developed countries (concerning more than 75% of the population aged 19–50 in the U.S.) [12]. In the human diet, most preformed VA occurs as retinyl palmitate (RP), while β-carotene (βC) is the most abundant proVA carotenoid [13]. The proportion of preformed VA and proVA carotenoids that we eat depends on our dietary habits. For example, in vegans, 100% of dietary VA originates from proVA carotenoids. A recent analysis of the results of 11 studies in eight developed countries (representing ≈ 120,000 participants) has shown that preformed VA intake accounted for about 65% of total VA intake, while provitamin A carotenoids represented 35% of total VA intake (βC: 86%; α-carotene: 10%; β-cryptoxanthin: 4% thereof, respectively) [13]. Although both preformed VA and proVA carotenoids can be metabolized to the three main active VA molecules recovered in the human body, i.e., RET, retinal and retinoic acid, the metabolic pathways by which each form of VA is metabolized are partly different until they are converted to retinal. This allows us to suggest that individuals, or populations, that possess different abilities to absorb or metabolize these two forms of VA, due to, e.g., genetic variations that modulate expression/activity of proteins involved in these pathways, are not able to similarly use these two forms of VA.

This review starts with a description of the fate of VA in the human body, from the food matrix in which it is ingested to extra-hepatic tissues, by going through its main storage organ: the liver. This allows us to identify candidate proteins, and thus candidate genes, that could explain the interindividual variability in blood and tissue concentrations of VA molecules. This review then lists the genetic variations that have been associated with the interindividual variability in VA blood concentration and bioavailability. The review finishes by listing the points to focus on in the forthcoming years to identify the main genetic variations that are involved in these phenotypes.

2. Metabolism of Vitamin A in the Gastrointestinal Lumen

Dietary preformed VA, which is chiefly RP, and dietary proVA carotenoids, which are chiefly βC, are both insoluble in water. Thus, although they can be ingested in very different food matrices, e.g., butter, liver or carrots, they are assumed to transfer, at least in part, from their food matrix to lipid droplets of dietary fat emulsions that are present in the gastrointestinal lumen during digestion [14–17] (Figure 1). This transfer, as well as the transfer of VA to mixed micelles, is modulated by numerous factors, e.g., food matrix, food processing, presence of fibers, lipids, etc. It is beyond the scope of this review to describe the current knowledge on all of these factors, but dedicated reviews can be found elsewhere [14,18]. This transfer can be facilitated by gastric and pancreatic enzymes that participate in food digestion, i.e., proteases, amylases and lipases. VA or proVA carotenoids transferred to lipid droplets are then assumed to transfer to mixed micelles, although a fraction might be solubilized by dietary proteins [19]. Again, this transfer is assumed to be facilitated by the action of digestive enzymes [20]. From this step on, RP and βC fates branch off. RP in mixed micelles and in emulsion lipid droplets is hydrolysed to RET by pancreatic lipase (encoded by *PNLIP*) and also to a lesser extent by pancreatic lipase-related protein-2 (encoded by *PNLIPRP2*) [15]. Moreover, the brush border membrane-associated enzyme phospholipase B, encoded by *PLB1*, has also been suggested to participate in RP hydrolysis [21]. It has been shown that inhibition of retinyl ester hydrolysis in the gut dramatically impairs RET absorption [22], adding evidence that retinyl ester hydrolysis is compulsory prior to RET absorption. βC is not significantly metabolized, or chemically modified, and stays as such in mixed micelles [16]. Then, mixed micelles transport RET and βC to the apical side of the enterocyte where they are taken up via both passive diffusion and facilitated transport (see the next section for a state of the art description of these mechanisms). Surprisingly, while two apical membrane proteins involved in the uptake of βC have been identified, the protein(s) involved in the uptake of RET has (have) not. Yet, it has been assumed for forty years that RET uptake is, at least partly, facilitated [23].

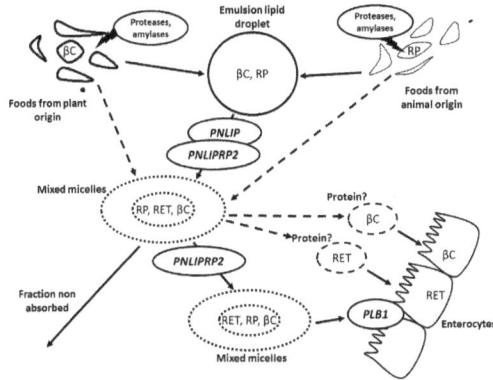

Figure 1. Proteins involved, or hypothesized to be involved, in vitamin A (VA) metabolism within the lumen of the upper gastrointestinal tract. βC: β-carotene and all other provitamin A carotenoids; PLB1: phospholipase B; PNLIP: pancreatic lipase; PNLIPRP2: pancreatic lipase-related protein 2; RET: retinol; RP: retinyl palmitate and all other retinyl esters. Proteins followed by a question mark have been hypothesized to be involved because RET and βC are not soluble in water, and thus, non-micellarized VA is assumed to be associated with proteins. A dotted arrow means the pathway is suspected to exist, but there is no evidence thereof yet.

3. Apical Uptake, Intracellular Metabolism and Basolateral Secretion of Vitamin A by the Intestinal Cell

Since mixed micelles are assumed to dissociate in the unstirred water layer adjacent to the enterocyte apical membrane [24], VA incorporated in mixed micelles, i.e., RET and βC, is supposed to reach the apical membrane as free molecules. However, the fact that scavenger-receptor class B-type I (SR-BI), which is encoded by *SCARB1*, facilitates in cell culture and in mice the uptake of several molecules with fairly different chemical structures, e.g., cholesterol [25], vitamin E [26], vitamin K [27] and carotenoids [28], does not fit with this assumption. Consequently, another hypothesis might be that this transporter interacts with mixed micelles rather than with free VA molecules and that micelle components and VA then diffuse to the apical membrane. The mechanisms by which these molecules cross this membrane and are secreted into the cytoplasm are not known. Several results suggest that both the SR-BI and CD36 molecule (CD36) are involved in proVA carotenoid uptake [28–31] (Figure 2), but not in that of RET [28]. Yet it is assumed, from the work of Hollander's group [23,32], that RET is absorbed, at least partly, by a saturable, protein-mediated passive absorption mechanism. This membrane protein remains to be identified.

After having crossed the apical membrane, RET and βC have to cross the polarized intestinal cell to be secreted at its basolateral side. The intracellular transport of RET is performed, at least partly, by the cellular retinol-binding protein type II (CRBPII), which is expressed solely in the adult intestine [33]. It is assumed that CRBPII transports RET to the sites where it is either oxidized to retinal and then to retinoic acid, which is involved in gene expression regulation in the enterocyte, or esterified to retinyl esters, a necessary step for its incorporation into chylomicrons. RET esterification, which occurs in the endoplasmic reticulum, has been shown to be performed by several enzymes. The main one, i.e., the enzyme that esterifies most RET in usual dietary conditions [34], is lecithin-retinol acyltransferase (LRAT), which uses RET bound to CRBPII as a substrate [35]. The other ones are acyl-CoA:retinol acyltransferases (ARAT) that esterify RET via an acyl-CoA-dependent process [34,35]. At least two enzymes that exhibit an ARAT activity are present in the enterocyte [34]. The main one is diacylglycerol acyltransferase 1 (DGAT1) [34], but there is likely at least another one. Indeed, since loss of DGAT1 activity does not completely impair RET esterification [36], this suggests that either LRAT is very efficient or, most likely, that another enzyme that exhibits an ARAT activity is present in the enterocyte [34]. The relative activity of these acyltransferases, which use different sources of intracellular fatty acids to esterify RET, i.e., LRAT uses fatty acids from intracellular membrane phospholipids, while DGAT1 and the other ARAT(s) use newly-absorbed fatty acids, is assumed to explain the variability in the pattern of retinyl esters synthetized after meals that provided a different amount and species of fatty acids [37]. Less is known about the intracellular transport and metabolism of βC in the enterocyte. Nevertheless, since it is assumed that it is not transported by CRBPII, another intracellular binding protein is likely to be involved [38]. This protein could be beta-carotene oxygenase 1 (BCO1), which is mainly located in the cytosol of mature enterocytes from the jejunum [39], because it is the main enzyme that cleaves βC [40–43], and it has a great affinity for βC. This intracellular transport protein could also be beta-carotene oxygenase 2 (BCO2), although it is apparently mainly located in mitochondria [44]. The intracellular βC transporter could also be a fatty acid binding protein (FABP), more likely liver FABP (L-FABP), which is also present in the intestine and which displays high-affinity binding for various hydrophobic ligands [45]. At this step, it is important to make clear that only a fraction of absorbed βC is metabolized in the enterocyte. The importance of this fraction, which was estimated at about 70% by using the stable isotope method [46], depends on the VA status of the body (see the next section). The fraction of non-metabolized βC is incorporated in nascent chylomicrons [47]. The exact mechanism of this incorporation is not known, but it is assumed that it involves enzymes/apoproteins responsible for the assembling of these triglyceride-rich lipoproteins, such as microsomal triglyceride transfer protein (MTP) and apoB48.

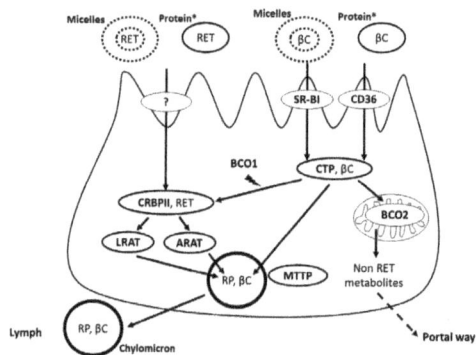

Figure 2. Proteins involved in vitamin A metabolism within the enterocyte. ARAT: acyl-CoA:retinol acyltransferases; βC: β-carotene and all other provitamin A carotenoids; BCO1: β-carotene oxygenase 1; BCO2: β-carotene oxygenase 2; CD36: cluster determinant 36; CRBPII: cellular retinol binding protein II; CTP: cellular transport protein (BCO1 and L-FABP are candidates); LRAT: lecithin retinol acyltransferase; MTTP: microsomal triglyceride transfer protein; RET: retinol; RP: retinyl palmitate and all other retinyl esters; SR-BI: scavenger receptor class B type I. It is assumed that there is an apical transporter of RET, but since it has not been identified, a question mark has been added.

The more apolar forms of VA present in the intestinal cell, i.e., RP and βC, are assumed to be mostly secreted in chylomicrons, while the less apolar forms, i.e., RET [48], retinoic acid and apocarotenoids, are assumed to be secreted in the portal blood. The relative proportion of VA secreted in these two pathways is not known, but we suggest that it depends on the relative activities of the enterocyte enzymes involved in VA metabolism.

4. Regulation of Vitamin A Absorption

It is now acknowledged that VA status regulates βC absorption and cleavage efficiency via a negative feedback loop: the higher the VA status, the lower βC absorption efficiency and cleavage, and inversely. The mechanism involves an intestinal transcription factor called intestine specific homeobox (ISX), which acts as a repressor of *SCARB1* and *BCO1* upon retinoic acid activation [49,50]. Following VA uptake, the intracellular concentration of retinoic acid increases leading to the induction of ISX gene expression. Consequently, less βC is taken up by the enterocyte, and less βC is converted to retinal. When the intracellular concentration of retinoic acid drops, which is assumed to be the case when the dietary VA intake is insufficient, ISX exerts less repressor activity towards *SCARB1* and *BCO1*, and consequently, βC uptake and conversion efficiency increase. This mechanism is thought to regulate the absorption and the cleavage efficiencies of other proVA carotenoids, as well, as they are also absorbed via SR-BI and cleaved by BCO1. A study in Zambian children with hypervitaminosis A supports this regulation. Indeed, these children had high serum carotenoid concentrations [51], and many of them experienced hypercarotenodermia during mango season, a period of high carotenoid intake. This might indicate that proVA carotenoid conversion to VA by BCO1 was more inhibited by the hypervitaminosis A than their absorption via SR-BI. This is not surprising as proVA carotenoids' absorption involves not only SR-BI, but also CD36, which is not assumed to be regulated by ISX. Finally, it is important to state that there is no study dedicated to assess whether VA status also modulates the absorption efficiency of preformed VA.

5. Postprandial Blood Transport of Newly-Absorbed Vitamin A from the Intestine to the Liver

The intestine is assumed to secrete most newly-absorbed VA into chylomicrons. The two main VA vitamers found in these triglyceride-rich lipoproteins are (i) RP [37], which comes either from RET re-esterification or from esterification of RET produced by enterocyte metabolism of βC, and (ii) βC that has not undergone cleavage by BCO1 or BCO2 in the enterocyte. Most of RET is secreted as retinyl esters in the chylomicrons, regardless of the chemical and physical form of administration [22]. Note that when a pharmacological dose of retinyl palmitate is ingested with a meal almost depleted in fat, chylomicrons can also contain a significant proportion of RET that has not undergone esterification in the enterocyte [37]. It has been shown that most RP and βC are not exchanged between lipoproteins and remain in chylomicron and their remnants during their intravascular metabolism [52,53]. Most VA incorporated into chylomicron remnants, which are produced during vascular lipolysis of chylomicron triglycerides by both lipoprotein lipase (LPL) and glycosylphosphatidylinositol anchored high density lipoprotein binding protein 1 (GPIHBP1) [54], is taken up by hepatocytes during the postprandial period [55]. Although most newly-absorbed VA is secreted into chylomicrons, it is assumed that the water-soluble VA metabolites, e.g., retinoic acid and apo-carotenals, could be secreted in the portal circulation and could then directly reach the liver.

6. Liver Metabolism of Vitamin A and Blood Transport of Vitamin A from the Liver to Extra-Hepatic Tissues

Liver is the main storage organ for VA (Figure 3). Indeed, it has been estimated that for healthy, well-nourished individuals, approximately 70% of VA present in the body is stored in the liver [56]. Following chylomicron-remnant uptake by the liver, which involves cell surface receptors, i.e., LDL-receptor, LDL-receptor related protein 1 (LRP1) and heparan sulfate proteoglycans (HSPGs) [54], it is assumed that chylomicron remnant RP and βC are released in hepatocytes during chylomicron remnant metabolism. They are then assumed to follow different metabolic pathways. RP is assumed to be hydrolyzed by a retinyl ester hydrolase (REH) to give RET. RET is then assumed to bind to cellular retinol-binding protein type I (CRBPI) [57] and be transported to either the site where it is transferred to retinol-binding protein 4 (RBP4) or to hepatic stellate cells where it is esterified by LRAT [58,59]. Interestingly though, hepatic LRAT expression is regulated by VA status [55]. This regulation likely involves retinoic acid and its response elements, i.e., retinoic acid receptor (RAR) and/or retinoid X receptor (RXR). This regulation is proposed to give rise to a positive feedback loop when cellular retinoic acid concentrations are high, turning on hepatic stellate cell LRAT expression [60] and increasing the synthesis of retinyl esters [56] in these cells [61,62], which are also called fat-storing cells, lipocytes or Ito cells. These cells store approximately 70%–90% of liver VA [56]. The mobilization of retinyl ester stores is performed by at least two lipases: adipose triglyceride lipase (ATGL) [63] and patatin-like phospholipase domain-containing 3 (PNPLA3) protein [64], which has also a triglyceride hydrolase activity [65,66]. Conversely to that of chylomicron RP, the fate of chylomicron βC in the liver is barely known. Indeed, how βC is released from chylomicrons and how it is transported into hepatocytes remains unanswered. Concerning its cleavage, it is assumed that it is either cleaved to retinal by BCO1, which is highly expressed in hepatic stellate cells [67], or BCO2, which is apparently more expressed in hepatocytes [67]. The fraction of βC that does not undergo this cleavage is either incorporated into very low density lipoproteins (VLDL), which are then secreted in the blood, or stored in lipid droplets in parenchymal cells and in hepatic stellate cells [67,68]. The mechanism involved in the mobilization of these βC stores is not known, but we hypothesize that it requires the hydrolysis of lipid droplet triglycerides.

The liver secretes VA either in the bile, as oxidized and/or conjugated metabolites [69,70], or in the blood. Two main forms of VA are secreted in the blood: RET and βC. RET is bound to serum retinol binding protein (sRBP, RBP4), which in turn binds to transthyretin (TTR), stabilizing the complex [71]. βC is incorporated in VLDL. RET associated with RBP4/TTR is taken up by two structurally-related membrane receptors: stimulated by retinoic acid 6 (STRA6) [72] and the recently discovered STRA6-like, also known as RBP4 receptor-2 (RBPR2) [73]. Retinol uptake via STRA6 depends on a functional coupling with intracellular LRAT [74]. STRA6 and RBPR2 exhibit different tissue expression patterns: STRA6 is expressed in numerous tissues, but not in liver and intestine, where RBPR2 is mostly expressed [73]. VLDL-βC and low density lipoprotein (LDL)-βC, which originate from VLDL metabolism, are most likely taken up via the LDL-receptor-dependent mechanisms [75], requiring the tissue/organs to express the LDL-receptor.

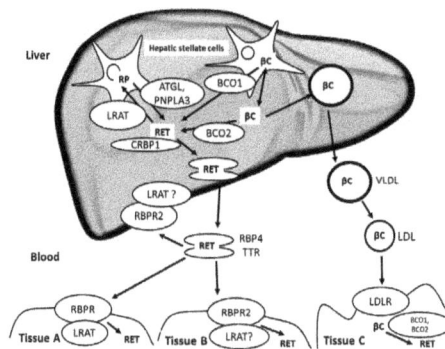

Figure 3. Proteins involved in the liver metabolism of vitamin A. ATGL: adipose triglyceride lipase; βC: β-carotene and all other provitamin A carotenoids; BCO1: β-carotene oxygenase 1; BCO2: β-carotene oxygenase 2; CD36: cluster determinant 36; CRBPI: cellular retinol binding protein I; LDLR: LDL receptor; LRAT: lecithin retinol acyltransferase; PNPLA3: patatin-like phospholipase domain-containing 3; RBPR2: RBP4 receptor-2; RBP4: serum retinol-binding protein; RBPR: RBP receptor (encoded by STRA6); RET: retinol; RP: retinyl palmitate and all other retinyl esters; TTR: transthyretin. The liver is the hub of vitamin A metabolism: it is the main organ that stores VA and distributes it to the peripheral tissues. VA reaches the liver mainly as retinyl esters, mainly RP, and provitamin A carotenoids, mainly βC, incorporated in chylomicrons following VA absorption. VA is then mostly stored in hepatic stellate cells. This figure shows the main proteins involved in the mobilization of the liver stores of VA and in the distribution of liver VA to peripheral tissues.

7. Vitamin A Metabolism in Extra-Hepatic Tissues

VA plays a critical role as a signaling molecule in most tissues [76,77] and chromophore in eyes [2–5]. The metabolism of VA in extra-hepatic tissues is assumed to involve pathways like those present in the liver, e.g., RET is assumed to give retinal, then retinoic acid; βC is assumed to be cleaved into retinal and/or apocarotenals, although some differences do exist. Another example concerns the hydrolysis of retinyl esters. Indeed, while hormone-sensitive lipase (HSL) is the predominant retinyl ester hydrolase in adipocytes [63,78], it is apparently not involved in retinyl ester hydrolysis in the liver [63]. Nevertheless, it is out of the topic of this review to comprehensively describe the metabolism of VA in all extra-hepatic tissues.

8. Physiological Regulation of Blood Vitamin A Concentrations

Numerous forms of VA circulate in human blood: RET, proVA carotenoids, retinyl esters, retinoic acid, retinyl-β-glucuronide, retinoyl-β-glucuronide [56]. Furthermore, the blood concentration of these various VA forms can significantly vary in the postprandial period as compared to the fasting state. Thus, when talking about the blood VA concentration, it is important to specify which VA molecule is meant and when its concentration is measured, i.e., in the fasting state or during the postprandial period. It is assumed that the blood concentration of these different forms of VA is differently regulated by our body. In this review, we have decided to focus on the regulation of the three main forms of VA, in terms of absolute concentration, recovered at fast and in the postprandial period, i.e., RET, βC and retinyl esters.

Concerning RET concentration, it is acknowledged that it is tightly regulated [79] with concentrations ranging from 2 to 4 μM at fast in adults [80]. Its concentration only changes in response to extreme VA dietary events or in disease states [79], and in the postprandial period when a meal rich in VA is provided to subjects deficient in VA. This last observation is assumed to be due to the fact that when hepatic VA stores are very low, free RBP accumulates in the liver [81]. When a high amount of VA then reaches the liver, usually following the consumption of a high dose of VA, it binds the free RBP accumulated, and it is quickly released in the blood, leading to a transitory increase in blood RET [82]. This has led to developing two tests that are used to evaluate the VA status: the relative dose response (RDR) test [82,83] and the modified relative dose response test (MRDR) [84,85].

Regarding the βC blood concentration, it is acknowledged that there is no direct regulation. Indeed, this form of VA is found in all lipoprotein classes [86–88], including chylomicrons during the postprandial period when a meal containing βC is ingested. Thus, blood concentration of βC depends on: (1) the state at which the blood is collected, i.e., at fast or in the postprandial period; (2) the amount of βC that was ingested in the previous meal; and (3) on the metabolism of lipoproteins in which it is incorporated and, thus, on the regulation of lipoprotein metabolism.

Concerning retinyl esters, although it has been suggested that some are recovered in VLDL and LDL [56], most of them are incorporated in chylomicrons after VA absorption and intestinal VA metabolism. Thus, it is assumed that there is no direct regulation of their blood concentration. Indeed, retinyl esters are assumed to stay within the chylomicrons during their blood metabolism, and thus, their blood concentration exhibits a bell-shaped curve [47] that closely mimics that of chylomicron triglycerides. For this reason, retinyl esters are assumed to be a valuable marker of chylomicrons and their remnants [89]. Thus, blood retinyl ester concentration during the postprandial period is assumed to be governed by the factors that regulate the metabolism of chylomicrons, i.e., those that govern their intestinal secretion, blood metabolism and uptake by the liver [54,90,91].

Overall, it can be concluded that blood VA concentration is modulated by the activity of numerous proteins, e.g., those that participate in the secretion and blood metabolism of chylomicrons and other lipoproteins, regarding βC and RP, and those that participate in the liver secretion and blood metabolism of RET.

9. Genetic Variations that Have Been Suggested to Modulate Blood Vitamin A Concentrations

The measurement of liver stores of VA is considered the gold standard to assess an individual's VA status. However, there is no non-invasive method to date, and thus, the use of alternative biomarkers is required (see [79] for a recent review thereof). Serum RET concentration is homeostatically regulated and only correlates with liver VA stores in the case of deficiency. Moreover, it can be affected by current or recent acute infections or chronic inflammation. Consequently, the World Health Organization does not recommend its use to assess the VA status of individuals, although it is still useful at the population level [92]. Retinol isotope dilution [93] is a quantitative and sensitive method to assess VA status over a wide range of liver VA stores. Since methods to assess VA status remain expensive, the use of GWAS to identify genetic variations associated with VA status is a great challenge, and consequently, the information on the influence of genetic variations on VA status is scarce. Only one study has reported the association of an SNP with liver stores of VA: Kovarova et al. [94] showed that an SNP in *PNPLA3*, a gene involved in the mobilization of retinyl esters stored in stellate cells [64], was associated with increased RP liver storage in a group of 42 patients undergoing liver surgery. Interestingly, the minor allele of the SNP is highly prevalent in populations from Latin American (about 70%), whereas it is found at a much lower frequency (around 20%) in populations from Europe and Africa [95]. We suggest that the effect of this SNP could be due both to a lower hydrolysis of liver RP, but also to a lower hydrolysis of intracellular triglycerides that solubilize RP. Indeed, it has been demonstrated that a loss-of-function mutation in *PNPLA3* impairs triglyceride hydrolysis [65] and promotes intracellular lipid accumulation by reducing the lipidation of VLDL [96]. Furthermore this mutation, as well as mutations in *ATGL*, which is the other lipase known to hydrolyze both RP and triglycerides [63], are genetic determinants of chronic liver diseases [97–99].

9.1. Genetic Variations Associated with Fasting Blood Vitamin A Concentrations

RET and βC are the two most concentrated VA forms in the fasting blood. Their concentration is used to assess VA or βC status, respectively. Although their usefulness for assessing the VA status of individuals is questionable, they are still acknowledged to provide valuable information on the VA status of a population [92]. Since populations with different dietary habits likely have different VA metabolism, because of adaptation and evolution, it is relevant to study the contribution of genetic variations to this phenomenon. Indeed, this might lead to provide recommended dietary allowances, or nutritional/cooking advice, more fitted to the genetic specificity of ethnic groups. Fewer than 10 studies are available on the effect of genetic variations on VA metabolism, and most of them are dedicated to associations with blood concentrations of RET or βC.

Concerning RET, the first study showing an association between a genetic variation and the blood concentration of its blood binding protein, i.e., RBP4, was published in 1995 [100]. It showed that genetic variations causing amino acid substitutions at position 84 of the TTR molecule (Ser84 and Asn84) led to substantial decreases in blood concentrations of RBP4. Four years later, two mutations in *RBP4* in two German sisters were associated with extremely low, i.e., <0.19 μmol/L, blood RET concentrations although the authors reported a partial cellular supply of retinol from circulating retinyl esters [101]. It was further shown that, although the mutant proteins can form complexes with retinol and TTR in vitro, the mutated retinol-RBP complexes are significantly less stable than normal retinol-RBP complexes, which in turn can lead to the lowering of plasma retinol and RBP concentrations [102]. A GWAS has confirmed that SNPs in the two genes encoding the proteins that transport RET in the blood, i.e., RBP4 and TTR, can significantly affect blood RET concentrations [103]. Nevertheless, it appears that fasting blood RET concentration can also be modulated by genetic variations in proteins/enzymes located in tissues. Indeed, an association between SNPs in *BCO1* and blood RET was found [104], suggesting that provitamin A carotenoids significantly participate in blood RET concentrations. Finally, a recent study has found an association between an SNP in *PNPLA3* and blood RET concentration in patients with non-alcoholic fatty liver disease or obesity [105]. Of note, the same SNP has been associated in another study with increased RP liver storage [94].

Concerning fasting blood βC concentration, one GWAS [106] and two candidate gene association studies [104,107] have shown that SNPs in *BCO1*, the main βC metabolizing enzyme, were associated with its circulating concentration. Candidate gene association studies have also found SNPs associated with blood βC concentration in three other genes. These genes were *LPL* [108], which encodes for lipoprotein lipase, a lipase involved in vascular metabolism of lipoproteins, which transport among other molecules βC, hepatic lipase (*HL)* [109], which encodes hepatic lipase, another vascular lipase involved in lipoprotein metabolism, and *SCARB1* [110], the gene that encodes for SR-BI, a membrane protein that participates in the cellular uptake of HDL [111], which can carry βC, and in the uptake of βC by enterocytes [28,30,112].

9.2. Genetic Variations Associated with Postprandial Blood Vitamin A Concentrations

Although the identification of genetic variations associated with fasting blood RET or proVA carotenoid concentrations is relevant to better understand VA metabolism, the application of the results to clinical practice or dietary recommendation is otherwise not straightforward due to two main reasons. First, as mentioned above, fasting blood RET concentration does not constitute a good biomarker of VA status of individuals due to its very tight homeostatic control. Second, since the highest risk factor for developing VA deficiency or insufficiency is usually low VA intakes and since proVA carotenoids display a wide-ranging bioavailability (data are lacking regarding preformed VA bioavailability), which is partly due to genetic variability, the fight against VA deficiency should rely on identifying tailored nutritional strategies, i.e., based on the assessment of the preformed VA/proVA carotenoid responder phenotype of a population/individual. For example, an individual or a group of individuals exhibiting VA deficiency (or at risk) with low capacity to absorb and/or convert proVA carotenoids should be given preformed VA supplements. The knowledge of a genotype associated with low fasting blood RET or proVA concentrations only provides little information regarding the best nutritional strategy to adopt to avoid VA deficiency, and it is thus more relevant to search for genetic variations associated with postprandial blood VA concentrations, a marker of the preformed VA/proVA carotenoid responder phenotype.

As stated above, in the postprandial period, blood can contain the three main forms of VA, depending on the source of VA that was ingested in the preceding meal and on the VA status of the subject. Indeed, following a meal containing only preformed VA, the blood contains RP incorporated in chylomicrons plus all of the other VA species that circulate at fast, i.e., mainly RET and proVA carotenoids. Following a meal containing proVA carotenoids, the blood contains RP plus the non-cleaved fraction of proVA carotenoids in chylomicrons, plus all of the other VA species that circulate at fast.

For the time being, there are only three studies dedicated to identifying genetic variations associated with postprandial blood VA concentration (Table 1). Since the measurement of this phenotype requires that volunteers stay in a clinical environment for several hours with repeated blood collections, the number of subjects included in this kind of study is usually relatively low (typically < 100). This precludes the use of GWAS, due to lack of power, and requires the use of candidate gene association studies to identify genetic variants involved. These studies were dedicated to βC metabolism and measured either postprandial chylomicron βC [113] or postprandial triglyceride-rich lipoprotein βC and RP concentrations [114,115] after test meals that provided βC. Thus, there is still no data on genetic variations associated with postprandial blood RP concentrations after a test meal rich in preformed VA. Consequently, it is obvious that the observations/conclusions presented in this chapter will be significantly improved in the future. In the study dedicated to identifying genetic variations associated with βC bioavailability [113], it was observed that the variability in the postprandial blood βC response (Area under the curve of the 0–8 h postprandial chylomicron βC concentrations) was associated with a combination of 25 SNPs in or near 12 candidate genes. Four of these genes were involved in the postprandial chylomicron triacylglycerol response in the same group of subjects [91], which was not surprising, as newly-absorbed βC is carried from the intestine to the liver via chylomicrons. Nevertheless, eight of these genes were specifically associated with the βC response. Possible explanations why these genes were associated with the βC response are discussed in the original paper [113]. Nevertheless, two associations deserve closer attention. The association with *ISX* confirms that genetic variations in this gene, which encodes a transcription factor involved in βC intestinal absorption and conversion, are key determinants of blood βC concentrations. Indeed, it was also reported in another study that an SNP in the ISX binding site in the *BCO1* promoter (rs6564851) was associated with decreased conversion rates of βC by 50% and increased fasting blood concentrations of βC [49]. The association with *BCO1* supports associations observed with postprandial βC and RP responses in other studies [114,115], confirming that this gene and its variations are key regulators of blood concentrations of these VA forms.

Table 1. Summary of SNPs associated with fasting blood vitamin A concentration or vitamin A bioavailability.

SNP/Mutation	Global MAF [1]	Nearest Gene	Trait	Reference	Study Type
(Ile59Asn) (rs121918584)	-	*RBP4*	FB-RET	[101,102]	CS
Gly75Asp (rs1218585)	0.115	*RBP4*	FB-RET	[101,102]	CS
c.248 + 1G>A	-	*RBP4*	FB-RET	[116]	CS
rs10882272	0.390	*RBP4*	FB-RET	[103]	GWAS
rs1667255	0.500	*TTR*	FB-RET	[103]	GWAS
rs738409	0.2622	*PNPLA3*	FB-RET	[105]	CGAS
rs6564851	0.476	*BCO1*	FB-βC	[104,106,107,114,117]	GWAS and CGAS
rs12926540	0.493	*BCO1*	FB-βC	[117]	GWAS
rs7501331	0.213	*BCO1*	FB-βC	[104,115]	CGAS
rs12934922	0.357	*BCO1*	FB-βC	[104,115]	CGAS
rs1800588	0.292	*HL*	FB-βC	[109]	CGAS
S447X	-	*LPL*	FB-βC	[108]	CGAS
SR-BI intron 5	-	*SCARB1*	FB-βC	[110]	CGAS
rs61932577	0.033	*SCARB1*	FB-βC/αC	[28]	CGAS
rs1984112	0.347	*CD36*	FB-βCryt/αC	[28]	CGAS
rs1761667	0.390	*CD36*	FB-βCryt/αC	[28]	CGAS
rs7755	0.388	*CD36*	FB-βCryt/αC	[28]	CGAS
rs10991408 *	0.116	*ABCA1*	βC-B [2]	[113]	CGAS
rs2791952 *	0.140	*ABCA1*	βC-B	[113]	CGAS
rs3887137 *	0.123	*ABCA1*	βC-B	[113]	CGAS
rs2278357	0.247	*ABCG5*	βC-B	[113]	CGAS
rs1042031 *	0.153	*APOB*	βC-B	[113]	CGAS
rs35364714 *	0.115	*APOB*	βC-B	[113]	CGAS
rs4643493 *	0.082	*APOB*	βC-B	[113]	CGAS
rs7196470	0.278	*BCO1*	βC-B	[113]	CGAS
rs1247620	0.137	*CXCL8*	βC-B	[113]	CGAS
rs1358594	0.291	*CXCL8*	βC-B	[113]	CGAS
rs6834586	0.221	*CXCL8*	βC-B	[113]	CGAS
rs3798709	0.252	*ELOVL2*	βC-B	[113]	CGAS
rs911196	0.252	*ELOVL2*	βC-B	[113]	CGAS
rs9468304	0.302	*ELOVL2*	βC-B	[113]	CGAS
rs16994824	0.206	*ISX*	βC-B	[113]	CGAS
rs202313	0.113	*ISX*	βC-B	[113]	CGAS
rs5755368	0.250	*ISX*	βC-B	[113]	CGAS
rs11857380 *	0.157	*LIPC*	βC-B	[113]	CGAS
rs12185072 *	0.198	*LIPC*	βC-B	[113]	CGAS
rs1869138 *	0.117	*LIPC*	βC-B	[113]	CGAS
rs8043708	0.237	*PKD1L2*	βC-B	[113]	CGAS
rs12139131	0.096	*RPE65*	βC-B	[113]	CGAS
rs4926340	0.093	*RPE65*	βC-B	[113]	CGAS
rs2501175	0.327	*SOD2*	βC-B	[113]	CGAS
rs946199 *	0.192	*TCF7L2*	βC-B	[113]	CGAS

[1] Abbreviations: CS: case subject(s) with very low vitamin A status; CGAS: candidate gene association study; GWAS: genome-wide association study; MAF: minor allele frequency, retrieved from the SNP database in PubMed (https://www.ncbi.nlm.nih.gov/pubmed?cmd=search); the gene official symbols are those found in PubMed and approved by the Hugo Gene Nomenclature Committee (available online: http://www.genenames.org/). FB-βC: fasting blood β-carotene concentration; FB-βCrypt/αC: fasting blood β-cryptoxanthin or α-carotene; FB-RET: fasting blood retinol concentration; βC-B: β-carotene bioavailability. [2] In this study, β-carotene bioavailability was estimated by measuring the postprandial chylomicron β-carotene response (0–8 h area under the curve) to a β-carotene containing test-meal. * These SNPs were associated with the variability of β-carotene bioavailability, but this association was likely due to their involvement in the postprandial metabolism of chylomicrons [91,113], which are the lipoparticles that carry newly-absorbed β-carotene from the intestine to the liver.

10. Other Genetic Variations that Could Be Involved in the Blood Concentration of Vitamin A

The few available studies reviewed in the two previous paragraphs highlights the tremendous work that remains to be done to identify all of the genetic variations associated with the concentration of the different forms of VA that circulate in the blood at fast and during the postprandial period. Furthermore, there is no study dedicated to identifying genetic variations that could modulate VA concentration in different tissues. It should also be reminded that, although SNPs represent >96% of polymorphisms [95], other genetic variations occur in DNA, e.g., copy number variants, insertion/deletion of some base pairs, as well as epigenetic modifications. A genetic score that would aim to predict concentrations of the different forms of VA in blood and in different tissues should therefore consider all of the genetic variations that can have a significant impact on these concentrations. Finally, association studies must be performed in different populations to be sure that the associations are not specific to some ethnic groups.

In summary, there is now enough evidence to state that blood, and likely tissue, concentrations of the different forms of VA, as well as VA bioavailability, are partly modulated by SNPs in several genes. However, much work remains to be done to obtain combinations of genetic variations (SNPs, but also other kinds of genetic variations) that will allow us to confidently predict the concentration of VA in the blood or in a target tissue of an individual by knowing his/her genotypes at these variations. Yet, the potential usefulness of this area of research is exciting regarding personalized nutrition and the fight against VA deficiency. Nevertheless, it should be reminded that genetics only represents one of the factors that affect VA concentration in blood and tissues, albeit stable over the lifespan, since other factors, such as VA dietary intake and factors that affect VA bioavailability (e.g., cooking practice), also affect this status. Thus, a prediction of VA concentration in blood and in various tissues should consider these variables, as well.

11. Conclusions

This review shows that genetic variations modulate both fasting blood retinol and βC concentrations and βC bioavailability. It also allows us to realize that a lot of work remains to be done to identify all the genetic variations that modulate these phenotypes and to propose a genetic test that will allow us to predict VA status or VA bioavailability in different ethnies.

Acknowledgments: This review is supported by the Micronutrients Genomics Project, which is a community-driven initiative to promote systematic capture, storage, management, analyses and dissemination of data and knowledge on micronutrient-genome interactions [118].

Author Contributions: Patrick Borel and Charles Desmarchelier have equally contributed to the writing of this review.

Conflicts of Interest: The authors declare no conflict of interest.

References

1. Rucker, R.B.; Suttie, J.W.; McCormick, D.B.; Machlin, L.J. *Handbook of Vitamins*, 3rd ed.; Marcel Dekker, Inc.: New York, NY, USA; Basel, Switzerland, 2001.
2. Dowling, J.E. George wald (1906-97)—Biologist who discovered the role of vitamin A in vision—Obituary. *Nature* **1997**, *387*, 356. [CrossRef] [PubMed]
3. Viewpoint, A.P.; Maumenee, A.E. The history of vitamin A and its ophthalmic implications. *Arch. Aphthalmol.* **1993**, *111*, 547–550.
4. Rando, R.R. The chemistry of vitamin A and vision. *Angew. Chem. Int. Ed. Engl.* **1990**, *29*, 461–480. [CrossRef]
5. Wright, C.B.; Redmond, T.M.; Nickerson, J.M. A history of the classical visual cycle. *Prog. Mol. Biol. Transl. Sci.* **2015**, *134*, 433–448. [PubMed]
6. Ross, A.C.; Gardner, E.M. The function of vitamin A in cellular growth and differentiation, and its roles during pregnancy and lactation. *Adv. Exp. Med. Biol.* **1994**, *352*, 187–200. [PubMed]
7. Love, J.M.; Gudas, L.J. Vitamin A, differentiation and cancer. *Curr. Opin. Cell Biol.* **1994**, *6*, 825–831. [CrossRef]

8. Zile, M.H. Function of vitamin A in vertebrate embryonic development. *J. Nutr.* **2001**, *131*, 705–708. [PubMed]
9. Clagett-Dame, M.; de Luca, H.F. The role of vitamin A in mammalian reproduction and embryonic development. *Annu. Rev. Nutr.* **2002**, *22*, 347–381. [CrossRef] [PubMed]
10. Goodman, D.S. Vitamin A and retinoids in health and disease. *N. Engl. J. Med.* **1984**, *310*, 1023–1031. [PubMed]
11. Mason, J.; Greiner, T.; Shrimpton, R.; Sanders, D.; Yukich, J. Vitamin A policies need rethinking. *Int. J. Epidemiol.* **2015**, *44*, 283–292. [CrossRef] [PubMed]
12. Troesch, B.; Hoeft, B.; McBurney, M.; Eggersdorfer, M.; Weber, P. Dietary surveys indicate vitamin intakes below recommendations are common in representative western countries. *Br. J. Nutr.* **2012**, *108*, 692–698. [CrossRef] [PubMed]
13. Weber, D.; Grune, T. The contribution of beta-carotene to Vitamin A supply of humans. *Mol. Nutr. Food Res.* **2012**, *56*, 251–258. [CrossRef] [PubMed]
14. Borel, P. Factors affecting intestinal absorption of highly lipophilic food microconstituents (fat-soluble vitamins, carotenoids and phytosterols). *Clin. Chem. Lab. Med.* **2003**, *41*, 979–994. [CrossRef] [PubMed]
15. Reboul, E.; Berton, A.; Moussa, M.; Kreuzer, C.; Crenon, I.; Borel, P. Pancreatic lipase and pancreatic lipase-related protein 2, but not pancreatic lipase-related protein 1, hydrolyze retinyl palmitate in physiological conditions. *Biochim. Biophys. Acta* **2006**, *1761*, 4–10. [CrossRef] [PubMed]
16. Tyssandier, V.; Reboul, E.; Dumas, J.F.; Bouteloup-Demange, C.; Armand, M.; Marcand, J.; Sallas, M.; Borel, P. Processing of vegetable-born carotenoids in the human stomach and duodenum. *Am. J. Physiol. Gastrointest. Liver Physiol.* **2003**, *284*, G913–G923. [CrossRef] [PubMed]
17. Borel, P.; Pasquier, B.; Armand, M.; Tyssandier, V.; Grolier, P.; Alexandre-Gouabau, M.C.; Andre, M.; Senft, M.; Peyrot, J.; Jaussan, V.; et al. Processing of Vitamin A and E in the human gastrointestinal tract. *Am. J. Physiol. Gastrointest. Liver Physiol.* **2001**, *280*, G95–G103. [PubMed]
18. Desmarchelier, C.; Borel, P. Overview of carotenoid bioavailability determinants: From dietary factors to host genetic variations. *Trends Food Sci. Technol.* **2017**, in press.
19. Mensi, A.; Borel, P.; Goncalves, A.; Nowicki, M.; Gleize, B.; Roi, S.; Chobert, J.M.; Haertle, T.; Reboul, E. Beta-lactoglobulin as a vector for beta-carotene food fortification. *J. Agric. Food Chem.* **2014**, *62*, 5916–5924. [CrossRef] [PubMed]
20. Tyssandier, V.; Lyan, B.; Borel, P. Main factors governing the transfer of carotenoids from emulsion lipid droplets to micelles. *Biochim. Biophys. Acta* **2001**, *1533*, 285–292. [CrossRef]
21. Rigtrup, K.M.; Kakkad, B.; Ong, D.E. Purification and partial characterization of a retinyl ester hydrolase from the brush border of rat small intestine mucosa: Probable identity with brush border phospholipase b. *Biochemistry (Mosc.)* **1994**, *33*, 2661–2666. [CrossRef]
22. Fernandez, E.; Borgstrom, B. Intestinal absorption of retinol and retinyl palmitate in the rat. Effects of tetrahydrolipstatin. *Lipids* **1990**, *25*, 549–552. [CrossRef] [PubMed]
23. Hollander, D.; Muralidhara, K.S. Vitamin a1 intestinal absorption in vivo: Influence of luminal factors on transport. *Am. J. Physiol. Gastrointest. Liver Physiol.* **1977**, *232*, E471–E477.
24. Porter, C.J.; Trevaskis, N.L.; Charman, W.N. Lipids and lipid-based formulations: Optimizing the oral delivery of lipophilic drugs. *Nat. Rev. Drug Discov.* **2007**, *6*, 231–248. [CrossRef] [PubMed]
25. Reboul, E.; Soayfane, Z.; Goncalves, A.; Cantiello, M.; Bott, R.; Nauze, M.; Terce, F.; Collet, X.; Comera, C. Respective contributions of intestinal niemann-pick c1-like 1 and scavenger receptor class b type i to cholesterol and tocopherol uptake: In vivo v. In vitro studies. *Br. J. Nutr.* **2012**, *107*, 1296–1304. [CrossRef] [PubMed]
26. Reboul, E.; Klein, A.; Bietrix, F.; Gleize, B.; Malezet-Desmoulins, C.; Schneider, M.; Margotat, A.; Lagrost, L.; Collet, X.; Borel, P. Scavenger receptor class b type i (sr-bi) is involved in vitamin e transport across the enterocyte. *J. Biol. Chem.* **2006**, *281*, 4739–4745. [CrossRef] [PubMed]
27. Goncalves, A.; Margier, M.; Roi, S.; Collet, X.; Niot, I.; Goupy, P.; Caris-Veyrat, C.; Reboul, E. Intestinal scavenger receptors are involved in vitamin k1 absorption. *J. Biol. Chem.* **2014**. [CrossRef] [PubMed]
28. Borel, P.; Lietz, G.; Goncalves, A.; Szabo de Edelenyi, F.; Lecompte, S.; Curtis, P.; Goumidi, L.; Caslake, M.J.; Miles, E.A.; Packard, C.; et al. Cd36 and sr-bi are involved in cellular uptake of provitamin A carotenoids by caco-2 and hek cells, and some of their genetic variants are associated with plasma concentrations of these micronutrients in humans. *J. Nutr.* **2013**, *143*, 448–456. [CrossRef] [PubMed]

29. During, A.; Dawson, H.D.; Harrison, E.H. Carotenoid transport is decreased and expression of the lipid transporters sr-bi, npc1l1, and abca1 is downregulated in caco-2 cells treated with ezetimibe. *J. Nutr.* **2005**, *135*, 2305–2312. [PubMed]

30. Van Bennekum, A.; Werder, M.; Thuahnai, S.T.; Han, C.H.; Duong, P.; Williams, D.L.; Wettstein, P.; Schulthess, G.; Phillips, M.C.; Hauser, H. Class b scavenger receptor-mediated intestinal absorption of dietary beta-carotene and cholesterol. *Biochemistry (Mosc.)* **2005**, *44*, 4517–4525. [CrossRef] [PubMed]

31. During, A.; Doraiswamy, S.; Harrison, E.H. Xanthophylls are preferentially taken up compared with beta-carotene by retinal cells via a srbi-dependent mechanism. *J. Lipid Res.* **2008**, *49*, 1715–1724. [CrossRef] [PubMed]

32. Hollander, D.; Wang, H.P.; Chu, C.Y.T.; Badawi, M.A. Preliminary characterization of a small intestinal binding component for retinol and fatty acids in the rat. *Life Sci.* **1978**, *23*, 1011–1018. [CrossRef]

33. Ong, D.E.; Page, D.L. Cellular retinol-binding protein (type two) is abundant in human small intestine. *J. Lipid Res.* **1987**, *28*, 739–745. [PubMed]

34. Wongsiriroj, N.; Piantedosi, R.; Palczewski, K.; Goldberg, I.J.; Johnston, T.P.; Li, E.; Blaner, W.S. The molecular basis of retinoid absorption: A genetic dissection. *J. Biol. Chem.* **2008**, *283*, 13510–13519. [CrossRef] [PubMed]

35. O'Byrne, S.M.; Wongsiriroj, N.; Libien, J.; Vogel, S.; Goldberg, I.J.; Baehr, W.; Palczewski, K.; Blaner, W.S. Retinoid absorption and storage is impaired in mice lacking lecithin:Retinol acyltransferase (lrat). *J. Biol. Chem.* **2005**, *280*, 35647–35657. [CrossRef] [PubMed]

36. Ables, G.P.; Yang, K.J.; Vogel, S.; Hernandez-Ono, A.; Yu, S.; Yuen, J.J.; Birtles, S.; Buckett, L.K.; Turnbull, A.V.; Goldberg, I.J.; et al. Intestinal dgat1 deficiency reduces postprandial triglyceride and retinyl ester excursions by inhibiting chylomicron secretion and delaying gastric emptying. *J. Lipid Res.* **2012**, *53*, 2364–2379. [CrossRef] [PubMed]

37. Sauvant, P.; Mekki, N.; Charbonnier, M.; Portugal, H.; Lairon, D.; Borel, P. Amounts and types of fatty acids in meals affect the pattern of retinoids secreted in human chylomicrons after a high-dose preformed vitamin A intake. *Metabolism* **2003**, *52*, 514–519. [CrossRef] [PubMed]

38. Reboul, E.; Borel, P. Proteins involved in uptake, intracellular transport and basolateral secretion of fat-soluble vitamins and carotenoids by mammalian enterocytes. *Prog. Lipid Res.* **2011**, *50*, 388–402. [CrossRef] [PubMed]

39. Duszka, C.; Grolier, P.; Azim, E.M.; Alexandre-Gouabau, M.C.; Borel, P.; Azais-Braesco, V. Rat intestinal beta-carotene dioxygenase activity is located primarily in the cytosol of mature jejunal enterocytes. *J. Nutr.* **1996**, *126*, 2550–2556. [PubMed]

40. Grolier, P.; Duszka, C.; Borel, P.; Alexandre-Gouabau, M.C.; Azais-Braesco, V. In vitro and in vivo inhibition of beta-carotene dioxygenase activity by canthaxanthin in rat intestine. *Arch. Biochem. Biophys.* **1997**, *348*, 233–238. [CrossRef] [PubMed]

41. Dela Sena, C.; Riedl, K.M.; Narayanasamy, S.; Curley, R.W., Jr.; Schwartz, S.J.; Harrison, E.H. The human enzyme that converts dietary provitamin A carotenoids to vitamin A is a dioxygenase. *J. Biol. Chem.* **2014**, *289*, 13661–13666. [CrossRef] [PubMed]

42. Dela Sena, C.; Narayanasamy, S.; Riedl, K.M.; Curley, R.W., Jr.; Schwartz, S.J.; Harrison, E.H. Substrate specificity of purified recombinant human beta-carotene 15,15'-oxygenase (bco1). *J. Biol. Chem.* **2013**, *288*, 37094–37103. [CrossRef] [PubMed]

43. Amengual, J.; Widjaja-Adhi, M.A.; Rodriguez-Santiago, S.; Hessel, S.; Golczak, M.; Palczewski, K.; von Lintig, J. Two carotenoid oxygenases contribute to mammalian provitamin A metabolism. *J. Biol. Chem.* **2013**, *288*, 34081–34096. [CrossRef] [PubMed]

44. Raghuvanshi, S.; Reed, V.; Blaner, W.S.; Harrison, E.H. Cellular localization of beta-carotene 15,15' oxygenase-1 (bco1) and beta-carotene 9',10' oxygenase-2 (bco2) in rat liver and intestine. *Arch. Biochem. Biophys.* **2015**, *572*, 19–27. [CrossRef] [PubMed]

45. Gajda, A.M.; Storch, J. Enterocyte fatty acid-binding proteins (fabps): Different functions of liver and intestinal fabps in the intestine. *Prostaglandins Leukot. Essent. Fatty Acids* **2015**, *93*, 9–16. [CrossRef] [PubMed]

46. Tang, G.; Qin, J.; Dolnikowski, G.G.; Russell, R.M. Short-term (intestinal) and long-term (postintestinal) conversion of beta-carotene to retinol in adults as assessed by a stable-isotope reference method. *Am. J. Clin. Nutr.* **2003**, *78*, 259–266. [PubMed]

47. Borel, P.; Grolier, P.; Mekki, N.; Boirie, Y.; Rochette, Y.; le Roy, B.; Alexandre-Gouabau, M.C.; Lairon, D.; Azais-Braesco, V. Low and high responders to pharmacological doses of beta-carotene: Proportion in the population, mechanisms involved and consequences on beta-carotene metabolism. *J. Lipid Res.* **1998**, *39*, 2250–2260. [PubMed]

48. Nayak, N.; Harrison, E.H.; Hussain, M.M. Retinyl ester secretion by intestinal cells: A specific and regulated process dependent on assembly and secretion of chylomicrons. *J. Lipid Res.* **2001**, *42*, 272–280. [PubMed]

49. Lobo, G.P.; Amengual, J.; Baus, D.; Shivdasani, R.A.; Taylor, D.; von Lintig, J. Genetics and diet regulate vitamin A production via the homeobox transcription factor isx. *J. Biol. Chem.* **2013**, *288*, 9017–9027. [CrossRef] [PubMed]

50. Lobo, G.P.; Hessel, S.; Eichinger, A.; Noy, N.; Moise, A.R.; Wyss, A.; Palczewski, K.; von Lintig, J. Isx is a retinoic acid-sensitive gatekeeper that controls intestinal beta,beta-carotene absorption and vitamin A production. *FASEB J.* **2010**, *24*, 1656–1666. [CrossRef] [PubMed]

51. Mondloch, S.; Gannon, B.M.; Davis, C.R.; Chileshe, J.; Kaliwile, C.; Masi, C.; Rios-Avila, L.; Gregory, J.F., 3rd; Tanumihardjo, S.A. High provitamin A carotenoid serum concentrations, elevated retinyl esters, and saturated retinol-binding protein in zambian preschool children are consistent with the presence of high liver vitamin A stores. *Am. J. Clin. Nutr.* **2015**, *102*, 497–504. [CrossRef] [PubMed]

52. Blomhoff, R.; Helgerud, P.; Dueland, S.; Berg, T.; Pedersen, J.I.; Norum, K.R.; Drevon, C.A. Lymphatic absorption and transport of retinol and vitamin d-3 from rat intestine. Evidence for different pathways. *Biochim. Biophys. Acta* **1984**, *772*, 109–116. [CrossRef]

53. Tyssandier, V.; Choubert, G.; Grolier, P.; Borel, P. Carotenoids, mostly the xanthophylls, exchange between plasma lipoproteins. *Int. J. Vitam. Nutr. Res.* **2002**, *72*, 300–308. [CrossRef] [PubMed]

54. Dallinga-Thie, G.M.; Franssen, R.; Mooij, H.L.; Visser, M.E.; Hassing, H.C.; Peelman, F.; Kastelein, J.J.; Peterfy, M.; Nieuwdorp, M. The metabolism of triglyceride-rich lipoproteins revisited: New players, new insight. *Atherosclerosis* **2010**, *211*, 1–8. [CrossRef] [PubMed]

55. Blomhoff, R.; Helgerud, P.; Rasmussen, M.; Berg, T.; Norum, K.R. In vivo uptake of chylomicron [3h]retinyl ester by rat liver: Evidence for retinol transfer from parenchymal to nonparenchymal cells. *Proc. Natl. Acad. Sci. USA* **1982**, *79*, 7326–7330. [CrossRef] [PubMed]

56. O'Byrne, S.M.; Blaner, W.S. Retinol and retinyl esters: Biochemistry and physiology. *J. Lipid Res.* **2013**, *54*, 1731–1743. [CrossRef] [PubMed]

57. Ong, D.E. Purufication and partial characterization of cellular retinol-binding protein from human liver. *Cancer Res.* **1982**, *42*, 1033–1037. [PubMed]

58. Ong, D.E.; MacDonald, P.N.; Gubitosi, A.M. Esterification of retinol in rat liver. *J. Biol. Chem.* **1988**, *263*, 5789–5796. [PubMed]

59. Rose, A.C. Retinol esterification by rat liver microsomes. *J. Biol. Chem.* **1982**, *257*, 2453–2459.

60. Nagatsuma, K.; Hayashi, Y.; Hano, H.; Sagara, H.; Murakami, K.; Saito, M.; Masaki, T.; Lu, T.; Tanaka, M.; Enzan, H.; et al. Lecithin: Retinol acyltransferase protein is distributed in both hepatic stellate cells and endothelial cells of normal rodent and human liver. *Liver Int.* **2009**, *29*, 47–54. [CrossRef] [PubMed]

61. Wake, K. Development of vitamin A-rich lipid droplets in multivesicular bodies or rat liver stellate cells. *J. Cell Biol.* **1974**, *63*, 683–691. [CrossRef] [PubMed]

62. Wake, K. Perisinusoidal stellate cells (fat-storing cells, interstitial cells, lipocytes), their related structure in and around the liver sinusoids, and vitamin A-storing cells in extrahepatic organs. *Int. Rev. Cytol.* **1980**, *66*, 303–353. [PubMed]

63. Taschler, U.; Schreiber, R.; Chitraju, C.; Grabner, G.F.; Romauch, M.; Wolinski, H.; Haemmerle, G.; Breinbauer, R.; Zechner, R.; Lass, A.; et al. Adipose triglyceride lipase is involved in the mobilization of triglyceride and retinoid stores of hepatic stellate cells. *Biochim. Biophys. Acta* **2015**, *1851*, 937–945. [CrossRef] [PubMed]

64. Pirazzi, C.; Valenti, L.; Motta, B.M.; Pingitore, P.; Hedfalk, K.; Mancina, R.M.; Burza, M.A.; Indiveri, C.; Ferro, Y.; Montalcini, T.; et al. Pnpla3 has retinyl-palmitate lipase activity in human hepatic stellate cells. *Hum. Mol. Genet.* **2014**, *23*, 4077–4085. [CrossRef] [PubMed]

65. Pingitore, P.; Pirazzi, C.; Mancina, R.M.; Motta, B.M.; Indiveri, C.; Pujia, A.; Montalcini, T.; Hedfalk, K.; Romeo, S. Recombinant pnpla3 protein shows triglyceride hydrolase activity and its i148m mutation results in loss of function. *Biochim. Biophys. Acta* **2014**, *1841*, 574–580. [CrossRef] [PubMed]

66. He, S.; McPhaul, C.; Li, J.Z.; Garuti, R.; Kinch, L.; Grishin, N.V.; Cohen, J.C.; Hobbs, H.H. A sequence variation (i148m) in pnpla3 associated with nonalcoholic fatty liver disease disrupts triglyceride hydrolysis. *J. Biol. Chem.* **2010**, *285*, 6706–6715. [CrossRef] [PubMed]

67. Shmarakov, I.; Fleshman, M.K.; D'Ambrosio, D.N.; Piantedosi, R.; Riedl, K.M.; Schwartz, S.J.; Curley, R.W., Jr.; von Lintig, J.; Rubin, L.P.; Harrison, E.H.; et al. Hepatic stellate cells are an important cellular site for beta-carotene conversion to retinoid. *Arch. Biochem. Biophys.* **2010**, *504*, 3–10. [CrossRef] [PubMed]

68. Lakshman, M.R.; Asher, K.A.; Attlesey, M.G.; Satchithanandam, S.; Mychkovsky, I.; Coutlakis, P.J. Absorption, storage, and distribution of beta-carotene in normal and beta-carotene-fed rats: Roles of parenchymal and stellate cells. *J. Lipid Res.* **1989**, *30*, 1545–1550. [PubMed]

69. Zachman, R.D.; Singer, M.B.; Olson, J.A. Biliary secretion of metabolites of retinol and of retinoic acid in the guinea pig and chick. *J. Nutr.* **1966**, *88*, 137–142. [PubMed]

70. Zachman, R.D.; Olson, J.A. Formation and enterohepatic circulation of water-soluble metabolites of retinol(vitamin A)in the rat. *Nature* **1964**, *201*, 1222–1223. [CrossRef] [PubMed]

71. Peterson, P.A. Characteristics of a vitamin A transporting protein complex occurring in human serum. *J. Biol. Chem.* **1971**, *246*, 34–43. [PubMed]

72. Kawaguchi, R.; Yu, J.; Honda, J.; Hu, J.; Whitelegge, J.; Ping, P.; Wiita, P.; Bok, D.; Sun, H. A membrane receptor for retinol binding protein mediates cellular uptake of vitamin A. *Science* **2007**, *315*, 820–825. [CrossRef] [PubMed]

73. Alapatt, P.; Guo, F.; Komanetsky, S.M.; Wang, S.; Cai, J.; Sargsyan, A.; Rodriguez Diaz, E.; Bacon, B.T.; Aryal, P.; Graham, T.E. Liver retinol transporter and receptor for serum retinol-binding protein (rbp4). *J. Biol. Chem.* **2013**, *288*, 1250–1265. [CrossRef] [PubMed]

74. Amengual, J.; Golczak, M.; Palczewski, K.; von Lintig, J. Lecithin:Retinol acyltransferase is critical for cellular uptake of vitamin A from serum retinol-binding protein. *J. Biol. Chem.* **2012**, *287*, 24216–24227. [CrossRef] [PubMed]

75. Thomas, S.E.; Harrison, E.H. Mechanisms of selective delivery of xanthophylls to retinal pigment epithelial cells by human lipoproteins. *J. Lipid Res.* **2016**, *57*, 1865–1878. [CrossRef] [PubMed]

76. Chambon, P. The molecular and genetic dissection of the retinoid signalling pathway. *Gene* **1993**, *135*, 223–228. [CrossRef]

77. Iskakova, M.; Karbyshev, M.; Piskunov, A.; Rochette-Egly, C. Nuclear and extranuclear effects of vitamin A. *Can. J. Physiol. Pharmacol.* **2015**, *93*, 1065–1075. [CrossRef] [PubMed]

78. Strom, K.; Gundersen, T.E.; Hansson, O.; Lucas, S.; Fernandez, C.; Blomhoff, R.; Holm, C. Hormone-sensitive lipase (hsl) is also a retinyl ester hydrolase: Evidence from mice lacking hsl. *FASEB J.* **2009**, *23*, 2307–2316. [CrossRef] [PubMed]

79. Tanumihardjo, S.A.; Russell, R.M.; Stephensen, C.B.; Gannon, B.M.; Craft, N.E.; Haskell, M.J.; Lietz, G.; Schulze, K.; Raiten, D.J. Biomarkers of nutrition for development (bond)-vitamin A review. *J. Nutr.* **2016**, *146*, 1816S–1848S. [CrossRef] [PubMed]

80. Herbeth, B.; Zittoun, J.; Miravet, L.; Bourgeay-Causse, M.; Carreguery, G.; Delacoux, E.; le Devehat, C.; Lemoine, A.; Mareschi, J.P.; Martin, J.; et al. Reference intervals for vitamins B1, B2, E, D, retinol, beta-carotene, and folate in blood: Usefulness of dietary selection criteria. *Clin. Chem.* **1986**, *32*, 1756–1759. [PubMed]

81. Muto, Y.; Smith, J.E.; Milch, P.O.; Goodman, D.S. Regulation of retinol-binding protein metabolism by vitamin A status in the rat. *J. Biol. Chem.* **1972**, *247*, 2542–2550. [PubMed]

82. Loerch, J.D.; Underwood, B.A.; Lewis, K.C. Response of plasma levels of vitamin A to a dose of vitamin A as an indicator of hepatic vitamin A reserves in rats. *J. Nutr.* **1979**, *109*, 778–786. [PubMed]

83. Olson, J.A. The reproducibility, sensitivity and specificity of the relative dose response (rdr) test for determining vitamin A status. *J. Nutr.* **1991**, *121*, 917–920. [PubMed]

84. Wahed, M.A.; Alvarez, J.O.; Khaled, M.A.; Mahalanabis, D.; Rahman, M.M.; Habte, D. Comparison of the modified relative dose response (mrdr) and the relative dose response (rdr) in the assessment of vitamin A status in malnourished children. *Am. J. Clin. Nutr.* **1995**, *61*, 1253–1256. [PubMed]

85. Tanumihardjo, S.A.; Olson, J.A. The reproducibility of the modified relative dose response (mrdr) assay in healthy individuals over time and its comparison with conjunctival impression cytology (cic). *Eur. J. Clin. Nutr.* **1991**, *45*, 407–411. [PubMed]

86. Borel, P.; Grolier, P.; Armand, M.; Partier, A.; Lafont, H.; Lairon, D.; Azais-Braesco, V. Carotenoids in biological emulsions: Solubility, surface-to-core distribution, and release from lipid droplets. *J. Lipid Res.* **1996**, *37*, 250–261. [PubMed]

87. Clevidence, B.A.; Bieri, J.G. Association of carotenoids with human plasma lipoproteins. *Methods Enzymol.* **1993**, *214*, 33–46. [PubMed]

88. Cornwell, D.G.; Kruger, F.A.; Robinson, H.B. Studies on the absorption of beta-carotene and the distribution of total carotenoid in human serum lipoproteins after oral administration. *J. Lipid Res.* **1962**, *3*, 65–70.

89. Berr, F.; Kern, F. Plasma clearance of chylomicrons labeled with retinyl palmitate in healthy human subjects. *J. Lipid Res.* **1984**, *25*, 805–812. [PubMed]

90. Perez-Martinez, P.; Delgado-Lista, J.; Perez-Jimenez, F.; Lopez-Miranda, J. Update on genetics of postprandial lipemia. *Atheroscler. Suppl.* **2010**, *11*, 39–43. [CrossRef] [PubMed]

91. Desmarchelier, C.; Martin, J.C.; Planells, R.; Gastaldi, M.; Nowicki, M.; Goncalves, A.; Valero, R.; Lairon, D.; Borel, P. The postprandial chylomicron triacylglycerol response to dietary fat in healthy male adults is significantly explained by a combination of single nucleotide polymorphisms in genes involved in triacylglycerol metabolism. *J. Clin. Endocrinol. Metab.* **2014**, *99*, E484–E488. [CrossRef] [PubMed]

92. World Health Organization. *Serum Retinol Concentrations for Determining the Prevalence of Vitamin A Deficiency in Populations. Vitamin and Mineral Nutrition Information System*; World Health Organization: Geneva, Swizerland, 2011.

93. Furr, H.C.; Green, M.H.; Haskell, M.; Mokhtar, N.; Nestel, P.; Newton, S.; Ribaya-Mercado, J.D.; Tang, G.; Tanumihardjo, S.; Wasantwisut, E. Stable isotope dilution techniques for assessing vitamin A status and bioefficacy of provitamin A carotenoids in humans. *Public Health Nutr.* **2005**, *8*, 596–607. [CrossRef] [PubMed]

94. Kovarova, M.; Konigsrainer, I.; Konigsrainer, A.; Machicao, F.; Haring, H.U.; Schleicher, E.; Peter, A. The genetic variant i148m in pnpla3 is associated with increased hepatic retinyl-palmitate storage in humans. *J. Clin. Endocrinol. Metab.* **2015**, *100*, E1568–E1574. [CrossRef] [PubMed]

95. Genomes Project, C.; Auton, A.; Brooks, L.D.; Durbin, R.M.; Garrison, E.P.; Kang, H.M.; Korbel, J.O.; Marchini, J.L.; McCarthy, S.; McVean, G.A.; et al. A global reference for human genetic variation. *Nature* **2015**, *526*, 68–74.

96. Pirazzi, C.; Adiels, M.; Burza, M.A.; Mancina, R.M.; Levin, M.; Stahlman, M.; Taskinen, M.R.; Orho-Melander, M.; Perman, J.; Pujia, A.; et al. Patatin-like phospholipase domain-containing 3 (pnpla3) i148m (rs738409) affects hepatic vldl secretion in humans and in vitro. *J. Hepatol.* **2012**, *57*, 1276–1282. [CrossRef] [PubMed]

97. Fischer, J.; Lefevre, C.; Morava, E.; Mussini, J.M.; Laforet, P.; Negre-Salvayre, A.; Lathrop, M.; Salvayre, R. The gene encoding adipose triglyceride lipase (pnpla2) is mutated in neutral lipid storage disease with myopathy. *Nat. Genet.* **2007**, *39*, 28–30. [CrossRef] [PubMed]

98. Dongiovanni, P.; Donati, B.; Fares, R.; Lombardi, R.; Mancina, R.M.; Romeo, S.; Valenti, L. Pnpla3 i148m polymorphism and progressive liver disease. *World J. Gastroenterol.* **2013**, *19*, 6969–6978. [CrossRef] [PubMed]

99. Trepo, E.; Romeo, S.; Zucman-Rossi, J.; Nahon, P. Pnpla3 gene in liver diseases. *J. Hepatol.* **2016**, *65*, 399–412. [CrossRef] [PubMed]

100. Waits, R.P.; Yamada, T.; Uemichi, T.; Benson, M.D. Low plasma concentrations of retinol-binding protein in individuals with mutations affecting position 84 of the transthyretin molecule. *Clin. Chem.* **1995**, *41*, 1288–1291. [PubMed]

101. Biesalski, H.K.; Frank, J.; Beck, S.C.; Heinrich, F.; Illek, B.; Reifen, R.; Gollnick, H.; Seeliger, M.W.; Wissinger, B.; Zrenner, E. Biochemical but not clinical vitamin A deficiency results from mutations in the gene for retinol binding protein. *Am. J. Clin. Nutr.* **1999**, *69*, 931–936. [PubMed]

102. Folli, C.; Viglione, S.; Busconi, M.; Berni, R. Biochemical basis for retinol deficiency induced by the i41n and g75d mutations in human plasma retinol-binding protein. *Biochem. Biophys. Res. Commun.* **2005**, *336*, 1017–1022. [CrossRef] [PubMed]

103. Mondul, A.M.; Yu, K.; Wheeler, W.; Zhang, H.; Weinstein, S.J.; Major, J.M.; Cornelis, M.C.; Mannisto, S.; Hazra, A.; Hsing, A.W.; et al. Genome-wide association study of circulating retinol levels. *Hum. Mol. Genet.* **2011**, *20*, 4724–4731. [CrossRef] [PubMed]

104. Hendrickson, S.J.; Hazra, A.; Chen, C.; Eliassen, A.H.; Kraft, P.; Rosner, B.A.; Willett, W.C. Beta-carotene 15,15′-monooxygenase 1 single nucleotide polymorphisms in relation to plasma carotenoid and retinol concentrations in women of european descent. *Am. J. Clin. Nutr.* **2012**, *96*, 1379–1389. [CrossRef] [PubMed]

105. Mondul, A.; Mancina, R.M.; Merlo, A.; Dongiovanni, P.; Rametta, R.; Montalcini, T.; Valenti, L.; Albanes, D.; Romeo, S. Pnpla3 i148m variant influences circulating retinol in adults with nonalcoholic fatty liver disease or obesity. *J. Nutr.* **2015**, *145*, 1687–1691. [CrossRef] [PubMed]

106. Ferrucci, L.; Perry, J.R.; Matteini, A.; Perola, M.; Tanaka, T.; Silander, K.; Rice, N.; Melzer, D.; Murray, A.; Cluett, C.; et al. Common variation in the beta-carotene 15,15′-monooxygenase 1 gene affects circulating levels of carotenoids: A genome-wide association study. *Am. J. Hum. Genet.* **2009**, *84*, 123–133. [CrossRef] [PubMed]

107. Yabuta, S.; Urata, M.; Wai Kun, R.Y.; Masaki, M.; Shidoji, Y. Common snp rs6564851 in the bco1 gene affects the circulating levels of beta-carotene and the daily intake of carotenoids in healthy Japanese women. *PLoS ONE* **2016**, *11*, e0168857. [CrossRef] [PubMed]

108. Herbeth, B.; Gueguen, S.; Leroy, P.; Siest, G.; Visvikis-Siest, S. The lipoprotein lipase serine 447 stop polymorphism is associated with altered serum carotenoid concentrations in the stanislas family study. *J. Am. Coll. Nutr.* **2007**, *26*, 655–662. [CrossRef] [PubMed]

109. Borel, P.; Moussa, M.; Reboul, E.; Lyan, B.; Defoort, C.; Vincent-Baudry, S.; Maillot, M.; Gastaldi, M.; Darmon, M.; Portugal, H.; et al. Human fasting plasma concentrations of vitamin e and carotenoids, and their association with genetic variants in apo c-iii, cholesteryl ester transfer protein, hepatic lipase, intestinal fatty acid binding protein and microsomal triacylglycerol transfer protein. *Br. J. Nutr.* **2009**, *101*, 680–687. [PubMed]

110. Borel, P.; Moussa, M.; Reboul, E.; Lyan, B.; Defoort, C.; Vincent-Baudry, S.; Maillot, M.; Gastaldi, M.; Darmon, M.; Portugal, H.; et al. Human plasma levels of vitamin e and carotenoids are associated with genetic polymorphisms in genes involved in lipid metabolism. *J. Nutr.* **2007**, *137*, 2653–2659. [PubMed]

111. Hoekstra, M. SR-BI as target in atherosclerosis and cardiovascular disease—A comprehensive appraisal of the cellular functions of SR-BI in physiology and disease. *Atherosclerosis* **2017**. [CrossRef] [PubMed]

112. Harrison, E.H. Mechanisms involved in the intestinal absorption of dietary vitamin A and provitamin A carotenoids. *Biochim. Biophys. Acta* **2012**, *1821*, 70–77. [CrossRef] [PubMed]

113. Borel, P.; Desmarchelier, C.; Nowicki, M.; Bott, R. A combination of single-nucleotide polymorphisms is associated with interindividual variability in dietary beta-carotene bioavailability in healthy men. *J. Nutr.* **2015**, *145*, 1740–1747. [CrossRef] [PubMed]

114. Lietz, G.; Oxley, A.; Leung, W.; Hesketh, J. Single nucleotide polymorphisms upstream from the beta-carotene 15,15′-monooxygenase gene influence provitamin A conversion efficiency in female volunteers. *J. Nutr.* **2012**, *142*, 161S–165S. [CrossRef] [PubMed]

115. Leung, W.C.; Hessel, S.; Meplan, C.; Flint, J.; Oberhauser, V.; Tourniaire, F.; Hesketh, J.E.; von Lintig, J.; Lietz, G. Two common single nucleotide polymorphisms in the gene encoding beta-carotene 15,15′-monooxygenase alter beta-carotene metabolism in female volunteers. *FASEB J.* **2009**, *23*, 1041–1053. [CrossRef] [PubMed]

116. Khan, K.N.; Carss, K.; Raymond, F.L.; Islam, F.; Nihr BioResource-Rare Diseases, C.; Moore, A.T.; Michaelides, M.; Arno, G. Vitamin A deficiency due to bi-allelic mutation of rbp4: There's more to it than meets the eye. *Ophthalmic Genet.* **2016**, 1–2. [CrossRef] [PubMed]

117. Wood, A.R.; Perry, J.R.; Tanaka, T.; Hernandez, D.G.; Zheng, H.F.; Melzer, D.; Gibbs, J.R.; Nalls, M.A.; Weedon, M.N.; Spector, T.D.; et al. Imputation of variants from the 1000 genomes project modestly improves known associations and can identify low-frequency variant—Phenotype associations undetected by hapmap based imputation. *PLoS ONE* **2013**, *8*, e64343. [CrossRef] [PubMed]

118. Van Ommen, B.; El-Sohemy, A.; Hesketh, J.; Kaput, J.; Fenech, M.; Evelo, C.T.; McArdle, H.J.; Bouwman, J.; Lietz, G.; Mathers, J.C.; et al. The micronutrient genomics project: A community-driven knowledge base for micronutrient research. *Genes Nutr.* **2010**, *5*, 285–296. [CrossRef] [PubMed]

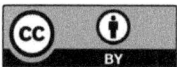

nutrients

Article

CYP1A2 Genotype Variations Do Not Modify the Benefits and Drawbacks of Caffeine during Exercise: A Pilot Study

Juan J. Salinero, Beatriz Lara, Diana Ruiz-Vicente, Francisco Areces, Carlos Puente-Torres, César Gallo-Salazar, Teodoro Pascual and Juan Del Coso *

Exercise Physiology Laboratory, Camilo José Cela University, Madrid 28692, Spain; jjsalinero@ucjc.edu (J.J.S.); blara@ucjc.edu (B.L.); diruiz@ucjc.edu (D.R.-V.); fareces@ucjc.edu (F.A.); carlos.puente@sek.es (C.P.-T.); cgallo@ucjc.edu (C.G.-S.); tpascual@ucjc.edu (T.P.)
* Correspondence: jdelcoso@ucjc.edu; Tel.: +34-918-153-131

Received: 7 December 2016; Accepted: 8 March 2017; Published: 11 March 2017

Abstract: Previous investigations have determined that some individuals have minimal or even ergolytic performance effects after caffeine ingestion. The aim of this study was to analyze the influence of the genetic variations of the CYP1A2 gene on the performance enhancement effects of ingesting a moderate dose of caffeine. In a double-blind randomized experimental design, 21 healthy active participants (29.3 ± 7.7 years) ingested 3 mg of caffeine per kg of body mass or a placebo in testing sessions separated by one week. Performance in the 30 s Wingate test, visual attention, and side effects were evaluated. DNA was obtained from whole blood samples and the CYP1A2 polymorphism was analyzed (rs762551). We obtained two groups: AA homozygotes ($n = 5$) and C-allele carriers ($n = 16$). Caffeine ingestion increased peak power (682 ± 140 vs. 667 ± 137 W; $p = 0.008$) and mean power during the Wingate test (527 ± 111 vs. 518 ± 111 W; $p < 0.001$) with no differences between AA homozygotes and C-allele carriers ($p > 0.05$). Reaction times were similar between caffeine and placebo conditions (276 ± 31 vs. 269 ± 71 milliseconds; $p = 0.681$) with no differences between AA homozygotes and C-allele carriers. However, 31.3% of the C-allele carriers reported increased nervousness after caffeine ingestion, while none of the AA homozygotes perceived this side effect. Genetic variations of the CYP1A2 polymorphism did not affect the ergogenic effects and drawbacks derived from the ingestion of a moderate dose of caffeine.

Keywords: genetics; cycling; ergogenic aid; side effects; performance

1. Introduction

The ergogenic effects of caffeine ingestion when consumed in low-to-moderate doses ($\sim$3–6 mg·kg^{-1} [1]) have been widely established in trained athletes. The scientific evidence regarding the performance-enhancing properties of caffeine has been found in short-term high-intensity sports modalities [2], team sports competitions [3–5], and endurance-based exercise [6,7]. Moreover, the pre-exercise ingestion of caffeine is effective in increasing physical performance in resistance activities [8,9]. Apart from the benefits related to physical performance, caffeine can also improve cognitive performance because it reduces simple and choice reaction times [10–12], increases alertness and concentration [13–15], and improves complex cognitive abilities [16]. Nevertheless, the ingestion of low-to-moderate doses of caffeine significantly increased the prevalence of side effects in the hours after ingestion, such as insomnia, activeness, and nervousness [17,18].

Multiple mechanisms have been proposed to explain the ergogenic effects of caffeine supplementation on sports performance [1,19]. Initially, it was believed that caffeine ingestion increased free fatty acid oxidation in skeletal muscle and, consequently, helped to spare muscle and liver glycogen [19].

However, this theory is not sound in explaining the ergogenicity of caffeine found in short-term, high-intensity exercise where muscle and liver glycogen are not depleted [19]. Another more plausible explanation for the mechanism behind caffeine ergogenicity is related to the known stimulation effect of this substance on the central nervous system. By acting antagonistically on adenosine receptors, caffeine inhibits the negative effects that adenosine induces on neurotransmission, arousal, and pain perception [19]. Apart from its effect on the central nervous system, the findings of previous studies involving caffeine ingestion and physical performance also indicate that this substance might have an effect on peripheral systems (e.g., skeletal muscle contraction and neuromuscular function) [1]. However, most of the peripheral effects of caffeine are rarely found in vivo and with normal plasma caffeine concentrations [20].

While most investigations have reported the benefits of caffeine on exercise activities in a group of individuals, some investigations have reported that not all individuals experience enhanced exercise performance after the ingestion of moderate doses of caffeine [2,21–23]. In fact, these investigations have identified individuals with minimal ergogenic effects, or even slightly declined exercise performance, after the intake of caffeine [2,21–23], suggesting the existence of different physiological responses to the intake of the same dose of caffeine. Although there is still no clear evidence, several researchers have suggested that the inter-individual differences in the ergogenicity derived from caffeine could be related to genetic polymorphisms associated with cytochrome P450 proteins, specifically the CYP1A2 enzyme. This hepatic enzyme is responsible for caffeine metabolism and catabolizes caffeine into paraxanthine and other dymethylxanthines [24]. A single nucleotide polymorphism (SNP) in the CYP1A2 gene (−163C>A; rs762551) is responsible for the ultra-fast CYP1A2*1F haplotype which confers a faster capacity to metabolize caffeine on AA homozygotes [25]. According to this notion, AA homozygotes could degrade caffeine into paraxanthine faster than CA and CC individuals [26] which, in turn, could produce a higher clearance of this substance from the blood. Thus, AA homozygotes in the CYP1A2 −163C>A would have reduced ergogenic effects from caffeine ingestion (e.g., non-responders).

Previous investigations have been aimed at determining the influence of the −163C>A SNP on the ergogenic effects of caffeine, although the outcomes of this research are inconsistent [27–29]. It has been found that C-allele carriers for this SNP (CC homozygotes and CA heterozygotes) experienced a greater improvement with caffeine (6 mg·kg^{-1}) than AA homozygotes during a 3 km cycling trial, which is in agreement with the mechanism that relates AA homozygosity with a higher caffeine metabolism/clearance [28]. However, AA homozygotes had greater ergogenicity compared to C-allele carriers after ingesting caffeine (6 mg·kg^{-1}) prior to a 40 km time trial [27]. It has even been found that the ergogenic effects of caffeine (~4 mg·kg^{-1}) are unmodified by the −163C>A SNP because the change in performance induced by caffeine was similar for AA homozygotes and C-allele carriers during a 15 min cycling test [29]. In light of the contradictory outcomes surrounding this topic, the aim of the present study is to provide additional information about the influence of genetic variations of the CYP1A2 gene on the physical and cognitive ergogenicity derived from caffeine ingestion. We hypothesized that AA homozygotes for the CYP1A2 −163C>A SNP would not obtain lessened ergogenic effects after caffeine ingestion when compared to the C-allele counterparts, indicating that the CYP1A2 genetic variations are responsible, in part, for the existence of caffeine non-responders.

2. Materials and Methods

2.1. Subjects

Twenty-one healthy active participants volunteered to participate in this study. They had a mean ± standard deviation (SD) age of 28.9 ± 7.3 years, body mass of 69.1 ± 10.2 kg, and height of 175 ± 9 cm. The study included seven women, always tested in the luteal phase. The participants had no physical limitations or musculoskeletal injuries that could affect the results of the study. In addition, participants were non-smokers, but light caffeine consumers (<60 mg per day, ~1 cup of coffee).

Participants were fully informed of any risks and discomforts associated with the experiments before giving their informed written consent to participate. The study was approved by the Camilo Jose Cela University Research Ethics Committee (Ethical approval code: CEI-UCJC CAFEGEN 2013/14), in accordance with the latest version of the Declaration of Helsinki.

2.2. Pre-Experimental Procedures

One week before the experimental trials, participants underwent a routine physical examination to ensure that they were in good health. After that, they were nude weighed ($\pm$ 50 g, Radwag, Radom, Poland) to individualize caffeine doses. Afterwards, a venous blood sample (5 mL) was obtained from an antecubital vein, inserted into a tube with ethylenediaminetetraacetic acid (EDTA) and refrigerated (4 °C). This sample was analyzed within the following 24-h to determine three SNPs of the CYP1A2 gene: -163C>A (rs762551) resulting in ultra-speed CYP1A2*1F; -3860G>A (rs2069514), responsible for defective allele CYP1A2*1C; and -729C>T (rs12720461) resulting in defective allele CYP1A2*1K. DNA quantification was analyzed with a spectrophotometer (Epoch TM, Biotek Instruments, Inc., Winooski, VT, USA), amplified by RT-PCR and fluorometric detection by an allele-specific TaqMan® probe in Real-Time PCR StepOne Plus (Applied Biosystems, Life Technologies, Thermo Fisher Scientific Inc., Waltham, MA, USA). Subsequently, after a standardized warm-up, participants performed a familiarization session with all of the tests included in the study. Comfortable seat height and handle bar position on the cycle ergometer were determined and recorded for later testing sessions. The day before the familiarization tests and in between the pre-experimental and experimental periods, participants were encouraged to avoid strenuous exercise and caffeine ingestion in any form (e.g., coffee, cola, energy drinks, etc.) and compliance was obtained by exercise and dietary records.

2.3. Experimental Design

A double-blind, placebo-controlled randomized experimental design was used in this study. Each participant performed two experimental trials at the same time of day (from 3 to 5 p.m.) and under laboratory-controlled conditions (~22 °C dry temperature; ~38% relative humidity). Participants ingested 3 mg of caffeine (BulkPowders, Colchester, Essex, UK) per kg of body mass (3 mg·kg^{-1}; 207 $\pm$ 30 mg) or the same dose of a placebo substance (e.g., cellulose; Guinama, Valencia, Spain). The experimental substances were provided in identical opaque gelatin capsules (Guinama, Valencia, Spain) to avoid identification, which were ingested with 200 mL of water. The capsule was ingested 60 min before the onset of the experimental trials to allow complete caffeine absorption [30]. The order of the experimental trials (e.g., caffeine or placebo) was randomized and counterbalanced. An alphanumeric code was assigned to each trial to blind participants and investigators to the substance tested in each session. This code was unveiled after the analysis of the variables. The experimental trials were separated by one week to allow complete caffeine washout and a complete recovery.

The day before each experimental trial, participants refrained from strenuous exercise and adopted a similar diet and fluid intake regimen. Participants were also instructed to have a light meal at least 3 h before the onset of the experimental trials. Participants arrived at the laboratory in the afternoon and ingested the capsule assigned for the trial. Afterwards, participants rested supine for 60 min to allow for caffeine absorption [20].

Visual attention test. Participants completed an 8 min visual attention test designed to assess simple reaction time and error cognitive processes (E-Prime, Psychology Software Tools Inc., Sharpsburg, PA, USA). For this test, each participant remained seated in front of a computer screen, with noise-cancelling headphones and with no other sensorial stimulus. For the duration of the test letters were displayed in the centre of the digital interface (in black over a white desktop) in a random order while participants had to press the space bar as fast as possible when the letter "X" appeared on the screen but only if this letter was preceded by the letter "O". The letters appeared only for 50 ms (stimulus exposure time) and the inter-stimuli time was set at 950 ms. Average reaction time and the number of correct answers/errors were registered for the total test and in four blocks of 2 min.

Wingate test. Participants performed a 10 min standardized warm-up on the cycle ergometer that included cycling at 50 W and three submaximal 10 s sprints. Then, a 30 s maximal all-out test was performed with a load that represented 7.5% of body mass, as previously described [31,32]. For this test, participants started from a stationary position with their dominant leg ready to pedal and they were told that "they had to pedal as fast as they could from the beginning and during the whole duration of the test". Standardized encouragement and feedback were given to the participants by the same experimenter who was blinded to the treatments and who verified that participants remained seated during the test. The seat and handlebar positions were standardized between trials. Both second-by-second and peak power output was calculated and registered throughout the test (SNT Medical, Cardgirus, Barcelona, Spain). In addition, the fatigue index was calculated as the decline from peak power to the lowest power produced during the test.

Perceptual evaluation and side effects. Ten minutes after the end of the Wingate test participants were required to fill out an ad hoc questionnaire that included queries about their self-perceived exertion and muscle power during the tests. This questionnaire included a one- to 10-point scale to assess each item, and participants were previously informed that one point meant minimal and 10 points meant maximal values. Participants were also asked to indicate on a yes/no scale whether they had felt any perceptible effect and to "guess" the substance that they had consumed in that particular experimental trial (e.g., caffeine or placebo). Participants were encouraged to go to bed at their habitual bedtime and to report any sleeping issues during the night. The morning following the experimental trial, participants were required to fill out a questionnaire that has been previously used to assess the perceptible side effects of caffeinated energy drinks in the sports context [17] and laboratory conditions [8]. This questionnaire included information about sleep quality, prevalence of gastrointestinal problems, muscular pain and headache, and self-perception of nervousness or increased activeness.

2.4. Statistical Analysis

Paired *t*-tests were used to determine the statistical significance of the differences between experimental conditions (caffeine vs. placebo), including all participants as a whole group. Two-way ANOVA (experimental treatment × group) with repeated measures were used to determine the statistical significance of the effects produced by the ingestion of caffeine in AA homozygotes and C allele carriers. A non-parametric test for dichotomous variables and related samples (McNemar test) was used to analyze side effects derived from the ingestion of each substance. The significance level was set at $p < 0.05$. The results are presented as means $\pm$ SD.

3. Results

All subjects were identical in $-3860G>A$ (rs2069514) and $-729C>T$ (rs12720461). In $-163C>A$ (rs762551), we obtained two groups: AA homozygotes ($n = 5$) and C-allele carriers ($n = 16$).

In comparison to the placebo, the ingestion of caffeine did not produce any measurable effect during the visual attention test (Table 1). On average, for the four test blocks, the reaction time was similar between placebo and caffeine (282 ± 42 vs. 275 ± 31 ms; $p = 0.31$). The number of errors during the visual attention test was very similar with the placebo and with the caffeine (9.1% vs. 13.6%; $p = 1.00$), and there were no differences between genotype groups in any variable measured during this test.

Table 1. Reaction times in the visual attention test with the ingestion of 3 mg·kg^{-1} of caffeine or a placebo for AA homozygotes and C-allele carriers.

Variable	Placebo	Caffeine	Mean Difference	95% Confidence Interval of the Difference	*p*
Reaction time stage 1 (ms)	275 ± 50	268 ± 39	−7	(−32; 18)	0.580
AA homozygotes	256 ± 58	284 ± 58	28	(−50; 107)	0.337
C allele carriers	280 ± 49	264 ± 34	−16	(−44; 13)	0.259
Reaction time stage 2 (ms)	280 ± 42	276 ± 35	−4	(−21; 13)	0.582
AA homozygotes	296 ± 76	287 ± 54	−9	(−104; 86)	0.780
C allele carriers	276 ± 32	273 ± 31	−3	(−19; 14)	0.725
Reaction time stage 3 (ms)	291 ± 59	278 ± 38	−13	(−36; 9)	0.226
AA homozygotes	304 ± 118	288 ± 66	−16	(−159; 127)	0.745
C allele carriers	288 ± 39	276 ± 30	−12	(−32; 6)	0.178
Reaction time stage 4 (ms)	283 ± 43	276 ± 34	−7	(−20; 7)	0.203
AA homozygotes	286 ± 59	288 ± 51	2	(−55; 59)	0.914
C allele carriers	282 ± 40	274 ± 30	−8	(−23; 6)	0.232
Reaction time Mean (ms)	282 ± 42	275 ± 31	−7.5	(−23; 8)	0.309
AA homozygotes	285 ± 75	287 ± 54	2	(−84; 87)	0.965
C allele carriers	281 ± 33	272 ± 23	−9	(−24; 4)	0.165

Data are mean ± SD for 21 healthy participants: AA homozygotes (*n* = 5) and C-allele carriers (*n* = 16).

Caffeine ingestion increased the mean power output (521 ± 115 W with caffeine vs. 511 ± 113 W with placebo; *p* < 0.001; Figure 1) and the peak power during the Wingate test (680 ± 146 W with caffeine vs. 663 ± 143 W with placebo; *p* = 0.01; Table 2). C-allele carriers had increased mean and peak power with the ingestion of caffeine, while AA homozygotes only increased their peak power significantly with the caffeine (Table 2 and Figure 2). Nevertheless, there were no significant differences for the ergogenic effect of caffeine between AA homozygotes and C-allele carriers, either in the peak power or in the mean power attained during the Wingate test (*p* > 0.05). Caffeine ingestion did not affect the fatigue index reached during the test (*p* = 0.57). The individual responses to caffeine ingestion for mean power attained in the Wingate test are depicted in Figure 3. Most of the AA homozygotes and C-allele carriers obtained greater mean power with caffeine ingestion (Figure 3), although some of them decreased their performance in the trial with caffeine (one AA homozygote and one C-allele carrier). The ingestion of caffeine did not affect the perception of muscle power and exertion during the test (*p* > 0.05; Table 2). Furthermore, the effects of caffeine on self-reported feelings of muscle power and fatigue were not evident in AA homozygotes or C-allele carriers (*p* > 0.05).

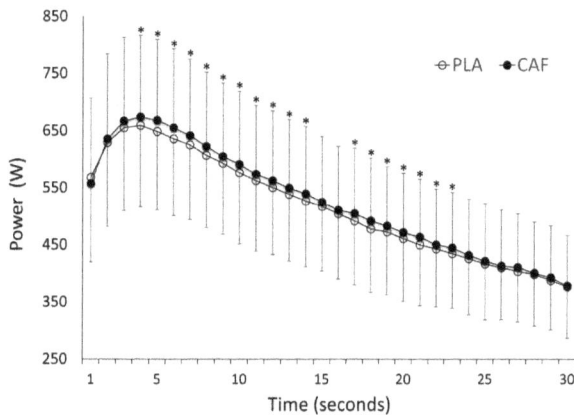

Figure 1. Power output during the Wingate test with the ingestion of caffeine or a placebo. Data are presented as mean ± SD from 21 healthy active participants. (*) Different from placebo condition (*p* < 0.05).

Table 2. Variables obtained during the Wingate test and subjective perception of muscle power and exertion with the ingestion of 3 mg·kg^{-1} of caffeine or a placebo for AA homozygotes and C-allele carriers.

Variable	Placebo	Caffeine	Mean Difference	95% IC for the Difference	*p*
Mean Power (W)	511 ± 113	521 ± 115 *	10	(5.3; 15.0)	0.000
AA homozygotes	494 ± 142	504 ± 140	9	(−0.9; 18.5)	0.120
C allele carriers	516 ± 107	527 ± 110 *	11	(4.6; 16.4)	0.002
Peak Power (W)	663 ± 143	680 ± 146 *	16	(3.7; 29.0)	0.014
AA homozygotes	637 ± 200	646 ± 201	9	(−0.9; 18.5)	0.065
C allele carriers	671 ± 128	690 ± 131 *	19	(1.9; 35.5)	0.031
Fatigue index (%)	44.2 ± 6.8	45.0 ± 7.2	0.8	(−2.0; 3.6)	0.571
AA homozygotes	42.3 ± 6.5	42.2 ± 6.7	−0.1	(−2.1; 1.8)	0.844
C allele carriers	44.8 ± 7.0	45.9 ± 7.3	1.1	(−2.7; 4.8)	0.555
Perceived power	6 ± 2	7 ± 2	1	(−0.3; 1.7)	0.158
AA homozygotes	6 ± 2	7 ± 2	1	(−2.6; 3.8)	0.634
C allele carriers	6 ± 2	7 ± 2	1	(−0.4; 1.9)	0.188
Perceived exertion	6 ± 2	6 ± 2	0	(−0.9; 1.1)	0.836
AA homozygotes	6 ± 1	6 ± 2	0	(−2.2; 3.0)	0.688
C allele carriers	6 ± 2	6 ± 2	0	(−1.2; 1.2)	1.000

Data are mean ± SD for 21 healthy participants: AA homozygotes (*n* = 5) and C-allele carriers (*n* = 16). (*) Different from placebo condition (*p* < 0.05).

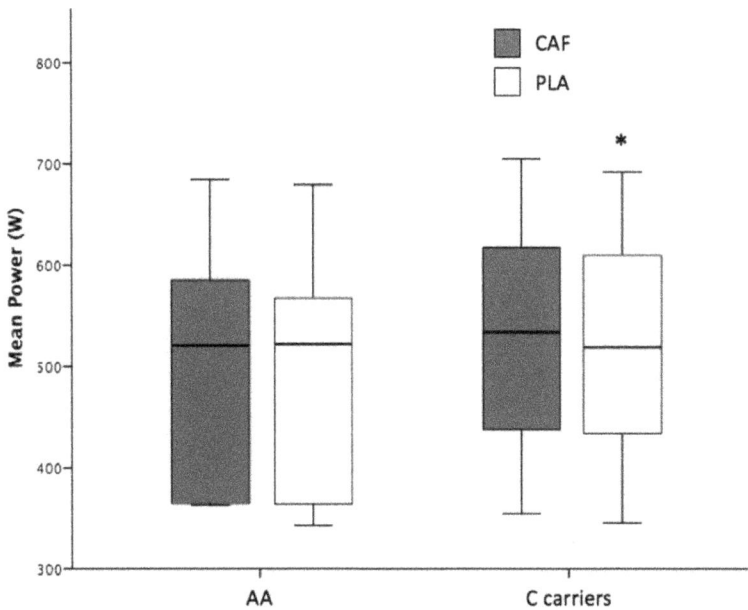

Figure 2. Mean power during the Wingate test with the ingestion of caffeine or a placebo in AA homozygotes (*n* = 5) and C-allele carriers (*n* = 16). (*) Different from placebo condition (*p* < 0.05).

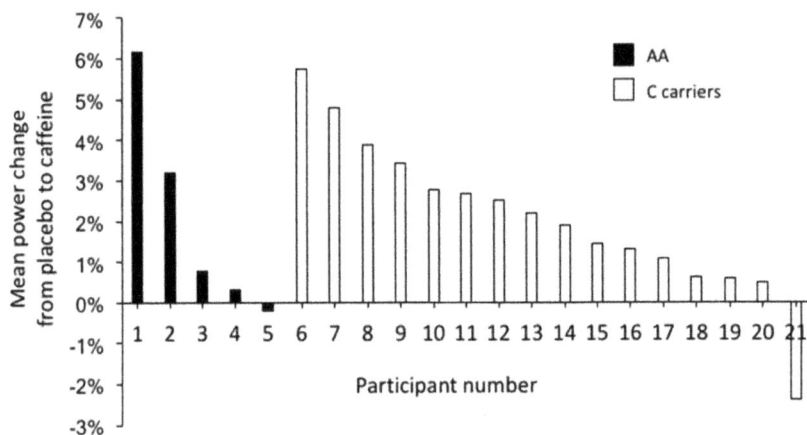

Figure 3. Individual responses during the Wingate test. Performance change from placebo condition to caffeine condition for AA homozygotes (*n* = 5) and C-allele carriers (*n* = 16).

Table 3 depicts the prevalence of side effects after the ingestion of caffeine or a placebo. There were no significant differences in the prevalence of side effects after the ingestion of caffeine and the ingestion of the placebo (Table 3; $p > 0.05$). Although the differences between AA homozygotes and C-allele carriers did not reach statistical significance in any of the side effects analyzed, 31.3% of C-allele carriers reported increased nervousness, while none of the AA homozygotes perceived this side effect.

Table 3. Prevalence of side effects with the ingestion of 3 mg·kg^{-1} of caffeine or a placebo for AA homozygotes and C-allele carriers.

Variable	Placebo Frequency (%)	Caffeine Frequency (%)
Nervousness	1 (4.8)	5 (23.8)
AA homozygotes	1 (20)	0 (0)
C allele carriers	0 (0)	5 (31.3)
Insomnia	3 (14.3)	7 (33.3)
AA homozygotes	0 (0)	2 (40.0)
C allele carriers	3 (18.8)	5 (31.3)
Gastrointestinal problems	0 (0)	3 (14.3)
AA homozygotes	0 (0)	1 (20.0)
C allele carriers	0 (0)	2 (12.5)
Activeness	3 (14.3)	6 (28.6)
AA homozygotes	2 (40.0)	1 (20.0)
C allele carriers	1 (6.3)	5 (31.3)
Irritability	0 (0)	2 (9.5)
AA homozygotes	0 (0)	0 (0)
C allele carriers	0 (0)	2 (12.5)
Muscular pain	4 (19)	3 (14.3)
AA homozygotes	0 (0)	0 (0)
C allele carriers	4 (25.0)	3 (18.8)
Headache	5 (23.8)	4 (19.0)
AA homozygotes	1 (20)	1 (20)
C allele carriers	4 (25.0)	3 (18.8)

Data are the percent of affirmative responses from 21 healthy active participants: AA homozygotes (*n* = 5) and C-allele carriers (*n* = 16).

4. Discussion

The aim of this study was to analyze the influence of genetic variations of the CYP1A2 gene on physical and cognitive ergogenicity derived from the ingestion of a moderate dose of caffeine. For this purpose, we analyzed three typical SNPs (−163C>A, −3860G>A, −729C>T) of the CYP1A2 gene in a group of healthy, active participants. Our data confirm that, for the whole group, 3 mg·kg^{-1} of caffeine was ergogenic during the Wingate test, although this dose of caffeine had no positive effects during a visual attention test. Furthermore, the side effects derived from the ingestion of caffeine were minimal when compared to the ingestion of a placebo. Interestingly, the ergogenic effects in the Wingate test found after caffeine ingestion were similarly present in both AA homozygotes and C-allele carriers of the CYP1A2 −163C>A polymorphism, while the prevalence of side effects in the hours following the caffeine intake were unaffected by the CYP1A2 genotype. All of this information suggests that CYP1A2 genetic variants had minimal influence on the benefits and drawbacks derived from caffeine ingestion, at least when ingested in a moderate dose.

Previous investigations have tried to determine the genetic influence of the CYP1A2 gene on the ergogenic or side effects derived from caffeine ingestion, based on previous reports in which the response to caffeine administration presented significant inter-individual differences [2,21]. However, the results of these pioneer investigations are controversial, at least for the −163C>A variations. Womack, Saunders, Bechtel, Bolton, Martin, Luden, Dunham and Hancock [27] found that trained cyclists with AA homozygosity for this SNP obtained an increased ergogenic effect from caffeine ingestion during a 40 km time trial when compared to the C-allele carrier counterparts. On the contrary, Pataky, Womack, Saunders, Goffe, D'Lugos, El-Sohemy and Luden [28] found that C allele carriers for −163C>A experienced greater ergogenic than AA homozygotes during a 3 km cycling time trial in recreational cyclist. Finally, Algrain, Thomas, Carrillo, Ryan, Kim, Lettan and Ryan [29] found that the ergogenic effect of caffeine did not differ across genotype groups in a 15 min maximal performance ride. Our data are in line with this last investigation because the variations in the −163C>A polymorphism did not affect the ergogenic effect obtained with the ingestion of a moderate dose of caffeine, at least in a short-duration maximal-intensity exercise test such as the 30 s Wingate test.

Caffeine seems to be highly ergogenic for short-term, high-intensity exercise ranging in duration from 60 to 180 s [19]. However, other traditional models examining power output (i.e., the 30 s Wingate test) have shown minimal effect or a failure to improve the performance after caffeine ingestion [19,33,34]. Thus, Goldstein, Ziegenfuss, Kalman, Kreider, Campbell, Wilborn, Taylor, Willoughby, Stout, Graves, Wildman, Ivy, Spano, Smith and Antonio [1] argued that current research is inconsistent when applied to strength and power activities. Magkos and Kavouras [20] reasoned that it may only be due to the difficulties in quantifying performance in such types of exercise, as well as to the minimal potential for improvement. Nevertheless, our data have shown that a dose of 3 mg·kg^{-1} of caffeine improved both peak and mean power during the test. Likewise, recent research has demonstrated an ergogenic effect in power activities, both in lower and upper limb exercises, such as power in half squats or bench presses, jumps, or repeated jumps in 15 s [2,5,8]. This ergogenic effect in anaerobic performance could be due to the influence of caffeine on the Na+/K+ pump, facilitating Na+/K+ATPase activity [19]. However, different researchers [1,19] have stated that the most likely mechanism of action related to caffeine ergogenicity is the inhibitory effect on adenosine, stimulating the central nervous system, thus leading to reduced pain perception while sustaining motor unit firing rates and neuro-excitability [19].

Our investigation is also innovative because it determines the influence of CYP1A2 genetic variants on caffeine ergogenicity during a cognitive-based test and the prevalence of side effects in the hours following its ingestion. Caffeine has been demonstrated to be effective to reduce the reaction time in simple choice tasks with doses of between 32 and 256 mg [10,11,35]. In addition, a dose of 5 mg·kg^{-1} improved the reaction time in non-fatigued conditions (e.g., previous to a simulated taekwondo contest [36]). On the other hand, Jacobson and Edgley [37] tested two different doses of caffeine, 300 and 600 mg, finding that only the lower dose of caffeine improved the reaction time.

In that investigation, the participants' mean body mass was 73 kg; thus, the doses investigated were ~4.1 mg·kg^{-1} and ~8.2 mg·kg^{-1}. Crowe et al. [38] found that caffeine did not improve cognitive performance (reaction time) when ingested at a higher dose (6 mg·kg^{-1} of caffeine). In the current investigation, the ingestion of caffeine was not effective to reduce the reaction time. Additionally, neither AA homozygotes nor C-allele carriers obtained reduced reaction times with the ingestion of caffeine. In any case, there is more information to determine the contradictory results found when testing caffeine in reaction time tests.

Previous research has shown that caffeine ingestion increased the prevalence of side effects, such as insomnia and nervousness [17]. The negative effect of caffeine on sleep quality has been mostly found in investigations in which caffeine was provided in the afternoon with less than six hours from caffeine ingestion to the onset of bedtime [4,39]. In this investigation, caffeine was provided in the afternoon, with ~7 h between ingestion and bedtime. However, there was no reported increased prevalence of insomnia (Table 3). The same as with the ergogenic effect of caffeine ingestion on physical performance, we expected an inter-individual variability in the prevalence of these adverse effects, especially related to the genetic variations of CYP1A2. We speculated that AA homozygotes would have faster caffeine metabolism, and so the effect on sleep quality could be minimized in subjects with this genetic variation. Nevertheless, our data showed that both AA homozygotes and C-allele carriers of the −163C>A polymorphism responded in a similar manner in the prevalence of insomnia.

The outcomes of the present investigation suggest that other individual factors must be responsible for the inter-individual differences in response to caffeine ingestion, such as other genes or other gene combinations. As caffeine ergogenicity has been mostly associated with the blockage of the "fatiguing" action of adenosine on its receptors, and variations of ADORA2A have been suggested as an explanation for the individual sensitivity to caffeine effects on sleep, anxiety, and cognitive performance [12,40,41]. However, there is no investigation that has determined the effect of ADORA2A polymorphisms on the ergogenicity of caffeine during exercise or sports activities.

This pilot study presents some limitations that might be discussed to improve the understanding of the outcomes. First, the sample size was small, which limits the generalization of the outcomes, especially for the AA homozygotes group. Second, the study sample included men and women; one might argue that the women's menstrual cycle could have interfered in the outcomes of the study. However, previous research has found that physiological/performance responses to caffeine ingestion are of similar magnitude for men and women [42], while perceived ergogenicity and the prevalence of side effects are also comparable between sexes [17]. Third, the dose used in the current study was moderate (3 mg·kg^{-1} of caffeine) and it is still possible that higher doses produce different ergogenic responses in AA homozygotes and C-allele carriers. Despite these limitations, we believe that this investigation provides new insights regarding the effect of the CYP1A2 genetic variants on the ergogenic effects of caffeine.

5. Conclusions

In summary, AA homozygotes and C-allele carriers for the CYP1A2 −163C>A SNP obtained an ergogenic effect of similar magnitude after the ingestion of 3 mg·kg^{-1} of caffeine: both groups of participants enhanced the power attained during the Wingate test, although this substance did not improve performance during a visual attention test. On the other hand, the ingestion of this dose of caffeine did not significantly influence the prevalence of side effects in the hours following the administration. Thus, the genetic variations of the CYP1A2 gene did not affect the ergogenicity or drawbacks derived from the ingestion of a moderate dose of caffeine (e.g., 3 mg·kg^{-1}). Further research is warranted to explain the inter-individual differences derived from caffeine ingestion and to elucidate the mechanism related to the existence of non-caffeine responders.

Acknowledgments: The authors wish to thank the subjects for their invaluable contribution to the study. The study was part of the CAFEGEN project financed by Ayudas a la Investigación Vicerrectorado Investigación from the Camilo Jose Cela University. This grant includes funds for covering the costs to publish in open access.

Author Contributions: J.J.S., B.L. and J.D.C. conceived and designed the experiments; J.J.S., B.L., D.R.V., C.G.S., C.P.T. and F.A. performed the experiments; J.D.C. prepared the caffeine doses and preserved the double-blind design; J.J.S., T.P. and B.L. analyzed the data; T.P. and J.D.C. contributed reagents/materials/analysis tools; J.J.S. and J.D.C. wrote the paper; all authors revised the manuscript.

Conflicts of Interest: The authors declare no conflict of interest.

References

1. Goldstein, E.R.; Ziegenfuss, T.; Kalman, D.; Kreider, R.; Campbell, B.; Wilborn, C.; Taylor, L.; Willoughby, D.; Stout, J.; Graves, B.S.; et al. International society of sports nutrition position stand: Caffeine and performance. *J. Int. Soc. Sports Nutr.* **2010**, *7*, 5. [CrossRef] [PubMed]

2. Lara, B.; Ruiz-Vicente, D.; Areces, F.; Abian-Vicen, J.; Salinero, J.J.; Gonzalez-Millan, C.; Gallo-Salazar, C.; Del Coso, J. Acute consumption of a caffeinated energy drink enhances aspects of performance in sprint swimmers. *Br. J. Nutr.* **2015**, *114*, 908–914. [CrossRef] [PubMed]

3. Del Coso, J.; Ramirez, J.A.; Munoz, G.; Portillo, J.; Gonzalez-Millan, C.; Munoz, V.; Barbero-Alvarez, J.C.; Munoz-Guerra, J. Caffeine-containing energy drink improves physical performance of elite rugby players during a simulated match. *Appl. Physiol. Nutr. Metab.* **2013**, *38*, 368–374. [CrossRef] [PubMed]

4. Lara, B.; Gonzalez-Millan, C.; Salinero, J.J.; Abian-Vicen, J.; Areces, F.; Barbero-Alvarez, J.C.; Munoz, V.; Portillo, L.J.; Gonzalez-Rave, J.M.; Del Coso, J. Caffeine-containing energy drink improves physical performance in female soccer players. *Amino Acids* **2014**, *46*, 1385–1392. [CrossRef] [PubMed]

5. Perez-Lopez, A.; Salinero, J.J.; Abian-Vicen, J.; Valades, D.; Lara, B.; Hernandez, C.; Areces, F.; Gonzalez, C.; Del Coso, J. Caffeinated energy drinks improve volleyball performance in elite female players. *Med. Sci. Sports Exerc.* **2015**, *47*, 850–856. [CrossRef] [PubMed]

6. Pitchford, N.W.; Fell, J.W.; Leveritt, M.D.; Desbrow, B.; Shing, C.M. Effect of caffeine on cycling time-trial performance in the heat. *J. Sci. Med. Sport* **2014**, *17*, 445–449. [CrossRef] [PubMed]

7. Hodgson, A.B.; Randell, R.K.; Jeukendrup, A.E. The metabolic and performance effects of caffeine compared to coffee during endurance exercise. *PLoS ONE* **2013**, *8*, e59561. [CrossRef] [PubMed]

8. Del Coso, J.; Salinero, J.J.; Gonzalez-Millan, C.; Abian-Vicen, J.; Perez-Gonzalez, B. Dose response effects of a caffeine-containing energy drink on muscle performance: A repeated measures design. *J. Int. Soc. Sports Nutr.* **2012**, *9*, 21. [CrossRef] [PubMed]

9. Duncan, M.J.; Stanley, M.; Parkhouse, N.; Cook, K.; Smith, M. Acute caffeine ingestion enhances strength performance and reduces perceived exertion and muscle pain perception during resistance exercise. *Eur. J. Sport Sci.* **2013**, *13*, 392–399. [CrossRef] [PubMed]

10. Giles, G.E.; Mahoney, C.R.; Brunye, T.T.; Gardony, A.L.; Taylor, H.A.; Kanarek, R.B. Differential cognitive effects of energy drink ingredients: Caffeine, taurine, and glucose. *Pharmacol. Biochem. Behav.* **2012**, *102*, 569–577. [CrossRef] [PubMed]

11. Haskell, C.F.; Kennedy, D.O.; Wesnes, K.A.; Scholey, A.B. Cognitive and mood improvements of caffeine in habitual consumers and habitual non-consumers of caffeine. *Psychopharmacology* **2005**, *179*, 813–825. [CrossRef] [PubMed]

12. Renda, G.; Committeri, G.; Zimarino, M.; Di Nicola, M.; Tatasciore, A.; Ruggieri, B.; Ambrosini, E.; Viola, V.; Antonucci, I.; Stuppia, L.; et al. Genetic determinants of cognitive responses to caffeine drinking identified from a double-blind, randomized, controlled trial. *Eur. Neuropsychopharmacol.* **2015**, *25*, 798–807. [CrossRef] [PubMed]

13. Lieberman, H.R.; Tharion, W.J.; Shukitt-Hale, B.; Speckman, K.L.; Tulley, R. Effects of caffeine, sleep loss, and stress on cognitive performance and mood during US Navy seal training. Sea-air-land. *Psychopharmacology* **2002**, *164*, 250–261. [CrossRef] [PubMed]

14. McLellan, T.M.; Kamimori, G.H.; Voss, D.M.; Bell, D.G.; Cole, K.G.; Johnson, D. Caffeine maintains vigilance and improves run times during night operations for special forces. *Aviat Space Environ. Med.* **2005**, *76*, 647–654. [PubMed]

15. McLellan, T.M.; Kamimori, G.H.; Voss, D.M.; Tate, C.; Smith, S.J. Caffeine effects on physical and cognitive performance during sustained operations. *Aviat Space Environ. Med.* **2007**, *78*, 871–877. [PubMed]

16. Hogervorst, E.; Bandelow, S.; Schmitt, J.; Jentjens, R.; Oliveira, M.; Allgrove, J.; Carter, T.; Gleeson, M. Caffeine improves physical and cognitive performance during exhaustive exercise. *Med. Sci. Sports Exerc.* **2008**, *40*, 1841–1851. [CrossRef] [PubMed]

17. Salinero, J.J.; Lara, B.; Abian-Vicen, J.; Gonzalez-Millan, C.; Areces, F.; Gallo-Salazar, C.; Ruiz-Vicente, D.; Del Coso, J. The use of energy drinks in sport: Perceived ergogenicity and side effects in male and female athletes. *Br. J. Nutr.* **2014**, *112*, 1494–1502. [CrossRef] [PubMed]

18. Tarnopolsky, M.A. Caffeine and creatine use in sport. *Ann. Nutr. Metab.* **2010**, *57*, 1–8. [CrossRef] [PubMed]

19. Davis, J.K.; Green, J.M. Caffeine and anaerobic performance: Ergogenic value and mechanisms of action. *Sports Med.* **2009**, *39*, 813–832. [CrossRef] [PubMed]

20. Magkos, F.; Kavouras, S.A. Caffeine use in sports, pharmacokinetics in man, and cellular mechanisms of action. *Crit. Rev. Food Sci. Nutr.* **2005**, *45*, 535–562. [CrossRef] [PubMed]

21. Skinner, T.L.; Jenkins, D.G.; Coombes, J.S.; Taaffe, D.R.; Leveritt, M.D. Dose response of caffeine on 2000-m rowing performance. *Med. Sci. Sports Exerc.* **2010**, *42*, 571–576. [CrossRef] [PubMed]

22. Meyers, B.M.; Cafarelli, E. Caffeine increases time to fatigue by maintaining force and not by altering firing rates during submaximal isometric contractions. *J. Appl. Physiol.* **2005**, *99*, 1056–1063. [CrossRef] [PubMed]

23. Doherty, M.; Smith, P.M.; Davison, R.C.; Hughes, M.G. Caffeine is ergogenic after supplementation of oral creatine monohydrate. *Med. Sci. Sports Exerc.* **2002**, *34*, 1785–1792. [CrossRef] [PubMed]

24. Perera, V.; Gross, A.S.; McLachlan, A.J. Measurement of CYP1A2 activity: A focus on caffeine as a probe. *Curr. Drug Metab.* **2012**, *13*, 667–678. [CrossRef] [PubMed]

25. Ghotbi, R.; Christensen, M.; Roh, H.K.; Ingelman-Sundberg, M.; Aklillu, E.; Bertilsson, L. Comparisons of CYP1A2 genetic polymorphisms, enzyme activity and the genotype-phenotype relationship in Swedes and Koreans. *Eur. J. Clin. Pharmacol.* **2007**, *63*, 537–546. [CrossRef] [PubMed]

26. Djordjevic, N.; Ghotbi, R.; Jankovic, S.; Aklillu, E. Induction of CYP1A2 by heavy coffee consumption is associated with the CYP1A2 -163C>A polymorphism. *Eur. J. Clin. Pharmacol.* **2010**, *66*, 697–703. [CrossRef] [PubMed]

27. Womack, C.J.; Saunders, M.J.; Bechtel, M.K.; Bolton, D.J.; Martin, M.; Luden, N.D.; Dunham, W.; Hancock, M. The influence of a CYP1A2 polymorphism on the ergogenic effects of caffeine. *J. Int. Soc. Sports Nutr.* **2012**, *9*, 7. [CrossRef] [PubMed]

28. Pataky, M.W.; Womack, C.J.; Saunders, M.J.; Goffe, J.L.; D'Lugos, A.C.; El-Sohemy, A.; Luden, N.D. Caffeine and 3-km cycling performance: Effects of mouth rinsing, genotype, and time of day. *Scand. J. Med. Sci. Sports* **2016**, *26*, 613–619. [CrossRef] [PubMed]

29. Algrain, H.; Thomas, R.; Carrillo, A.; Ryan, E.; Kim, C.; Lettan, R.; Ryan, E. The effects of a polymorphism in the cytochrome p450 CYP1A2 gene on performance enhancement with caffeine in recreational cyclists. *J. Caffeine Res.* **2015**, *6*, 1–6.

30. Armstrong, L.E. Caffeine, body fluid-electrolyte balance, and exercise performance. *Int. J. Sport Nutr. Exerc. Metab.* **2002**, *12*, 189–206. [CrossRef] [PubMed]

31. Attia, A.; Hachana, Y.; Chaabene, H.; Gaddour, A.; Neji, Z.; Shephard, R.J.; Chelly, M.S. Reliability and validity of a 20-s alternative to the wingate anaerobic test in team sport male athletes. *PLoS ONE* **2014**, *9*, e114444. [CrossRef] [PubMed]

32. Bar-Or, O. The wingate anaerobic test. An update on methodology, reliability and validity. *Sports Med.* **1987**, *4*, 381–394. [CrossRef] [PubMed]

33. Collomp, K.; Ahmaidi, S.; Audran, M.; Chanal, J.L.; Prefaut, C. Effects of caffeine ingestion on performance and anaerobic metabolism during the wingate test. *Int. J. Sports Med.* **1991**, *12*, 439–443. [CrossRef] [PubMed]

34. Greer, F.; McLean, C.; Graham, T.E. Caffeine, performance, and metabolism during repeated wingate exercise tests. *J. Appl. Physiol.* **1998**, *85*, 1502–1508. [PubMed]

35. Lieberman, H.R.; Wurtman, R.J.; Emde, G.G.; Roberts, C.; Coviella, I.L. The effects of low doses of caffeine on human performance and mood. *Psychopharmacology* **1987**, *92*, 308–312. [CrossRef] [PubMed]

36. Santos, V.G.; Santos, V.R.; Felippe, L.J.; Almeida, J.W., Jr.; Bertuzzi, R.; Kiss, M.A.; Lima-Silva, A.E. Caffeine reduces reaction time and improves performance in simulated-contest of taekwondo. *Nutrients* **2014**, *6*, 637–649. [CrossRef] [PubMed]

37. Jacobson, B.H.; Edgley, B.M. Effects of caffeine on simple reaction time and movement time. *Aviat Space Environ. Med.* **1987**, *58*, 1153–1156. [PubMed]

38. Crowe, M.J.; Leicht, A.S.; Spinks, W.L. Physiological and cognitive responses to caffeine during repeated, high-intensity exercise. *Int. J. Sport Nutr. Exerc. Metab.* **2006**, *16*, 528–544. [CrossRef] [PubMed]

39. Del Coso, J.; Portillo, J.; Munoz, G.; Abian-Vicen, J.; Gonzalez-Millan, C.; Munoz-Guerra, J. Caffeine-containing energy drink improves sprint performance during an international rugby sevens competition. *Amino Acids* **2013**, *44*, 1511–1519. [CrossRef] [PubMed]

40. Retey, J.V.; Adam, M.; Khatami, R.; Luhmann, U.F.; Jung, H.H.; Berger, W.; Landolt, H.P. A genetic variation in the adenosine A2A receptor gene (adora2a) contributes to individual sensitivity to caffeine effects on sleep. *Clin. Pharmacol. Ther.* **2007**, *81*, 692–698. [CrossRef] [PubMed]

41. Alsene, K.; Deckert, J.; Sand, P.; de Wit, H. Association between A2A receptor gene polymorphisms and caffeine-induced anxiety. *Neuropsychopharmacology* **2003**, *28*, 1694–1702. [CrossRef] [PubMed]

42. Kashuba, A.D.; Bertino, J.S., Jr.; Kearns, G.L.; Leeder, J.S.; James, A.W.; Gotschall, R.; Nafziger, A.N. Quantitation of three-month intraindividual variability and influence of sex and menstrual cycle phase on CYP1A2, N-acetyltransferase-2, and xanthine oxidase activity determined with caffeine phenotyping. *Clin. Pharmacol. Ther.* **1998**, *63*, 540–551. [CrossRef]

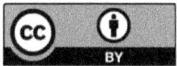

nutrients

MDPI

Article

High Fat Diets Sex-Specifically Affect the Renal Transcriptome and Program Obesity, Kidney Injury, and Hypertension in the Offspring

You-Lin Tain [1,2], Yu-Ju Lin [3], Jiunn-Ming Sheen [1], Hong-Ren Yu [1], Mao-Meng Tiao [1], Chih-Cheng Chen [1], Ching-Chou Tsai [3], Li-Tung Huang [1,4] and Chien-Ning Hsu [5,6,*]

[1] Department of Pediatrics, Kaohsiung Chang Gung Memorial Hospital and Chang Gung University College of Medicine, Kaohsiung 833, Taiwan; tainyl@hotmail.com (Y.-L.T.); ray.sheen@gmail.com (J.-M.S.); yuu2004taiwan@yahoo.com.tw (H.-R.Y.); tmm@cgmh.org.tw (M.-M.T.); charllysc@cgmh.org.tw (C.-C.C.); litung.huang@gmail.com (L.-T.H.)

[2] Institute for Translational Research in Biomedicine, Kaohsiung Chang Gung Memorial Hospital and Chang Gung University College of Medicine, Kaohsiung 833, Taiwan

[3] Department of Obstetrics and Gynecology, Kaohsiung Chang Gung Memorial Hospital and Chang Gung University College of Medicine, Kaohsiung 833, Taiwan; lyu015ster@gmail.com (Y.-J.L.); nick@cgmh.org.tw (C.-C.T.)

[4] Department of Traditional Chinese Medicine, Chang Gung University, Linkow 244, Taiwan

[5] Department of Pharmacy, Kaohsiung Chang Gung Memorial Hospital, Kaohsiung 833, Taiwan

[6] School of Pharmacy, Kaohsiung Medical University, Kaohsiung 807, Taiwan

* Correspondence: chien_ning_hsu@hotmail.com; Tel.: +886-975-368-975; Fax: +886-7733-8009

Received: 19 February 2017; Accepted: 24 March 2017; Published: 3 April 2017

Abstract: Obesity and related disorders have increased concurrently with an increased consumption of saturated fatty acids. We examined whether post-weaning high fat (HF) diet would exacerbate offspring vulnerability to maternal HF-induced programmed hypertension and kidney disease sex-specifically, with a focus on the kidney. Next, we aimed to elucidate the gene–diet interactions that contribute to maternal HF-induced renal programming using the next generation RNA sequencing (NGS) technology. Female Sprague-Dawley rats received either a normal diet (ND) or HF diet (D12331, Research Diets) for five weeks before the delivery. The offspring of both sexes were put on either the ND or HF diet from weaning to six months of age, resulting in four groups of each sex (maternal diet/post-weaning diet; $n = 5$–7/group): ND/ND, ND/HF, HF/ND, and HF/HF. Post-weaning HF diet increased bodyweights of both ND/HF and HF/HF animals from three to six months only in males. Post-weaning HF diet increased systolic blood pressure in male and female offspring, irrespective of whether they were exposed to maternal HF or not. Male HF/HF offspring showed greater degrees of glomerular and tubular injury compared to the ND/ND group. Our NGS data showed that maternal HF diet significantly altered renal transcriptome with female offspring being more HF-sensitive. HF diet induced hypertension and renal injury are associated with oxidative stress, activation of renin-angiotensin system, and dysregulated sodium transporters and circadian clock. Post-weaning HF diet sex-specifically exacerbates the development of obesity, kidney injury, but not hypertension programmed by maternal HF intake. Better understanding of the sex-dependent mechanisms that underlie HF-induced renal programming will help develop a novel personalized dietary intervention to prevent obesity and related disorders.

Keywords: clock gene; developmental origins of health and disease (DOHaD); high-fat diet; hypertension; next generation sequencing; nitric oxide; kidney disease; oxidative stress; renin-angiotensin system

---

1. Introduction

The growing prevalence of obesity has a profound impact on worldwide health, including risk of hypertension and kidney disease. Obesity may originate from the early life. Pre- and post-natal nutrition together influence developmental programming, leading to disease in adulthood [1]. Obesity and related disorders have increased concurrently with an increased consumption of saturated fatty acids [2]. High-fat (HF) diets have been generally used to generate animal models for obesity and related disorders [3–5]. In this regard, maternal HF intake leads to a variety of chronic diseases in adult offspring, including obesity, hypertension, and kidney disease [3,4,6,7].

The kidney controls blood pressure (BP) and plays a crucial role in the development of hypertension [8], thus renal programming is considered a key mechanism for programmed hypertension and kidney disease [8–11]. A number of mechanisms have been proposed to interpret renal programming, including oxidative stress, inappropriate activation of the renin-angiotensin system (RAS), and impaired tubular sodium handling [8–11]. Additionally, renal circadian clocks are involved in the sodium balance and BP control [12]. Disturbances of circadian clocks increase the risk of a variety of metabolic diseases [13]. Despite a previous study showing that HF diet causes dysregulated circadian clock in the liver and kidney [14], exactly how the circadian clock is programmed by maternal and post-weaning HF intake is unclear. Given that HF diet has been reported to mediate oxidative stress, RAS, sodium transporters, and circadian clock [5,14–16], we hypothesized that post-weaning HF intake enhances offspring vulnerability to maternal HF-induced programmed hypertension and kidney disease via mediating these mechanisms described above.

Sex differences have been observed in obesity, hypertension, and kidney disease [17–19]. However, it is unclear whether sex differences exist in maternal HF plus post-weaning HF consumption induced hypertension and kidney injury. Previously, our study showed that prenatal dexamethasone induced programmed hypertension and alterations of renal transcriptome in a sex-specific manner [20]. Additionally, we demonstrated that post-weaning HF diet exacerbated hypertension programmed by early dexamethasone exposure in adult male offspring [21]. However, to what extent maternal HF diet adversely affects the kidney to post-weaning HF intake in adult offspring and whether there exists sex-specific susceptibility is unclear. Although nutrigenetics and nutrigenomics have been introduced to understand existing interactions between genes and diets [22,23], very limited studies have analyzed the transcriptome of the offspring kidneys in response to maternal diets and examined their relationships to programmed hypertension and kidney disease [24,25]. We, hence, further employed the whole-genome RNA next-generation sequencing (NGS) to quantify the abundance of RNA transcripts in the one-week-old offspring kidney from maternal exposure to HF diet.

2. Materials and Methods

2.1. Experimental Design

This study was carried out in strict accordance with the recommendations of the Guide for the Care and Use of Laboratory Animals of the National Institutes of Health. The protocol was approved by the Institutional Animal Care and Use Committee of the Kaohsiung Chang Gung Memorial Hospital. Virgin Sprague-Dawley (SD) rats (BioLASCO Taiwan Co., Ltd., Taipei, Taiwan) were housed and maintained in a facility accredited by the Association for Assessment and Accreditation of Laboratory Animal Care International. International. The rats were exposed to a 12 h light/12 h dark cycle. Male SD rats were caged with female rats until mating was confirmed by examining vaginal plug.

Female rats were weight-matched and assigned to receive either a normal diet with regular rat chow (ND; Fwusow Taiwan Co., Ltd., Taichung, Taiwan; 52% carbohydrates, 23.5% protein, 4.5% fat, 10% ash, and 8% fiber) or high-fat hypercaloric diet (HF; D12331, Research Diets, Inc., New Brunswick, NJ, USA; 58% fat (hydrogenated coconut oil) plus high sucrose (25% carbohydrate)) ad libitum for 5 weeks before mating and during gestation and lactation. After birth, litters were culled to give equal numbers of males and females for a total of eight pups to standardize the received quantity of milk and maternal pup care. Three male and three female offspring from each group (control and HF) were killed at 1 week of age. Their kidneys were isolated for NGS analysis. The remaining offspring were assigned to four experimental groups of each sex (maternal diet/post-weaning diet; n = 5–7/group): ND/ND, ND/HF, HF/ND, and HF/HF. The offspring of both sexes were weaned at 3 weeks of age, and onto either the normal diet (ND) or HF diet ad libitum from weaning to 6 months of age. BP was measured in conscious rats at 4, 8, 12, 16, 20, and 24 weeks of age by using an indirect tail-cuff method (BP-2000, Visitech Systems, Inc., Apex, NC, USA) after systematically trained. To ensure accuracy and reproducibility, the rats were acclimated to restraint and tail-cuff inflation for 1 week before the experiment, and measurements were taken at 1:00 PM to 5:00 PM each day. Rats were placed on the specimen platform, and their tails were passed through tail cuffs and secured in place with tape. After a 10-minute warm up period, 10 preliminary cycles were performed to allow the rats to adjust to the inflating cuff. For each rat, 5 measurements were recorded at each time point as previously described [20]. Three stable consecutive measures were taken and averaged.

At 6 months of age, offspring were sacrificed in the early light phase of the light–dark cycle. Rats were anesthetized by intraperitoneally injecting ketamine (50 mg/kg body weight) and xylazine (10 mg/kg body weight) and were euthanized by intraperitoneally injecting an overdose of pentobarbital. The midline of the abdomen was opened. The aorta was cannulated with a 20–23-gauge butterfly needle, blood samples were collected, the vena cava was cut, and PBS was perfused until the kidneys were blanched. Kidneys were harvested after perfusion, divided into cortex and medulla, and stored at −80 °C for further analysis.

2.2. Biochemical Analysis

The blood concentrations of total cholesterol, high-density lipoprotein (HDL), triglyceride, glucose, and aspartate transaminase (AST) and alanine aminotransferase (ALT) activities were determined by a standard autoanalyzer (Hitachi model 7450, Tokyo, Japan). Intraperitoneal glucose tolerance test (IPGTT) was performed as previously described [26]. After an 8-h fast, blood samples were collected at five time points: before injection and at 15, 30, 60, and 120 min after the intraperitoneal injection of glucose (2 g/kg body weight). Plasma glucose levels were immediately measured using the enzymatic (hexokinase) method with a glucose assay kit. Plasma NOx ($NO^- + NO3^-$) levels were measured by the Griess reaction as previously described [27].

2.3. Histology and Morphometric Study

Histology was performed on 4 μm sections of formalin-fixed kidney, blocked in paraffin wax and stained with periodic acid-Schiff (PAS). The level of renal injury was assessed on a blinded basis by calculating glomerular and tubulointerstitial injuries that we described previously [27]. Up to one hundred glomeruli were scored based on the 0 to 4+ injury scale, to calculate the glomerular injury score. Tubulointerstitial injury (TI) scores were based on the presence of tubular cellularity, basement membrane thickening, dilation, atrophy, sloughing, or interstitial widening. TI scores were graded as follows: 0, no changes; grade 1, <10% TI involvement; grade 2, 10%–25% TI involvement; grade 3, 25%–50% TI involvement; grade 4, 50%–75% TI involvement; and grade 5, 75%–100% TI involvement.

2.4. Detection of L-arginine, L-citrulline, ADMA, and SDMA by HPLC

Plasma L-arginine, L-citrulline, and asymmetric dimethylarginine (ADMA, an endogenous inhibitor of nitric oxide synthase) levels were measured using high-performance liquid chromatography (HP series 1100; Agilent Technologies Inc., Santa Clara, CA, USA) with the o-phtalaldehyde-3-mercaptoprionic acid derivatization reagent described previously [28]. Standards contained concentrations of 1–100 mM L-arginine, 1–100 mM L-citrulline, 0.5–5 mM ADMA, and 0.5–5 mM SDMA. The recovery rate was approximately 95%.

2.5. Next-Generation Sequencing and Analysis

As we described previously [24], kidney cortex samples (n = 3/group) were pooled for whole-genome RNA NGS analysis and performed by Welgene Biotech Co., Ltd. (Taipei, Taiwan). All procedures were performed according to the Illumina protocol. For all samples, library construction was performed using the TruSeq RNA Sample Prep Kit v2 for ~160 bp (single-end) sequencing and the Solexa platform. Gene expression was quantified as fragment per kilobase of exon per million mapped fragment (FPKM). Cufflink v 2.1.1 and CummeRbund v 2.0.0 (Illumina Inc., San Diego, CA, USA) were used to perform statistical analyses of the gene expression profiles. Gene Ontology (GO) term enrichment and fold enrichment or depletion for gene lists of significantly up- and down regulated genes in kidney were determined. The reference genome and gene annotations were retrieved from Ensembl database. GO analysis for significant genes was performed using Kyoto Encyclopedia of Genes and Genomes (KEGG) and NIH DAVID Bioinformatics Resources 6.8 (NIH, Bethesda, MD, USA) to identify regulated biological themes [29].

2.6. Quantitative Real-time Polymerase Chain Reaction (PCR)

RNA was extracted using TRIzol reagent treated with DNase I (Ambion, Austin, TX, USA) to remove DNA contamination, and reverse transcribed with random primers (Invitrogen, Carlsbad, CA, USA) [28]. RNA concentration and quality were checked by measuring optical density at 260 and 280 nm. The complementary DNA (cDNA) product was synthesized using a MMLV Reverse Transcriptase (Invitrogen). Two-step quantitative real-time PCR was conducted using the QuantiTect SYBR Green PCR Kit (Qiagen, Valencia, CA, USA) and the iCycler iQ Multi-color Real-Time PCR Detection System (Bio-Rad, Hercules, CA, USA). First, the kidney fibrotic markers, extracellular matrix collagen I and α-smooth muscle actin (α-SMA) were analyzed. Next, components of RAS analyzed in this study included renin (*Ren*); (pro)renin receptor (*Atp6ap2*), angiotensinogen (*Agt*), angiotensin converting enzyme-1 and -2 (*Ace* and *Ace2*), angiotensin II type 1 and 2 receptor (*Agtr1a* and *Agtr2*), and angiotensin (1–7) receptor *Mas1*. Moreover, several core clock genes in the feedback loop were studied, including *Clock* and *Bmal1* of the positive limb; and *Cry1*, *Cry2*, *Per1*, *Per2*, and *Per3* of the negative limb. In addition to these, other clock genes or clock-controlled genes, such as *Ck1e* and *Nr1d1* were analyzed. The 18S rRNA gene (*Rn18s*) was used as a reference. Sequences of primers used in this study are provided in Table 1. All samples were run in duplicate. To quantify the relative gene expression, the comparative threshold cycle (CT) method was employed. For each sample, the average CT value was subtracted from the corresponding average r18S value, calculating the ΔCT. ΔΔCT was calculated by subtracting the average control ΔCT value from the average experimental ΔCT. The fold-increase of the experimental sample relative to the control was calculated using the formula $2^{-\Delta\Delta CT}$.

2.7. Western Blot

Western blot analysis was performed as previously described [28]. Sodium hydrogen exchanger type 3 (NHE3), Na$^+$/Cl$^-$ cotransporter (NCC), Na-K-2Cl cotransporter (NKCC2), and Na$^+$/K$^+$-ATPase a 1 subunit (NaKATPase) were analyzed by incubating the samples overnight with the following antibodies: rabbit anti-rat antibody for NHE3 (1:1000 dilution; Alpha Diagnostic Intl Inc., San Antonio, TX, USA), rabbit anti-rat antibody for NCC (1:2000 dilution; Merck Millipore, Billerica, MA, USA), rabbit anti-rat antibody for NKCC2 (1:1000 dilution; Alpha Diagnostic Intl Inc.), and mouse antibody for NaKATPase (1:10,000 dilution; Abcam, Cambridge, MA, USA). Bands of interest were visualized using ECL reagents (PerkinElmer, Waltham, MA, USA) and quantified by densitometry (Quantity One Analysis software; Bio-Rad), as integrated optical density (IOD) after subtraction of background. The IOD was factored for Ponceau red staining to correct for any variations in total protein loading. The protein abundance was represented as IOD/PonS.

Table 1. Quantitative real-time polymerase chain reaction primers sequences.

Gene	Forward	Reverse
Collagen I	5 aggcataaagggtcatcgtg 3	5 accgttgagtccatctttgc 3
α-SMA	5 gaccctgaagtatccgatagaaca 3	5 cacgcgaagctcgttatagaag 3
Ren	5 aacattaccagggcaactttcact 3	5 accccttcatggtgatctg 3
Atp6ap2	5 gaggcagtgaccctcaacat 3	5 ccctcctcacacaacaaggt 3
Agt	5 gcccaggtcgcgatgat 3	5 tgtacaagatgctgagtgaggcaa 3
Ace	5 caccggcaaggtctgctt 3	5 cttggcatagtttcgtgaggaa 3
Ace2	5 acccttcttacatcagccctactg 3	5 tgtccaaaacctaccccacatat 3
Agtr1a	5 gctgggcaacgagtttgtct 3	5 cagtccttcagctggatcttca 3
Agtr1b	5 caatctggctgtggctgactt 3	5 tgcacatcacaggtccaaaga 3
Mas1	5 catctctcctctcggctttgtg 3	5 cctcatccggaagcaaagg 3
Clock	5 ccactgtacaatacgatggtgatctc 3	5 tgcggcatactggatggaat3
Bmal1	5 attccagggggaaccaga 3	5 gaaggtgatgaccctcttatcct 3
Per1	5 gcttgtgtggactgtggtagca 3	5 gccccaatccatccagttgt 3
Per2	5 catctgccacctcagactca 3	5 ctggtgtgacttgtatcactgct 3
Per3	5 tggccacagcatcagtaca 3	5 tacactgctggcactgcttc 3
Cry1	5 atcgtgcgcatttcacatac 3	5 tccgccattgagttctatgat 3
Cry2	5 gggagcatcagcaacacag 3	5 gcttccagcttgcgtttg 3
Ck1e	5 gcctctatcaacacccacct 3	5 ggagcccaggttgaagtaca 3
Nr1d1	5 ctactggctccctcacccagga 3	5 gacactcggctgctgtcttcca 3
Rn18s	5 gccgcggtaattccagctcca 3	5 cccgcccgctcccaagatc 3

α-SMA = α-smooth muscle actin, Ren = Renin, Atp6ap2 = Prorenin receptor (PRR), Agt = Angiotensinogen (AGT), Ace = Angiotensin converting enzyme (ACE), Ace2 = Angiotensin converting enzyme-2 (ACE2), Agtr1a = Angiotensin II type 1 receptor (AT1R), Agtr2 = Angiotensin II type 2 receptor (AT2R), Clock = Circadian locomotor output cycles kaput, Bmal1 = Brain and muscle aryl-hydrocarbon receptor nuclear translocator-like 1, Per1 = Period 1, Per2 = Period 2, Per3 =Period 3, Cry1 = Cryptochrome 1, Cry2 = Cryptochrome 2, Ck1e = Casein kinase 1 epsilon, Nr1d1 = Nuclear receptor subfamily 1, group D member 1 (also known as Rev-Erb-alpha), Rn18s = 18S ribosomal RNA (r18S).

2.8. Immunohistochemistry Staining for 8-OHdG

8-Hydroxydeoxyguanosine (8-OHdG) is a DNA oxidation product that was measured to assess DNA damage. Paraffin-embedded tissue sectioned at a thickness of 2 μm was deparaffinized in xylene and rehydrated in a graded ethanol series to phosphate-buffered saline. Immunohistochemical staining was performed using anti-8-OHdG antibody (1:2500; Santa Cruz Biotechnology, Dallas, TX, USA) with a SuperSensitive polymer-horseradish peroxidase immunohistochemistry detection kit (BioGenex, San Ramon, CA, USA) as we described previously [27]. Identical staining without the primary antibody was used as a negative control.

2.9. Statistical Analysis

All data are expressed as mean ± SEM. Parameters were compared using two-way analysis of variance (ANOVA) followed by a Tukey's post hoc test for multiple comparisons. Weights, metabolic and plasma parameters among the groups were further analyzed by one-way ANOVA with a Tukey's post hoc test. A *P*-value < 0.05 was considered statistically significant. All analyses were performed using the Statistical Package for the Social Sciences software (SPSS Inc., Chicago, IL, USA).

3. Results

3.1. Morphological Features and Biochemistry

There were no differences in the litter size (ND = 14 ± 0.8; HF = 15.5 ± 0.8) and ratio of male-to-female pups (ND vs. HF = 0.84 vs. 1.14). One male pup died at Postnatal Day 5 in the ND/ND group, while the mortality rate was 0% in the other groups. The birth body weight was lower in HF offspring compared to ND offspring in both sexes (Figure 1A). HF offspring born with intrauterine growth restriction (IUGR) continued to have lower body weight until one month of age in both sexes (Figure 1B). In males, post-weaning HF diet increased BW of both ND/HF and HF/HF animals from three to six months (Figure 1C). In contrast, significant BW gain was not shown in female offspring fed with HF diet (Figure 1D).

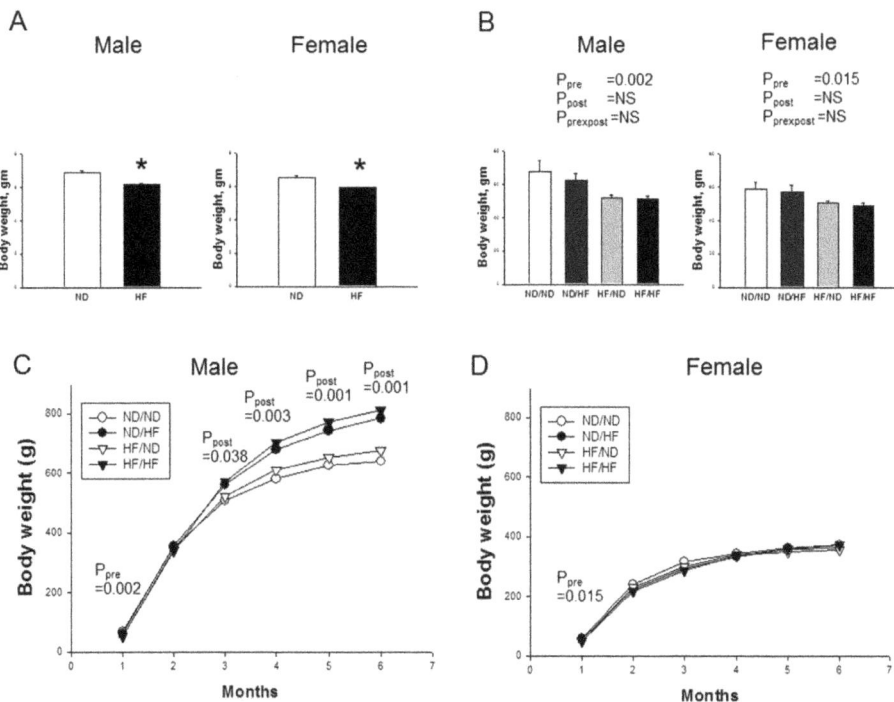

Figure 1. Effects of maternal and postnatal high-fat (HF) diet on bodyweight in: (**A**) neonates; (**B**) male and female offspring at one month of age; and (**C**) male offspring; and (**D**) female offspring from one to six months. * $p < 0.05$ vs. HF; Pre × Post, interaction of pre × post; NS, not significant; N (pups/L) = 5-7/3 per group.

At six months of age, either maternal or post-weaning HF has no effect on kidney weight of each sex. There was a significant effect of post-weaning HF diet on the kidney weight-to-body weight ratio in males ($P_{post} < 0.01$). As compared to ND/ND group, both maternal and post-weaning HF intake increased plasma levels of AST and ALT in both sexes (Table 2). Male offspring exposed to post-weaning HF consumption showed highest plasma levels of total cholesterol among the four groups. There was little measurable effect of either maternal or post-weaning HF diet on plasma levels of triglyceride, HDL, and glucose in offspring of both sexes. In female offspring, plasma triglyceride levels were higher in HF/ND group than those in ND/HF group. The increase in the glucose area under curve (AUC) after an IPGTT was found in ND/HF group compared to controls in females.

Table 2. Weights and metabolic parameters in offspring at six months of age.

Groups		ND/ND	ND/HF	HF/ND	HF/HF	*p* Value		
Number		M = 6; F = 6	M = 6; F = 6	M = 6; F = 6	M = 7; F = 6	Pre	Post	Pre × Post
Body weight (g)	Male	641 ± 39	785 ± 39 *	677 ± 21	813 ± 41*,$	NS	0.001	NS
	Female	372 ± 17	362 ± 19	355 ± 14	372 ± 10	NS	NS	NS
Left kidney (LK) weight (g)	Male	2.16 ± 0.14	2.12 ± 0.08	2.26 ± 0.08	2.08 ± 0.07	NS	NS	NS
	Female	1.28 ± 0.04	1.45 ± 0.1	1.37 ± 0.05	1.38 ± 0.01	NS	NS	NS
LK weight/ 100 g BW	Male	0.34 ± 0.02	0.27 ± 0.01 *	0.33 ± 0.01 #	0.26 ± 0.01*,$	NS	<0.001	NS
	Female	0.35 ± 0.02	0.4 ± 0.02	0.39 ± 0.01	0.37 ± 0.01	NS	NS	0.021
AST (U/L)	Male	88 ± 11	308 ± 58 *	82 ± 10 #	145 ± 19 #	0.019	<0.001	0.028
	Female	73 ± 3	160 ± 24	83 ± 12	82 ± 8	0.026	0.007	0.006
ALT (U/L)	Male	27 ± 3	196 ± 52 *	23 ± 2 #	66 ± 17 #	0.031	0.002	0.041
	Female	19 ± 2	67 ± 13	22 ± 3	30 ± 4	0.026	0.001	0.009
Total cholesterol (mg/dL)	Male	71 ± 8	82 ± 7	58 ± 5	65 ± 5	0.027	NS	NS
	Female	81 ± 9	95 ± 4	104 ± 7	95 ± 16	NS	NS	NS
Triglyceride (mg/dL)	Male	101 ± 26	61 ± 13	105 ± 9	87 ± 12	NS	NS	NS
	Female	97 ± 23	58 ± 9	120 ± 23 #	60 ± 8	NS	NS	NS
HDL (mg/dL)	Male	43 ± 4	49 ± 6	34 ± 4	42 ± 4	NS	NS	NS
	Female	39 ± 4	52 ± 2	59 ± 4	58 ± 10	NS	NS	NS
Glucose (mg/dL)	Male	81 ± 2	91 ± 3	93 ± 4	81 ± 3	NS	NS	NS
	Female	75 ± 4	76 ± 1	73 ± 2	62 ± 3 #	NS	NS	NS
IPGTT (AUC, mg/dL·120 min)	Male	22,071 ± 1354	23,923 ± 2345	23,498 ± 2286	25,922 ± 1973	-	-	-
	Female	26,420 ± 1406	31,389 ± 1773 *	26,890 ± 1820	26,949 ± 2416	-	-	-

AST, aspartate transaminase; ALT, alanine aminotransferase; HDL, high-density lipoprotein; IPGTT, intraperitoneal glucose tolerance test; AUC, area under curve; ND, normal diet; HF, high-fat diet; NS, not significant; -, not done; * $P < 0.05$ vs. ND/ND; # $P < 0.05$ vs. ND/HF; $ $P < 0.05$ vs. HF/ND; N (pups/L) = 5-7/3 per group.

3.2. Blood Pressure and Renal Outcome

Longitudinal measurement of systolic BP from four to 24 weeks of age showed that post-weaning HF diet increased SBP in male (Figure 2A, $P_{post} = 0.001$) and female offspring (Figure 2B, $P_{post} < 0.001$), irrespective of whether they were offspring of dams with maternal HF or not.

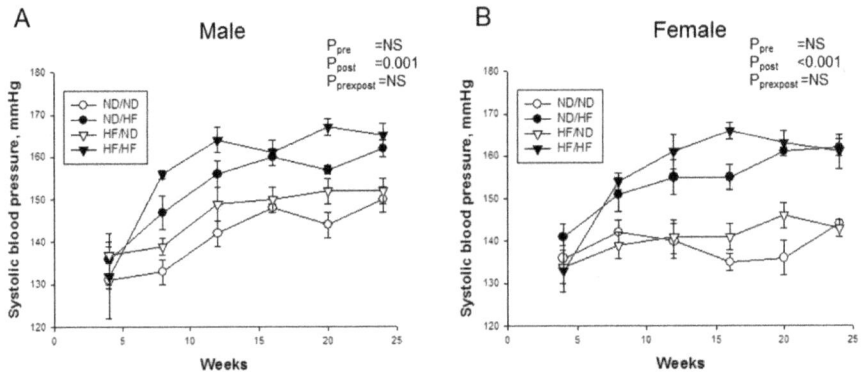

Figure 2. Effects of maternal and postnatal high-fat (HF) diet on systolic blood pressure in: (**A**) male; and (**B**) female offspring from four to 24 weeks. Pre × Post, interaction of pre × post; NS, not significant; N (pups/L) = 5-7/3 per group.

Consistent with previous reports [30,31], male offspring exposed to post-weaning HF showed glomerulosclerosis, segmental necrosis, thickening in the basal membrane of glomeruli and tubules, dilatation in glomerular capillaries, and tubular dilatation (Figure 3A). Maternal and post-weaning HF were associated with greater degrees of glomerular (Figure 3B, $P_{pre} = 0.03$ and $P_{post} = 0.007$) and tubulointerstitial injury (Figure 3C, $P_{pre} = 0.005$ and $P_{post} = 0.005$) in male offspring kidneys than those in females. Consistent with the histologic findings, compared with the ND/ND group, HF/HF group exhibited significantly increased extracellular matrix mRNA expression of collagen I and α-smooth muscle actin (α-SMA) (Figure 3D,E) in males. Additionally, maternal and post-weaning

HF synergistically caused a higher creatinine level in HF/HF group compared with ND/ND group in males. (Figure 3F, $P_{prexpost}$ = 0.011). However, plasma creatinine level was not different among the four groups in females. These data demonstrated that maternal and post-weaning HF-induced kidney injury mainly in male but not female offspring at 24 weeks of age.

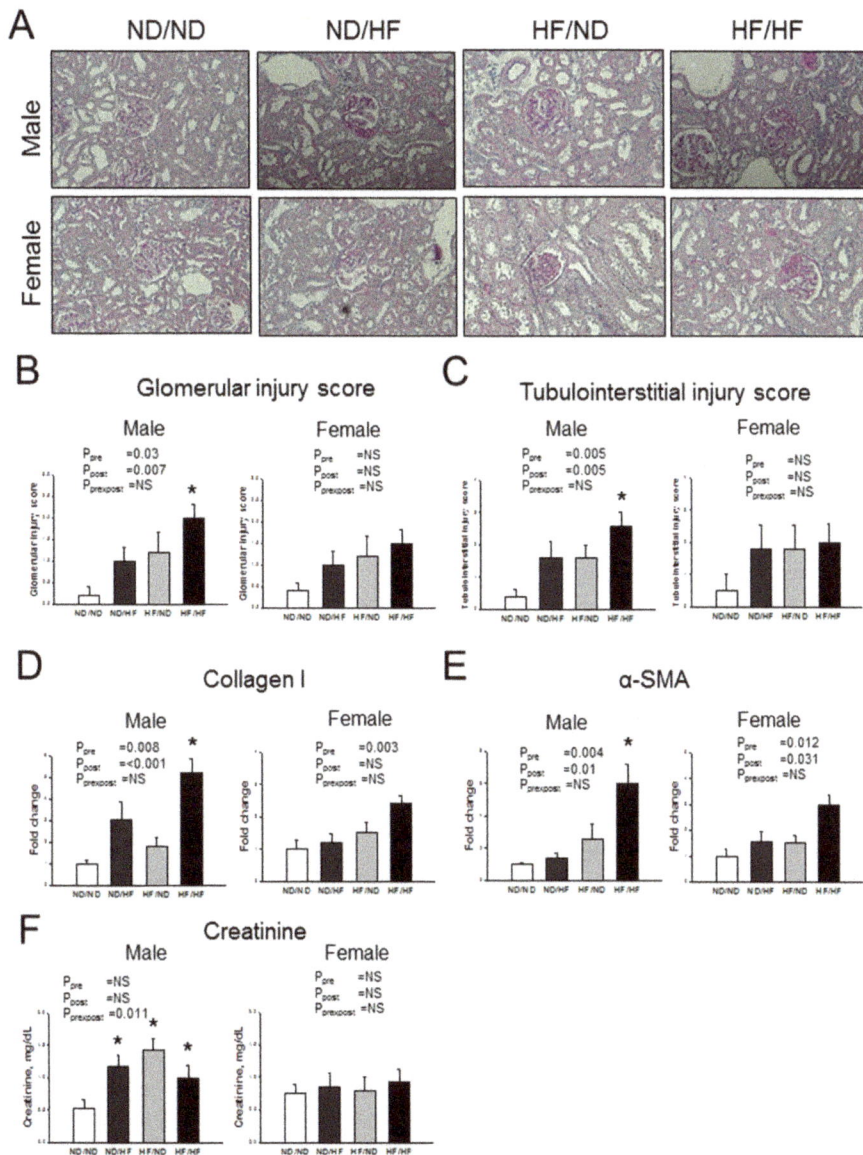

Figure 3. Maternal and post-weaning HF diet induced greater degrees of kidney injury in male than female offspring. Effects of maternal and post-weaning HF diet on: (**A**) morphological changes; (**B**) glomerular injury; (**C**) tubulointerstitial injury; (**D**) mRNA expression of collagen I; (**E**) α-smooth muscle actin (α-SMA); and (**F**) creatinine level. Pre × Post, interaction of pre × post; NS, not significant; * $p < 0.05$ vs. ND/ND; N (pups/L) = 5-7/3 per group.

3.3. Renal Transcriptome

We next analyzed differential gene expression induced by maternal HF consumption in the kidney. Among the differential expressed genes (DEGs), a total of 21 genes (five up- and 16 downregulated genes by male HF versus male ND, Table S1) met the selection criteria of: (i) genes that changed by FPKM > 0.3; and (ii) minimum of twofold difference in normalized read counts between group. As shown in Table S2, a total of 251 DEGs (154 up- and 97 downregulated genes by female HF versus female ND) were noted in response to maternal HF exposure in female offspring. Among them, a total of nine shared genes were identified: *Afp, Cubn, Dgkg, Kcnj15, Lrp2, Slc4a4, Slc6a19, Slc15a1,* and *Stra6*. The DEGs between males and females were further analyzed. There were 91 (67 male-biased genes vs. 24 female-biased genes) and nine (two male-biased genes vs. seven female-biased genes) genes by male versus female that reached a minimum of twofold difference between sexes in the ND group (Table S3) and HF group (Table S4), respectively.

We next used DAVID v6.8 [29] to find functionally related gene groups and gain biological insight from our gene lists. We found one and five signaling pathways identified as the significant KEGG pathways in the male and female offspring kidneys exposed to maternal HF, respectively (Table 3). These KEGG pathways include oxidative phosphorylation, protein digestion and absorption, metabolic pathways, ribosome, and cardiac muscle contraction. Even though none of these genes were related to regulation of BP by GO analysis, we observed four genes with at least twofold difference between HF vs. control in female: *Agtr1b* (fold change (FC) = 4.4) and *Ace* (FC = 0.3) in the RAS, *Ddah1* (FC = 0.3) in the NO system, and *Slc12a3* (FC = 0.3) belonging to sodium transporters.

Table 3. Significantly regulated Kyoto Encyclopedia of Genes and Genomes (KEGG) pathways in the one-week-old offspring kidneys exposed to maternal high-fat (HF) consumption.

KEGG Pathway	Count	Gene Symbol	*p*-Value	Benjamini
Male				
Protein digestion and absorption	2	*Slc15a1, Slc6a19*	5.6×10^{-2}	5.6×10^{-2}
Female				
Oxidative phosphorylation	5	*Atp5j2, Atp6v0d2, Ndufa5, Cox6c, Cox7c*	1.6×10^{-2}	1.6×10^{-2}
Protein digestion and absorption	4	*Slc15a1, Slc6a19, Slc7a7, Slc7a8*	2.2×10^{-2}	2.2×10^{-2}
Metabolic pathways	16	*Dhcr24, Abat, Atp5j2, Atp6v0d2, C1qalt1c1, Mgat4c, Ndufa5, Alox15, Cyp24a1, Cox6c, Cox7c, Dse, Dqkq, Gatm, Hykk, Polr2k*	2.3×10^{-2}	2.3×10^{-2}
Ribosome	5	*Mrpl33, Mrps18c, Rpl22l1, Rpl30, LOC100362027*	2.9×10^{-2}	2.9×10^{-2}
Cardiac muscle contraction	3	*Cacna2d2, Cox6c, Cox7c*	9.9×10^{-2}	9.9×10^{-2}

The top results, sorted by enrichment probability value and the Benjamini–Hochberg multiple testing correction for each Kyoto Encyclopedia of Genes and Genomes (KEGG) pathway, are reported.

Because oxidative stress, RAS pathway, and sodium transporters are involved in renal programming [8–11], and because our NGS data demonstrated that some components of these pathways were altered in response to maternal HF intake, we further investigated these pathways to elucidate underlying mechanisms related to programmed hypertension and kidney disease.

3.4. Oxidative Stress and Nitric Oxide Pathway

We evaluated oxidative stress in the kidney by immunostaining 8-OHdG, an oxidative DNA damage marker. As shown in Figure 4, immunostaining of both cytoplasmic and nuclear 8-OHdG in the glomeruli and renal tubules indicated little staining in the ND/ND group, an intermediate level of staining in the ND/HF as well as HF/ND groups, and intense staining in the HF/HF group in males. Unlike males, females showed little 8-OHdG staining in the ND/HF, HF/ND, and HF/HF groups.

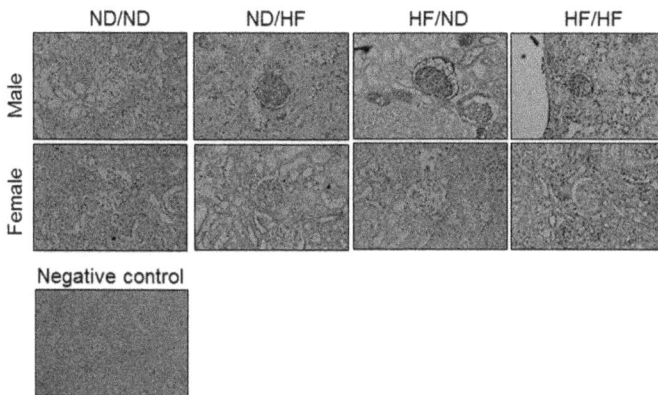

Figure 4. Light micrographs illustrating immunostaining for 8-OHdG in the offspring kidney (400×).

The link between oxidative stress and NO deficiency in programmed hypertension and kidney disease has been recognized [10,11]. We, hence, further investigated whether HF diet induced an imbalance in the NO pathway (Table 4). Plasma level of L-citrulline, a precursor of L-arginine, was higher in post-weaning HF treated groups in both sexes. Either maternal or post-weaning HF diet decreased plasma L-arginine level in males (P_{pre}=0.041 and P_{post} < 0.001), while only post-weaning HF had an effect to reduce plasma L-arginine level in females (P_{post} = 0.027). Although maternal HF increased plasma ADMA level in males (P_{pre} = 0.001), there was a significant effect of post-weaning HF with decreased plasma ADMA level in males (P_{post} = 0.003) and females (P_{post} = 0.001). Maternal HF induced a higher plasma SDMA, an indirect inhibitor of nitric oxide synthase, level in HF/ND group compared to ND/ND in males. Post-weaning HF caused a reduction of plasma SDMA level in females. In male offspring, post-weaning HF diet induced a lower L-arginine-to-ADMA ratio (P_{post} < 0.001), a marker representing NO bioavailability, which was accompanied by an interaction between maternal and post-weaning HF ($P_{prexpost}$ = 0.011). Similarly, post-weaning HF decreased plasma NOx level in males (P_{post} = 0.001). Taken together, our findings suggest sex-dependent renal programming associated with a greater degree of oxidative stress and a lower NO bioavailability in male than in female offspring kidney in response to HF consumption.

Table 4. Plasma levels of L-arginine, L-citrulline, ADMA, SDMA, and NO in offspring at six months of age.

Groups		ND/ND	ND/HF	HF/ND	HF/HF	P Value		
Number		M = 5; F = 6	M = 6; F = 6	M = 6; F = 6	M = 7; F = 6	Pre	Post	Pre × Post
L-Citrulline (μM)	Male	42.4 ± 2.2	42.0 ± 2.0	41.6 ± 1.6	46.2 ± 1.9	NS	NS	NS
	Female	48.7 ± 4.1	61.7 ± 9.5	44.5 ± 4.8	62.9 ± 4.7	NS	0.019	NS
L-Arginine (μM)	Male	168.0 ± 15.9	46.1 ± 12.8 *	172.0 ± 9.5 [#]	101.8 ± 15.5	0.041	<0.001	NS
	Female	152.4 ± 27.7	120.8 ± 23.4	179.0 ± 10.2	119.6 ± 5.2	NS	0.027	NS
ADMA (μM)	Male	1.02 ± 0.03	0.92 ± 0.03	1.23 ± 0.03 [#]	1.03 ± 0.07	0.001	0.003	NS
	Female	1.45 ± 0.09	1.25 ± 0.07	1.38 ± 0.03	1.1 ± 0.04 *,[S]	NS	0.001	NS
SDMA (μM)	Male	0.43 ± 0.03	0.55 ± 0.02	0.67 ± 0.03 *	0.53 ± 0.02	0.001	NS	<0.001
	Female	0.72 ± 0.08	0.65 ± 0.03	0.68 ± 0.05	0.5 ± 0.03 *	NS	0.028	NS
L-Arginine-to-ADMA ratio (μM/μM)	Male	165.7 ± 15.1	49.7 ± 13.9 *	138.6 ± 7.7 [#]	101.7 ± 17.6 *	NS	<0.001	0.011
	Female	107.2 ± 20.8	93.3 ± 16.0	129.1 ± 9.6	107.9 ± 3.0	NS	NS	NS
NOx (NO2− + NO−) (μM)	Male	218.6 ± 15.1	167.5 ± 5.1	195.7 ± 6.6	178 ± 7.4	NS	0.001	NS
	Female	172.8 ± 16.5	161.5 ± 17.6	161.5 ± 6.5	159.1 ± 24.5	NS	NS	NS

ADMA, asymmetric dimethylarginine; SDMA, symmetric dimethylarginine; ND, normal diet; HF, high-fat diet; Pre × Post, interaction of pre × post; NS, not significant; * $P < 0.05$ vs. ND/ND; [#] $P < 0.05$ vs. ND/HF; [S] $P < 0.05$ vs. HF/ND; N (pups/L) = 5-7/3 per group.

3.5. RAS and Sodium Transporters

We evaluated the renal mRNA expression of RAS components (Figure 5). Renal mRNA expression of *Ren* was higher in the HF/HF group than in ND/ND group. In females, HF/HF group had higher mRNA expression of *Atp6ap2* in the kidney compared to ND/ND group. Maternal HF significantly increased *Agt* expression in both sexes. In females, both maternal and post-weaning HF significantly increased the renal mRNA expression of *Ace* in the ND/HF, HF/ND, and HF/HF groups compared with those in ND/ND group (Figure 5B). However, downstream signals of the RAS, such as *Agtr1a*, *Agtr1b*, and *Mas1*, were not different among the four groups of both sexes.

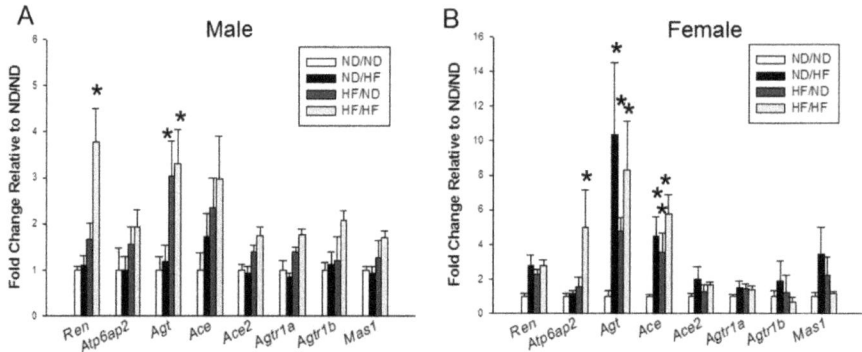

Figure 5. Effects of maternal and postnatal high-fat diet (HF) on gene expression of RAS components in: (**A**) male; and (**B**) female offspring. * $p < 0.05$ vs. ND/ND.

Additionally, we analyzed the levels of sodium transporters and found that renal levels of NHE3, NCC, NKCC2, and NaKATPase were not different among the four groups in males (Figure 6). However, maternal and post-weaning HF similarly increased renal NHE3, NCC, and NKCC2 protein levels in females.

3.6. Clock and Clock-Controlled Genes

Figure 7 represents clock and clock-controlled gene expression in offspring kidney. Maternal HF diet significantly upregulated mRNA expression of the positive element *Baml*, negative elements (*Cry1* and *Per2*), and clock-controlled gene (*Ck1e* and *Nr1d1*) in females. In males, clock and clock-controlled genes tended to be unaltered in response to maternal HF consumption. Post-weaning HF diet significantly downregulated mRNA level of most clock and clock-controlled genes in the males (All $P_{post} < 0.05$), with the exception of *Cry1* and *Cry2*. In females, post-weaning HF diet led to the downregulation of the *Baml, Ck1e, Cry1,* and *Per1*.

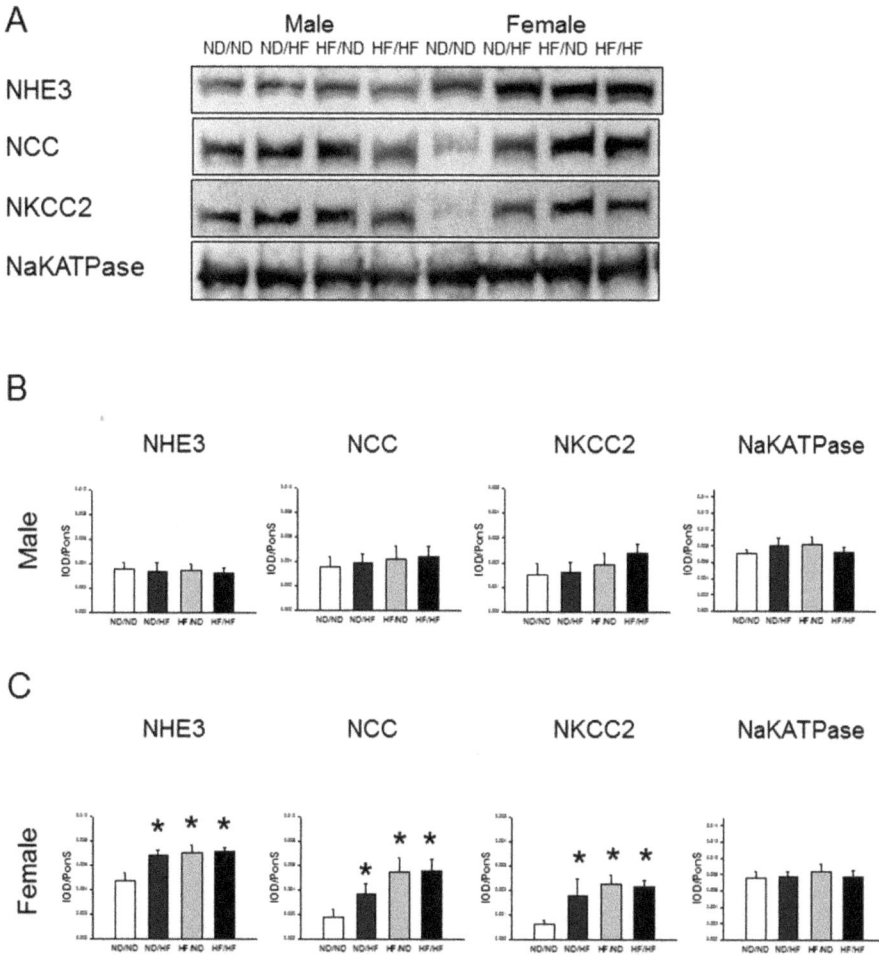

Figure 6. Effects of maternal and postnatal high-fat diet (HF) on sodium transporters expression in male and female offspring. (**A**) Representative Western blots of NHE3 (90 kDa), NCC (130 kDa), NKCC2 (160 kDa), and NaKATPase (112 kDa) of six-month-old male and female offspring. Relative abundance of renal cortical NHE3, NCC, NKCC2, NaKATPase as quantified in: male (**B**); and female (**C**) offspring. * $p < 0.05$ vs. ND/ND.

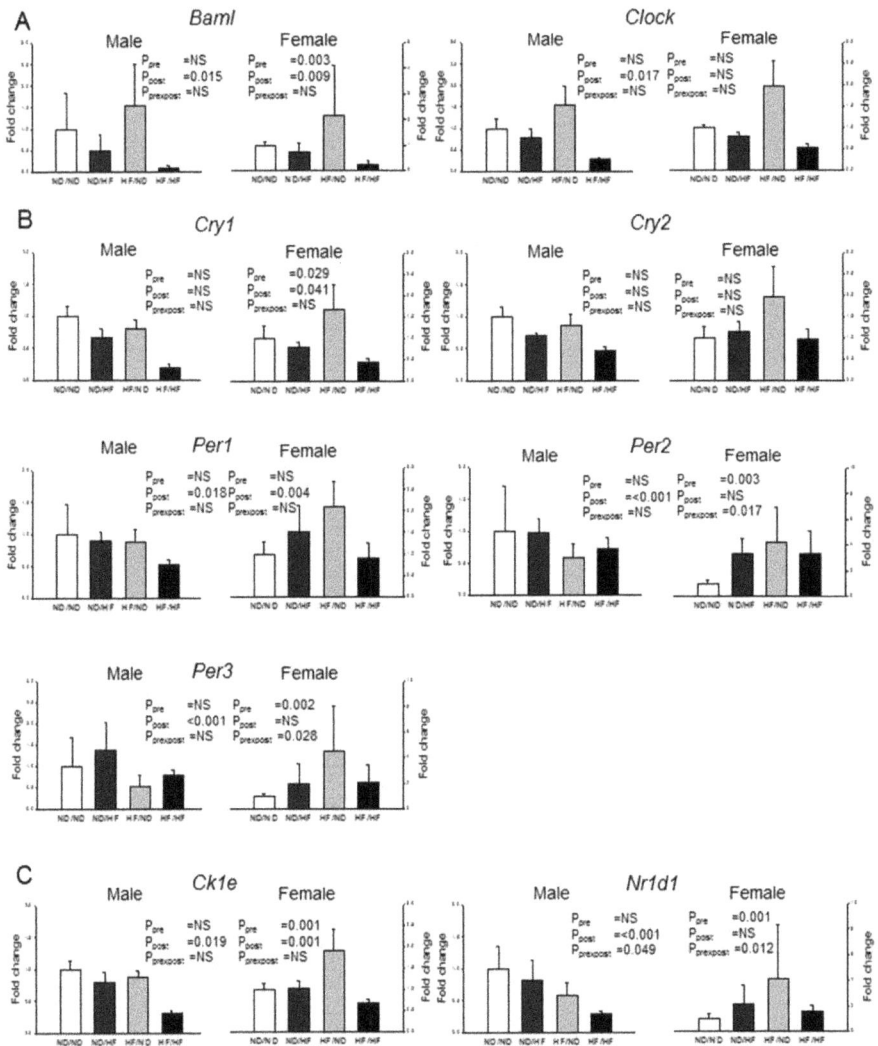

Figure 7. Effects of maternal and postnatal high-fat diet (HF) on mRNA levels of clock genes in male and female offspring kidneys. Relative fold changes of: (**A**) positive element *Baml* and *Clock*; (**B**) negative elements *Cry1*, *Per2*, and *Per3*; and (**C**) clock-controlled gene *Ck1e* and *Nr1d1* as quantified. Pre × Post, interaction of pre × post; NS, not significant; N (pups/L) = 5-7/3 per group.

4. Discussion

This study provides insight into several sex-specific mechanisms by which maternal and post-weaning HF intake causes different renal and metabolic outcomes in adult offspring. The key findings are the following: (1) post-weaning HF diet increased body weight only in male offspring; (2) post-weaning HF diet increased systolic blood pressure in both sexes; (3) males were more vulnerable to kidney damage compared to females in response to maternal and post-weaning HF intake; (4) maternal HF altered renal transcriptome in a sex specific fashion as demonstrated by 21 and 251 DEGs in male and female offspring, respectively; (5) maternal and post-weaning HF diet-induced hypertension and renal injury relevant to oxidative stress, RAS, and sodium transporters;

and (6) maternal and post-weaning HF differentially regulated renal clock-controlled genes in a sex specific manner.

We observed that maternal HF caused IUGR offspring continued to have lower body weight until one month of age in both sexes. Previous reports demonstrated that IUGR offspring, particularly those with rapid catch-up growth, have a higher risk of adult obesity and metabolic syndrome [32,33]. Although HF diets are often used to promote obesity in rodents, some authors did not find statistically differences in body weight [5]. In the present study, maternal HF elicited little effect on metabolic syndrome-like conditions (e.g., obesity and lipids) on the HF/ND offspring. However, post-weaning HF has a differential impact on the development of obesity and liver steatosis in both sexes. In males, ND/HF and HF/HF group became obese over time, with significantly elevated plasma ASL and ALT levels at six months of age. Nevertheless, post-weaning HF increased ASL and ALT levels but not body weights in female offspring. In lines with an earlier review showing that sex differences exist in obesity-related disorders [19], our results indicate that male offspring are predisposed to obesity and liver steatosis in response to HF consumption. Additionally, we observed that females exposed to HF intake tend to elicit an increased glucose AUC in IPGTT, which support the idea that impaired glucose tolerance is more prevalent in women [19].

Although HF diets are associated with hypertension [5], the observations of maternal HF-induced hypertension in offspring are varied [6]. Maternal HF induced responses of BP include an increase [34,35], decrease [36], or no change [34], mainly depending on strain, sex, age, measuring method, and different fatty acids compositions. In this work, we did not observe an impact from maternal HF on the development of hypertension in each sex. However, we noted that post-weaning HF similarly increased BP in either ND/HF or HF/HF group of both sexes. Previously, we and others showed pre- and post-natal insults could be independently or synergistically contributing to renal programming and programmed hypertension [8,10,20,28]. Our current study demonstrated that maternal HF did not either intensify or lessen post-weaning HF induced programmed hypertension in both sexes.

Renal injury has been reported in offspring exposed to maternal or post-weaning HF diets [24,25,32]. Consistent with previous reports showing fibrotic and epithelial-to-mesenchymal transition (EMT) markers were augmented by HF intake [30,31,37], we found that maternal and post-weaning HF increased mRNA expression of collagen I and α-SMA in the offspring kidneys of both sexes. Noteworthy, male offspring exposed to maternal plus post-weaning HF showed greater degrees of glomerular and tubulointerstitial injury and worse renal function compared to females.

There is emerging evidence that sex differences exist in the fetal programming of kidney disease [11,38], showing that males are more vulnerable than females. The important sex-dependent differences in the developmental programming of diseases seem to be related to sex hormones [38]. Previous studies furthermore indicated that estrogen helped to protect against kidney disease while testosterone shown to be harmful to kidney health [38,39]. Whether sex hormones influence the vulnerability to protect female offspring against HF-induced programmed kidney disease deserves further clarification. Our findings in conjunction with others indicate that male offspring tend to be more vulnerable to HF-induced renal injury than females [30,31].

In line with previous studies [24,40,41], our NGS data illustrated that maternal nutrition has great effects on renal transcriptome in the developing kidney. We observed that maternal HF intake induces significant changes in renal transcriptome with female offspring being more HF-sensitive. Although sex differences have been observed in developmental programming of obesity and kidney disease [17,19], our study is the first to show sex differences of maternal HF-induced changes with a focus on renal transcriptome. Our findings are consistent with previous studies showing that more genes in the placenta were affected in females than in males in different models of nutritional programming [42,43]. Since we found that female offspring are more resilient to HF-induced obesity and kidney disease, it is possible that the increased female sensitivity to maternal HF diet might buffer the deleterious effects, resulting in a better adaptation and less impact of programming in adulthood.

Our NGS data demonstrated ~20 genes in five KEGG pathways were significantly regulated in female in response to maternal HF consumption. Except defect in *Slc6a19* (encodes an amino acid transporter B°AT1) has been linked to hypertension [44], most genes are not relevant to hypertension and kidney disease. Additional studies are needed to determine whether these genes are common genes in the development of hypertension and kidney disease in other programming models.

Emerging evidence demonstrated that an early shift in the NO-ROS balance toward reduced NO bioavailability links to programmed hypertension and kidney disease in later life [8,10,11,45]. Oxidative stress has been demonstrated as a key mediator in the pathogenesis of obesity and related disorders [5,40]. In this work, several lines of evidence implicated the role of ADMA-NO pathway related oxidative stress on programmed hypertension and kidney disease induced by HF intake. First, post-weaning HF reduced plasma level of L-arginine, a substrate for nitric oxide synthase, level in both sexes. Second, there was a significant effect of maternal and post-weaning HF with increased plasma SDMA (an indirect inhibitor of nitric oxide synthase) level and decreased L-arginine-to-ADMA ratio (a marker representing NO bioavailability) in males. Third, post-waning HF decreased plasma NOx level in male offspring. Fourth, our NGS data identified the oxidative phosphorylation is a significantly regulated KEGG pathway. As known, defective oxidative phosphorylation-induced oxidative stress play a key role in many obesity-related disorders [46]. Last, maternal and post-weaning HF increased the degrees of oxidative stress damage represented as 8-OHdG IHC staining in male offspring, which is associated with a worse renal outcome. Thus, our results demonstrated that maternal and post-weaning HF diets-induced hypertension and kidney injury along with the ROS-NO imbalance. Since sex-specific NO availability might be involved in the development of hypertension [38], and since we noted post-weaning HF induced sex-specific changes in NO availability but not BP in each sex, our findings suggested that hypertension in response to post-weaning HF intake might be independent of NO pathway in males.

Next, we observed that HF consumption induced sex-specific alterations of the RAS and sodium transporters. However, the renoprotective mechanisms of female refractory to HF-induced kidney injury might not be related to the RAS and sodium transporters. Despite our previous study suggest sex-dependent renal programming within the RAS underling the programmed hypertension in a rat model of prenatal dexamethasone exposure [21], our present study showed that there was no sex difference on the most components of RAS in response to HF exposure. Additionally, maternal and post-weaning HF increased several sodium transporters in the female kidney, including NHE3, NCC, and NKCC2. Given that most sodium transporters are clock-controlled genes [47], and that increased expression of sodium transporters triggers programmed hypertension in various models [8,48], our observations suggest HF-induced disturbed circadian clock may induce sodium transporters to trigger sodium retention, contributing to the development of hypertension in females. However, whether HF-induced programming of kidney disease in males attributed to dysregulated RAS and sodium transporters deserve further elucidation.

In agreement with previous studies showing that HF diets alter circadian clock function [13,49], we observed that maternal HF diet upregulated mRNA expression of the positive element (*Baml*) and negative elements (*Cry1* and *Per2*) in females. In contrast, post-weaning HF diet led to the downregulation of the *Baml*, *Ck1e*, *Cry1*, and *Per1* in female offspring kidneys. Emerging evidence suggested that clock genes such as *Baml*, *Ck1e*, *Cry1*, *Per1* and *Per2* play an integral role in the development of hypertension and kidney disease [50,51]. Our data would support the concept that disturbed circadian clock in the kidney, induced by maternal or post-weaning HF, may contribute to the substantial renal injury and elevation of BP. A previous report showed that the kidney is less sensitive to feeding cues compared with other tissues [52]. Our data demonstrated that the effects of HF intake on renal clock genes have a distinct sex-specific bias, with female offspring being more HF-sensitive.

Our study has a few limitations. First, we did not examine other organs involved in obesity related diseases. The differential effects of maternal and post-weaning HF on male and female offspring may be derived from other tissues, such as the liver, fatty tissues, and vasculature. Another limitation is that clock genes expression was measured only at one point, it is not possible to infer whether the differences among the experimental groups are due to differences in gene expression degree or to a phase shift. Since HF-induced renal injury reported was related to renal accumulation of lipid in adult rats [53], additional studies are needed to elucidate whether this mechanism plays a crucial role in programmed kidney disease. Furthermore, we did not examine alterations of renal transcriptome in different windows of exposure to HF. Given that the interactions between genes and diet vary during different developmental windows, whether HF consumption leads to differentially regulated genes between diverse windows of exposure is worthy of further study. Finally, it should be noted that different nutritional insults might not use the same pathway to induce hypertension and kidney injury. Therefore, further studies should be performed using other models to determine whether the oxidative stress, RAS, sodium transporters, and circadian clock are common targets for preventing hypertension and kidney disease.

5. Conclusions

Thus, we conclude that maternal and post-weaning HF diet have sex-specific influences on the development of obesity, kidney injury, and hypertension. Maternal HF diet induces significant alterations in renal transcriptome with female offspring being more sensitive. Our data suggested an association among oxidative stress, RAS, sodium transporters, and circadian clock, which involved in the HF-induced hypertension and kidney injury in adult offspring. Most importantly, the coupling of maternal and post-weaning HF consumption aggravates obesity and kidney damage in males, which is associated with sex-specific renal programming. With better understanding of the sex-specific gene–diet interactions that underlie maternal and post-weaning HF-induced renal programming, our results can aid in developing effective personalized reprogramming strategies to prevent obesity and related disorders.

Supplementary Materials: The following are available online at www.mdpi.com/2072-6643/9/4/357/s1, Table S1: List of the 21 differentially expressed genes that are induced by maternal high-fat (HF) exposure in 1-week-old male offspring kidney, Table S2: List of the 251 differentially expressed genes that are induced by maternal high-fat (HF) exposure in 1-week-old female offspring kidney, Table S3: List of the 91 differentially expressed genes in the kidney of control male offspring vs. control female offspring at 1 week of age, Table S4: List of the 9 differentially expressed genes in the kidney of maternal high-fat (HF)-treated male offspring vs. maternal HF-treated female offspring at 1 week of age.

Acknowledgments: This work was supported by the Grants CMRPG8F0161 and CMRPG8F0121 from Chang Gung Memorial Hospital, Kaohsiung, Taiwan.

Author Contributions: You-Lin Tain contributed to concept generation, data interpretation, drafting of the manuscript, critical revision of the manuscript and approval of the article; Yu-Ju Lin contributed to data interpretation, critical revision of the manuscript and approval of the article; Jiunn-Ming Sheen contributed to data interpretation and approval of the article; Hong-Ren Yu contributed to data interpretation and approval of the article; Mao-Meng Tiao contributed to data interpretation and approval of the article; Chih-Cheng Chen contributed to data interpretation and approval of the article; Ching-Chou Tsai contributed to data interpretation and approval of the article; Li-Tung Huang contributed to critical revision of the manuscript and approval of the article; and Chien-Ning Hsu contributed to concept generation, data interpretation, critical revision of the manuscript and approval of the article.

Conflicts of Interest: The authors declare no conflict of interest.

References

1. Vickers, M.H. Early life nutrition, epigenetics and programming of later life disease. *Nutrients* **2014**, *6*, 2165–2178. [CrossRef] [PubMed]
2. Misra, A.; Singhal, N.; Khurana, L. Obesity, the metabolic syndrome, and type 2 diabetes in developing countries: Role of dietary fats and oils. *J. Am. Coll. Nutr.* **2010**, *29*, 289S–301S. [CrossRef] [PubMed]
3. Buettner, R.; Parhofer, K.G.; Woenckhaus, M.; Wrede, C.E.; Kunz-Schughart, L.A.; Schölmerich, J.; Bolheimer, L.C. Defining high-fat-diet rat models: Metabolic and molecular effects of different fat types. *J. Mol. Endocrinol.* **2006**, *36*, 485–501. [CrossRef] [PubMed]

4.   Buettner, R.; Schölmerich, J.; Bollheimer, L.C. High-fat diets: Modeling the metabolic disorders of human obesity in rodents. *Obesity* **2007**, *15*, 798–808. [CrossRef] [PubMed]

5.   Kakimoto, P.A.; Kowaltowski, A.J. Effects of high fat diets on rodent liver bioenergetics and oxidative imbalance. *Redox Biol.* **2016**, *8*, 216–225. [CrossRef] [PubMed]

6.   Williams, L.; Seki, Y.; Vuguin, P.M.; Charron, M.J. Animal models of in utero exposure to a high fat diet: A review. *Biochim. Biophys. Acta* **2014**, *1842*, 507–519. [CrossRef] [PubMed]

7.   Zhou, D.; Pan, Y.X. Pathophysiological basis for compromised health beyond generations: Role of maternal high-fat diet and low-grade chronic inflammation. *J. Nutr. Biochem.* **2015**, *26*, 1–8. [CrossRef] [PubMed]

8.   Paixão, A.D.; Alexander, B.T. How the kidney is impacted by the perinatal maternal environment to develop hypertension. *Biol. Reprod.* **2013**, *89*, 144. [CrossRef] [PubMed]

9.   Luyckx, V.A.; Bertram, J.F.; Brenner, B.M.; Fall, C.; Hoy, W.E.; Ozanne, S.E.; Vikse, B.E. Effect of fetal and child health on kidney development and long-term risk of hypertension and kidney disease. *Lancet* **2013**, *382*, 273–283. [CrossRef]

10. Tain, Y.L.; Joles, J.A. Reprogramming: A preventive strategy in hypertension focusing on the kidney. *Int. J. Mol. Sci.* **2015**, *17*, E23. [CrossRef] [PubMed]

11. Tain, Y.L.; Hsu, C.N. Developmental origins of chronic kidney disease: Should we focus on early life? *Int. J. Mol. Sci.* **2017**, *18*, 381. [CrossRef] [PubMed]

12. Tokonami, N.; Mordasini, D.; Pradervand, S.; Centeno, G.; Jouffe, C.; Maillard, M.; Bonny, O.; Gachon, F.; Gomez, R.A.; Sequeira-Lopez, M.L.; et al. Local renal circadian clocks control fluid-electrolyte homeostasis and BP. *J. Am. Soc. Nephrol.* **2014**, *25*, 1430–1439. [CrossRef] [PubMed]

13. Feng, D.; Lazar, M.A. Clocks, metabolism, and the epigenome. *Mol. Cell* **2012**, *47*, 158–167. [CrossRef] [PubMed]

14. Hsieh, M.C.; Yang, S.C.; Tseng, H.L.; Hwang, L.L.; Chen, C.T.; Shieh, K.R. Abnormal expressions of circadian-clock and circadian clock-controlled genes in the livers and kidneys of long-term, high-fat-diet-treated mice. *Int. J. Obes.* **2010**, *34*, 227–239. [CrossRef] [PubMed]

15. Roberts, C.K.; Barnard, R.J.; Sindhu, R.K.; Jurczak, M.; Ehdaie, A.; Vaziri, N.D. Oxidative stress and dysregulation of NAD(P)H oxidase and antioxidant enzymes in diet-induced metabolic syndrome. *Metabolism* **2006**, *55*, 928–934. [CrossRef] [PubMed]

16. Riazi, S.; Tiwari, S.; Sharma, N.; Rash, A.; Ecelbarger, C.M. Abundance of the Na-K-2Cl cotransporter NKCC2 is increased by high-fat feeding in Fischer 344 X Brown Norway (F1) rats. *Am. J. Physiol. Renal Physiol.* **2009**, *296*, F762–F770. [CrossRef] [PubMed]

17. Perucca, J.; Bouby, N.; Valeix, P.; Bankir, L. Sex difference in urine concentration across differing ages, sodium intake, and level of kidney disease. *Am. J. Physiol. Regul. Integr. Comp. Physiol.* **2007**, *292*, R700–R705. [CrossRef] [PubMed]

18. Sandberg, K.; Ji, H. Sex differences in primary hypertension. *Biol. Sex Differ.* **2012**, *3*, 7. [CrossRef] [PubMed]

19. Mauvais-Jarvis, F. Sex differences in metabolic homeostasis, diabetes, and obesity. *Biol. Sex Differ.* **2015**, *6*, 14. [CrossRef] [PubMed]

20. Tain, Y.L.; Sheen, J.M.; Yu, H.R.; Chen, C.C.; Tiao, M.M.; Hsu, C.N.; Lin, Y.J.; Kuo, K.C.; Huang, L.T. Maternal melatonin therapy rescues prenatal dexamethasone and postnatal high-fat diet induced programmed hypertension in male rat offspring. *Front. Physiol.* **2015**, *6*, 377. [CrossRef] [PubMed]

21. Tain, Y.L.; Wu, M.S.; Lin, Y.J. Sex differences in renal transcriptome and programmed hypertension in offspring exposed to prenatal dexamethasone. *Steroids* **2016**, *115*, 40–46. [CrossRef] [PubMed]

22. Corella, D.; Ordovas, J.M. Nutrigenomics in cardiovascular medicine. *Circ. Cardiovasc. Genet.* **2009**, *2*, 637–651. [CrossRef] [PubMed]

23. Juma, S.; Imrhan, V.; Vijayagopal, P.; Prasad, C. Prescribing personalized nutrition for cardiovascular health: Are we ready? *J. Nutrigenet. Nutrigenomics* **2014**, *7*, 153–160. [CrossRef] [PubMed]

24. Tain, Y.L.; Hsu, C.N.; Chan, J.Y.; Huang, L.T. Renal transcriptome analysis of programmed hypertension induced by maternal nutritional insults. *Int. J. Mol. Sci.* **2015**, *16*, 17826–17837. [CrossRef] [PubMed]

25. Tain, Y.L.; Chan, J.Y.; Hsu, C.N. Maternal fructose intake affects transcriptome changes and programmed hypertension in offspring in later life. *Nutrients* **2016**, *8*, 757. [CrossRef] [PubMed]

26. Sheen, J.M.; Hsieh, C.S.; Tain, Y.L.; Li, S.W.; Yu, H.R.; Chen, C.C.; Tiao, M.M.; Chen, Y.C.; Huang, L.T. Programming effects of prenatal glucocorticoid exposure with a postnatal high-fat diet in diabetes mellitus. *Int. J. Mol. Sci.* **2016**, *17*, E533. [CrossRef] [PubMed]

27. Tain, Y.L.; Hsieh, C.S.; Lin, I.C.; Chen, C.C.; Sheen, J.M.; Huang, L.T. Effects of maternal L-citrulline supplementation on renal function and blood pressure in offspring exposed to maternal caloric restriction: The impact of nitric oxide pathway. *Nitric Oxide* **2010**, *23*, 34–41. [CrossRef] [PubMed]

28. Tain, Y.L.; Lee, W.C.; Leu, S.; Wu, K.; Chan, J. High salt exacerbates programmed hypertension in maternal fructose-fed male offspring. *Nutr. Metab. Cardiovasc. Dis.* **2015**, *25*, 1146–1151. [CrossRef] [PubMed]

29. NIH DAVID Bioinformatics Resources 6.8. Available online: Https://david.ncifcrf.gov/ (accessed on 9 January 2017).

30. Jackson, C.M.; Alexander, B.T.; Roach, L.; Haggerty, D.; Marbury, D.C.; Hutchens, Z.M.; Flynn, E.R.; Maric-Bilkan, C. Exposure to maternal overnutrition and a high-fat diet during early postnatal development increases susceptibility to renal and metabolic injury later in life. *Am. J. Physiol. Renal Physiol.* **2012**, *302*, F774–F783. [CrossRef] [PubMed]

31. Aliou, Y.; Liao, M.C.; Zhao, X.P.; Chang, S.Y.; Chenier, I.; Ingelfinger, J.R.; Zhang, S.L. Post-weaning high-fat diet accelerates kidney injury, but not hypertension programmed by maternal diabetes. *Pediatr. Res.* **2016**, *79*, 416–424. [CrossRef] [PubMed]

32. Férézou-Viala, J.; Roy, A.F.; Sérougne, C.; Gripois, D.; Parquet, M.; Bailleux, V.; Gertler, A.; Delplanque, B.; Djiane, J.; Riottot, M.; Taouis, M. Long-term consequences of maternal high-fat feeding on hypothalamic leptin sensitivity and diet-induced obesity in the offspring. *Am. J. Physiol. Regul. Integr. Comp. Physiol.* **2007**, *293*, R1056–R1062. [CrossRef] [PubMed]

33. Howie, G.J.; Sloboda, D.M.; Kamal, T.; Vickers, M.H. Maternal nutritional history predicts obesity in adult offspring independent of postnatal diet. *J. Physiol.* **2009**, *587*, 905–915. [CrossRef] [PubMed]

34. Khan, I.Y.; Taylor, P.D.; Dekou, V.; Seed, P.T.; Lakasing, L.; Graham, D.; Dominiczak, A.F.; Hanson, M.A.; Poston, L. Gender-linked hypertension in offspring of lard-fed pregnant rats. *Hypertension* **2003**, *41*, 168–175. [CrossRef] [PubMed]

35. Armitage, J.A.; Lakasing, L.; Taylor, P.D.; Balachandran, A.A.; Jensen, R.I.; Dekou, V.; Ashton, N.; Nyengaard, J.R.; Poston, L. Developmental programming of aortic and renal structure in offspring of rats fed fat-rich diets in pregnancy. *J. Physiol.* **2005**, *565*, 171–184. [CrossRef] [PubMed]

36. Mitra, A.; Alvers, K.M.; Crump, E.M.; Rowland, N.E. Effect of high-fat diet during gestation, lactation, or postweaning on physiological and behavioral indexes in borderline hypertensive rats. *Am. J. Physiol. Regul. Integr. Comp. Physiol.* **2009**, *296*, R20–R28. [CrossRef] [PubMed]

37. Matsuda, S.; Arai, T.; Iwata, K.; Oka, M.; Nagase, M. A high-fat diet aggravates tubulointerstitial but not glomerular lesions in obese Zucker rats. *Kidney Int.* **1999**, *71*, S150–S152. [CrossRef]

38. Tomat, A.L.; Salazar, F.J. Mechanisms involved in developmental programming of hypertension and renal diseases. Gender differences. *Horm. Mol. Biol. Clin. Investig.* **2014**, *18*, 63–77. [CrossRef] [PubMed]

39. Elliot, S.J.; Berho, M.; Korach, K.; Doublier, S.; Lupia, E.; Striker, G.E.; Karl, M. Gender-specific effects of endogenous testosterone: Female alpha-estrogen receptor-deficient C57Bl/6J mice develop glomerulosclerosis. *Kidney Int.* **2007**, *72*, 464–472. [CrossRef] [PubMed]

40. Tain, Y.L.; Wu, K.L.; Lee, W.C.; Leu, S.; Chan, J.Y. Maternal fructose-intake-induced renal programming in adult male offspring. *J. Nutr. Biochem.* **2015**, *26*, 642–650. [CrossRef] [PubMed]

41. Tain, Y.L.; Lee, C.T.; Huang, L.T. Long-term effects of maternal citrulline supplementation on renal transcriptome prevention of nitric oxide depletion-related programmed hypertension: The impact of gene-nutrient interactions. *Int. J. Mol. Sci.* **2014**, *15*, 23255–23268. [CrossRef] [PubMed]

42. Mao, J.; Zhang, X.; Sieli, P.T.; Falduto, M.T.; Torres, K.E.; Rosenfeld, C.S. Contrasting effects of different maternal diets on sexually dimorphic gene expression in the murine placenta. *Proc. Natl. Acad. Sci. USA* **2010**, *107*, 5557–5562. [CrossRef] [PubMed]

43. Cox, L.A.; Li, C.; Glenn, J.P.; Lange, K.; Spradling, K.D.; Nathanielsz, P.W.; Jansson, T. Expression of the placental transcriptome in maternal nutrient reduction in baboons is dependent on fetal sex. *J. Nutr.* **2013**, *143*, 1698–1708. [CrossRef] [PubMed]

44. Pinto, V.; Pinho, M.J.; Soares-da-Silva, P. Renal amino acid transport systems and essential hypertension. *FASEBJ.* **2013**, *27*, 2927–2938. [CrossRef] [PubMed]

45. Tain, Y.L.; Hsu, C.N. Targeting on asymmetric dimethylarginine-related nitric oxide-reactive oxygen species imbalance to reprogram the development of hypertension. *Int. J. Mol. Sci.* **2016**, *17*, E2020. [CrossRef] [PubMed]

46. Cheng, Z.; Ristow, M. Mitochondria and metabolic homeostasis. *Antioxid. Redox Signal.* **2013**, *19*, 240–242. [CrossRef] [PubMed]

47. Bonny, O.; Vinciguerra, M.; Gumz, M.L.; Mazzoccoli, G. Molecular bases of circadian rhythmicity in renal physiology and pathology. *Nephrol. Dial. Transplant.* **2013**, *28*, 2421–2431. [CrossRef] [PubMed]

48. Paauw, N.D.; van Rijn, B.B.; Lely, A.T.; Joles, J.A. Pregnancy as a critical window for blood pressure regulation in mother and child: Programming and reprogramming. *Acta Physiol.* **2017**, *219*, 241–259. [CrossRef] [PubMed]

49. Oosterman, J.E.; Kalsbeek, A.; la Fleur, S.E.; Belsham, D.D. Impact of nutrients on circadian rhythmicity. *Am. J. Physiol. Regul. Integr. Comp. Physiol.* **2015**, *308*, R337–R350. [CrossRef] [PubMed]

50. Firsov, D.; Bonny, O. Circadian regulation of renal function. *Kidney Int.* **2010**, *78*, 640–645. [CrossRef] [PubMed]

51. Richards, J.; Diaz, A.N.; Gumz, M.L. Clock genes in hypertension: Novel insights from rodent models. *Blood Press. Monit.* **2014**, *19*, 249–254. [CrossRef] [PubMed]

52. Wu, T.; Fu, O.; Yao, L.; Sun, L.; Zhuge, F.; Fu, Z. Differential responses of peripheral circadian clocks to a short-term feeding stimulus. *Mol. Biol. Rep.* **2012**, *39*, 9783–9789. [CrossRef] [PubMed]

53. Kume, S.; Uzu, T.; Araki, S.; Sugimoto, T.; Isshiki, K.; Chin-Kanasaki, M.; Sakaguchi, M.; Kubota, N.; Terauchi, Y.; Kadowaki, T.; Haneda, M.; Kashiwagi, A.; Koya, D. Role of altered renal lipid metabolism in the development of renal injury induced by a high-fat diet. *J. Am. Soc. Nephrol.* **2007**, *18*, 2715–2723. [CrossRef] [PubMed]

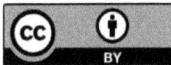

nutrients

MDPI

Commentary

Translation of Nutritional Genomics into Nutrition Practice: The Next Step

Chiara Murgia * and Melissa M. Adamski

Department of Nutrition, Dietetics and Food, Monash University, Notting Hill, VIC 3168, Australia;
melissa.adamski@monash.edu
* Correspondence: chiara.murgia@monash.edu; Tel.: +61-03-9902-4264

Received: 17 March 2017; Accepted: 4 April 2017; Published: 6 April 2017

Abstract: Genetics is an important piece of every individual health puzzle. The completion of the Human Genome Project sequence has deeply changed the research of life sciences including nutrition. The analysis of the genome is already part of clinical care in oncology, pharmacology, infectious disease and, rare and undiagnosed diseases. The implications of genetic variations in shaping individual nutritional requirements have been recognised and conclusively proven, yet routine use of genetic information in nutrition and dietetics practice is still far from being implemented. This article sets out the path that needs to be taken to build a framework to translate gene–nutrient interaction studies into best-practice guidelines, providing tools that health professionals can use to understand whether genetic variation affects nutritional requirements in their daily clinical practice.

Keywords: nutrigenetics; nutritional genomics; dietetics; best-practice

It is common for nutrition professionals to experience that the same dietary intervention and management strategy produce very different outcomes in different people. An overwhelming number of observations support the evidence that genetic background has a key role to play in individual response to diet and life-style, and in shaping individual nutritional requirements [1]. Proof of concept of these statements came from the well-described examples of inborn metabolic syndromes caused by single gene mutations affecting specific metabolic pathways. These syndromes are often successfully controlled with targeted dietary management which is able to prevent serious health consequences [2].

Phenylketonuria (PKU) is a rare inborn syndrome caused by a mutation in a single gene that encodes for the enzyme phenylalanine hydroxylase. The liver of PKU mutation carriers in homozygosis are unable to break down phenylalanine and are consequently unable to metabolise food that contains this amino acid. PKU was one of the first genetic conditions to be identified, and it is the result of a mutation in gene coding for an enzyme involved in a key step of a metabolic pathway; to date, the only effective management for PKU patients is a carefully tailored low protein diet [3]. Common polymorphisms (frequency > 1%) can also determine dietary requirements, for example, lactose intolerance is caused by the progressive reduction of the expression of the gene coding for the enzyme lactase due to a variant in the regulatory region of the gene. Carriers of these high frequency variants develop adverse symptoms if they consume milk or other lactose-rich dairy products [4]. These very well characterised examples show how the idea of changing, even dramatically, the diet of individuals carrying specific genetic variants is a common dietetic practice; so is the knowledge that foods, such as milk, that are highly nutritious for some, need to be consumed with care by others. The examples reported are relatively simple: a specific nutritional requirement is the consequence of a mutation or variation in a single gene. However, most of the time, the reality of nutrition and dietetic practice is more complicated. The metabolism of each nutrient involves the activity of several enzymes, each one encoded by a gene that is present in the population with multiple allelic variants; each of them potentially contributing to the absorption and utilisation of nutrients, ultimately affecting their requirements [5,6]. More than one genetic polymorphism is generally responsible for affecting the requirements of a nutrient or the predisposition to a chronic pathology. Indeed, it is now evident that even in traditionally classified monogenic conditions such as PKU, the penetrance and severity of the symptoms are determined by other gene variants, each one contributing with a specific effect size; in real life, every phenotype is produced by a combination of gene variants [3].

The completion of the Human Genome Project (HGP) [7] held the promise of resolving the complexity of individual responses to diet and the sometimes ineffectiveness of "one size fits all" public health guidelines for individuals, revealing the role of genetics in shaping nutritional requirements. The potential applications to nutrition of this invaluable tool were apparent since the genome was mapped. The first articles discussing nutrigenomics and nutrigenetics were published less than a year after the first draft and an initial analysis of the human DNA sequence was made available. Several papers discussed the potential impact of this new information on nutrition practice [7–9]. Since then, many authors have outlined how this new area of science may impact on nutrition practice. They have discussed what would be needed in terms of training and required knowledge for nutrition professionals, potential ethical, legal and social impacts on practice and other impacts on nutrition [10–12]. However, fifteen years and hundreds of publications later, the gap between the experimental and epidemiologic evidence and health practice is not yet closed [13]. The information provided by the HGP and the resources developed since its publication were applied in hundreds of studies; a PubMed search performed on 16 March 2017, using the search term "nutrigenomics OR nutrigenetics OR nutritional genomics" resulted in 2888 hits. While these papers/research are essential for understanding the impact of this new information on nutrition science and identifying what is needed to successfully put it into practice, progress in actually interpreting/translating the current evidence into useful information for healthcare professionals has yet to be seen. The importance of the genotype information is not the only factor that complicates this translation into practice; the discovery of other levels of control to dietary phenotyping, including environment-modulated epigenome and the intestinal microbiome are other complicating factors [14,15].

To translate genetic information into evidence-based nutritional recommendations, clear summaries and critical analysis of the current evidence base of identified polymorphisms and their interaction with nutrition and health need to be provided, including their effect size. This will allow healthcare professionals to more easily understand the relationship with nutrient metabolism, and whether there is any robust evidence for an intervention. First, the results in systematic reviews and meta-analysis need to be collated and second, user-friendly computational tools that can integrate the complex genetic and epigenetics information need to be built, integrating it with clinical and biochemical biomarkers. This approach has achieved a promising step toward with Eran Segal's group at Weizemann Institute. This important study developed an algorithm that integrates blood parameters, dietary habits, anthropometrics, physical activity, and gut microbiota to predict blood glucose response to meals with different contents of carbohydrates [16]. However, this complex tool does not take genetics or epigenetics into consideration.

A limited number of papers have reviewed the evidence in regards to specific areas of nutrigenetics in an attempt to collate and build the literature base [6,17–19]. This is one step closer to the inclusion of genetic variability as an important component and the translation of evidence into practice—but it is only the beginning.

Health professionals require clear best-practice guidelines to be able to translate the evidence into nutrition advice. In general, to guide nutrition and dietetic practice, nutrition research is regularly reviewed and analysed by experts to provide summaries of the latest evidence to guide practice. For example, the National Health and Medical Research Council in Australia provides guidance for the recommended nutrient intake along with summaries of the latest available evidence [20]. These are updated by expert working groups at regular periods to ensure up-to-dateness. Other countries also conduct similar research and translation [21,22]. These guidelines assist nutrition professionals in providing current, evidence-based recommendations. Similar processes occur in other health disciplines, where evidenced-based guidelines are developed, and regularly reviewed and updated to guide healthcare and medical professionals' practice.

Nutritionists and dietitians were identified as prime candidates to provide advice on nutrition and genetics, but the development of guidelines and evidence summaries for these professionals has been scarce [23]. Currently, nutrition professionals are expected to search, critically analyse and translate the findings into practice; for many, this may provide a challenge, especially since extensive genetic and genomic training is not a traditional area of training for nutrition professionals [24,25]. Assessments of the literature in regards to gene–nutrient interactions, similar to the Dietary Reference Intakes (DRIs) (USA) and Nutrient Reference Values (NRVs) (Australia), must be performed in order to translate nutritional genomics into clinical practice. We need to use the experience to build a framework to translate gene–nutrient interaction studies into usable guidelines and provide answers to nutrition professionals looking to understand whether genetic variation affects nutritional requirements. These assessments of the literature should be carried out by expert working groups comprising of geneticists, bioinformaticians, nutritionists, dietitians and clinical geneticists.

While the science of nutritional genomics continues to demonstrate potential individual responses to nutrition, the complex nature of gene, nutrition and health interactions continues to provide a challenge for healthcare professionals to analyse, interpret and apply to patient recommendations. Evidenced-based summaries and interpretations of the current literature base urgently need to be developed by expert working teams of both genetic experts and nutrition experts. These summaries can then provide the basis for the development of best-practice guidelines for nutrition professionals for use in clinical practice.

Author Contributions: Chiara Murgia and Melissa M. Adamski conceived and wrote the manuscript.

Conflicts of Interest: The authors declare no conflict of interest.

References

1. Fenech, M.; El-Sohemy, A.; Cahill, L.; Ferguson, L.R.; French, T.A.; Tai, E.S.; Milner, J.; Koh, W.P.; Xie, L.; Zucker, M.; et al. Nutrigenetics and nutrigenomics: Viewpoints on the current status and applications in nutrition research and practice. *J. Nutrigenet. Nutr.* **2011**, *4*, 69–89. [CrossRef] [PubMed]

2. Boyer, S.W.; Barclay, L.J.; Burrage, L.C. Inherited metabolic disorders: Aspects of chronic nutrition management. *Nutr. Clin. Pract.* **2015**, *30*, 502–510. [CrossRef] [PubMed]

3. Scriver, C.R. The pah gene, phenylketonuria, and a paradigm shift. *Hum. Mutat.* **2007**, *28*, 831–845. [CrossRef] [PubMed]

4. Deng, Y.; Misselwitz, B.; Dai, N.; Fox, M. Lactose intolerance in adults: Biological mechanism and dietary management. *Nutrients* **2015**, *7*, 8020–8035. [CrossRef] [PubMed]

5. Frazier-Wood, A.C. Dietary patterns, genes, and health: Challenges and obstacles to be overcome. *Curr. Nutr. Rep.* **2015**, *4*, 82–87. [CrossRef] [PubMed]

6. Day, K.J.; Adamski, M.M.; Dordevic, A.L.; Murgia, C. Genetic variations as modifying factors to dietary zinc requirements—A systematic review. *Nutrients* **2017**, *9*, 148. [CrossRef] [PubMed]

7. Lander, E.S.; Linton, L.M.; Birren, B.; Nusbaum, C.; Zody, M.C.; Baldwin, J.; Devon, K.; Dewar, K.; Doyle, M.; FitzHugh, W.; et al. Initial sequencing and analysis of the human genome. *Nature* **2001**, *409*, 860–921. [CrossRef] [PubMed]

8. Elliott, R.; Ong, T.J. Nutritional genomics. *BMJ-Brit. Med. J.* **2002**, *324*, 1438–1442. [CrossRef]

9. Van Ommen, B.; Stierum, R. Nutrigenomics: Exploiting systems biology in the nutrition and health arena. *Curr. Opin. Biotech.* **2002**, *13*, 517–521. [CrossRef]

10. DeBusk, R. Diet-related disease, nutritional genomics, and food and nutrition professionals. *J. Am. Diet. Assoc.* **2009**, *109*, 410–413. [CrossRef] [PubMed]

11. DeBusk, R.M.; Fogarty, C.P.; Ordovas, J.M.; Kornman, K.S. Nutritional genomics in practice: Where do we begin? *J. Am. Diet. Assoc.* **2005**, *105*, 589–598. [CrossRef] [PubMed]

12. Rosen, R.; Earthman, C.; Marquart, L.; Reicks, M. Continuing education needs of registered dietitians regarding nutrigenomics. *J. Am. Diet. Assoc.* **2006**, *106*, 1242–1245. [CrossRef] [PubMed]

13. Ferguson, J.F.; Allayee, H.; Gerszten, R.E.; Ideraabdullah, F.; Kris-Etherton, P.M.; Ordovas, J.M.; Rimm, E.B.; Wang, T.J.; Bennett, B.J. Nutrigenomics, the Microbiome, and Gene-Environment Interactions: New Directions in Cardiovascular Disease Research, Prevention, and Treatment. *Circ. Cardiovasc. Genet.* **2016**, *9*, 291–313. [CrossRef] [PubMed]

14. Dey, M. Toward a personalized approach in prebiotics research. *Nutrients* **2017**, *9*, 92. [CrossRef] [PubMed]

15. Sharma, U.; Rando, O.J. Metabolic inputs into the epigenome. *Cell Metab.* **2017**, *25*, 544–558. [CrossRef] [PubMed]

16. Zeevi, D.; Korem, T.; Zmora, N.; Israeli, D.; Rothschild, D.; Weinberger, A.; Ben-Yacov, O.; Lador, D.; Avnit-Sagi, T.; Lotan-Pompan, M.; et al. Personalized nutrition by prediction of glycemic responses. *Cell* **2015**, *163*, 1079–1094. [CrossRef] [PubMed]

17. Kanoni, S.; Nettleton, J.A.; Hivert, M.F.; Ye, Z.; van Rooij, F.J.; Shungin, D.; Sonestedt, E.; Ngwa, J.S.; Wojczynski, M.K.; Lemaitre, R.N.; et al. Total zinc intake may modify the glucose-raising effect of a zinc transporter (SLC30A8) variant: A 14-cohort meta-analysis. *Diabetes* **2011**, *60*, 2407–2416. [CrossRef] [PubMed]

18. Shaghaghi, M.A.; Kloss, O.; Eck, P. Genetic variation in human vitamin c transporter genes in common complex diseases. *Adv. Nutr.* **2016**, *7*, 287–298. [CrossRef] [PubMed]

19. Colson, N.J.; Naug, H.L.; Nikbakht, E.; Zhang, P.; McCormack, J. The impact of mthfr 677 C/Tgenotypes on folate status markers: A meta-analysis of folic acid intervention studies. *Eur. J. Nutr.* **2017**, *56*, 247–260. [CrossRef] [PubMed]

20. Nutrient Reference Values. Available online: https://www.nrv.gov.au/ (accessed on 15 March 2017).

21. Food and Nutrition Board, Institute of Medicine (I.o.M). Available online: http://nationalacademies.org/hmd/about-hmd/leadership-staff/hmd-staff-leadership-boards/food-and-nutrition-board.aspx (accessed on 15 March 2017).

22. Scientific Advisory Committee on Nutrition (SACN), U.K.G. Available online: https://www.gov.uk/government/groups/scientific-advisory-committee-on-nutrition (accessed on 15 March 2017).

23. Kicklighter, J.R.; Dorner, B.; Hunter, A.M.; Kyle, M.; Pflugh Prescott, M.; Roberts, S.; Spear, B.; Hand, R.K.; Byrne, C. Visioning report 2017: A preferred path forward for the nutrition and dietetics profession. *J. Acad. Nutr. Diet.* **2017**, *117*, 110–127. [CrossRef] [PubMed]

24. Collins, J.; Bertrand, B.; Hayes, V.; Li, S.X.; Thomas, J.; Truby, H.; Whelan, K. The application of genetics and nutritional genomics in practice: An international survey of knowledge, involvement and confidence among dietitians in the US, Australia and the UK. *Genes Nutr.* **2013**, *8*, 523–533. [CrossRef] [PubMed]

25. Li, S.X.; Collins, J.; Lawson, S.; Thomas, J.; Truby, H.; Whelan, K.; Palermo, C. A preliminary qualitative exploration of dietitians' engagement with genetics and nutritional genomics: Perspectives from international leaders. *J. Allied Health* **2014**, *43*, 221–228. [PubMed]

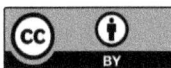

nutrients

Article

Novel Genetic Variants Associated with Child Refractory Esophageal Stricture with Food Allergy by Exome Sequencing

Min Yang [1,*], Min Xiong [2], Huan Chen [1], Lanlan Geng [1], Peiyu Chen [1], Jing Xie [1], Shui Qing Ye [2], Ding-You Li [3,*] and Sitang Gong [1,*]

[1]   Department of Gastroenterology, Guangzhou Women and Children's Medical Center,
     Guangzhou Medical University, 9 Jinsui Road, Guangzhou 510623, China; mandy1005@163.com (H.C.);
     genglan_2001@hotmail.com (L.G.); chenpei.y@163.com (P.C.); xiejing616@126.com (J.X.)
[2]   Division of Experimental and Translational Genetics, Children's Mercy Hospital,
     University of Missouri Kansas City School of Medicine, 2401 Gillham Road, Kansas City, MO 64108, USA;
     mxiong2@cmh.edu (M.X.); sqye@cmh.edu (S.Q.Y.)
[3]   Division of Gastroenterology, Children's Mercy Hospital,
     University of Missouri Kansas City School of Medicine, 2401 Gillham Road, Kansas City, MO 64108, USA
*   Correspondence: ymlyxw@hotmail.com (M.Y.); dyli@cmh.edu (D.-Y.L.); sitangg@126.com (S.G.);
     Tel.: +86-135-6010-1008 (M.Y.); +1-816-983-6770 (D.-Y.L.); +86-139-2600-2111 (S.G.)

Received: 26 January 2017; Accepted: 13 April 2017; Published: 15 April 2017

Abstract: Background: Refractory esophageal stricture (RES) may be attributed to food allergy. Its etiology and pathogenesis are not fully understood. Identification of novel genetic variants associated with this disease by exome sequencing (exome-seq) may provide new mechanistic insights and new therapeutic targets. Methods: To identify new and novel disease-associating variants, whole-exome sequencing was performed on an Illumina NGS platform in three children with RES as well as food allergy. Results: A total of 91,024 variants were identified. By filtering out 'normal variants' against those of the 1000 Genomes Project, we identified 12,741 remaining variants which are potentially associated with RES plus food allergy. Among these variants, there are 11,539 single nucleotide polymorphisms (SNPs), 627 deletions, 551 insertions and 24 mixture variants. These variants are located in 1370 genes. They are enriched in biological processes or pathways such as cell adhesion, digestion, receptor metabolic process, bile acid transport and the neurological system. By the PubMatrix analysis, 50 out of the top 100 genes, which contain most variants, have not been previously associated with any of the 17 allergy-associated diseases. These 50 genes represent newly identified allergy-associated genes. Those variants of 627 deletions and 551 insertions have also not been reported before in RES with food allergy. Conclusions: Exome-seq is potentially a powerful tool to identify potential new biomarkers for RES with food allergy. This study has identified a number of novel genetic variants, opening new avenues of research in RES plus food allergy. Additional validation in larger and different patient populations and further exploration of the underlying molecular mechanisms are warranted.

Keywords: children; exome-seq; food allergy; genetic variants; refractory esophageal stricture

1. Introduction

Benign esophageal stricture in children may be caused by caustic ingestion, peptic ulcer disease, congenital anomaly and esophageal surgery [1]. Endoscopic balloon dilatation is safe and effective in the majority of children with esophageal stricture [2]. Refractory esophageal stricture (RES) refers to those that do not respond to repeated dilations, which may be attributed to food allergy. There have been reports that cow's milk protein allergy may develop after gastrointestinal surgeries or injuries, possibly due to a disruption of the mucosal barrier [3–5]. We speculated that genetic susceptibility contributes to the development of food allergy in children with RES. The aim of this study was to use whole-exome sequencing to identify potential new underlying genetic variants in those children.

2. Methods

2.1. Patients

The institutional ethics committee of Guangzhou Women and Children's Medical Center approved this study protocol (20170301).

We included three children diagnosed with RES and multiple food allergies (Table 1). Patients' clinical features, laboratory tests and treatment outcomes were reviewed. After initial clinical evaluation, patients underwent endoscopic examination to assess for esophageal stricture. Subsequent endoscopic balloon dilatation was performed according to the standard protocol. Balloon dilatation was repeated based upon the patient's symptom of dysphagia. All three patients were considered refractory to esophageal balloon dilatations and were found to have a positive serum IgE (sIgE) response to milk, eggs and peanuts. After treatment with dietary allergen exclusion, all patients showed clinical improvement and resolution of esophageal stricture.

Table 1. Characteristics of children with refractory esophageal strictures. EBD: esophageal balloon dilatation; sIgE: serum IgE.

Case	1	2	3
Age (years)	12	2.5	4
Sex	male	male	male
Age at stricture diagnosis	8 years	1 month	2 years
Cause	Caustic agent	Post-surgery (esophageal atresia)	Post-surgery (Hiatal hernia)
Initial stenosis diameter (mm)	1	5	<1
EBD (times)	18	7	6
Esophageal mucosal eosinophil/hpf	9	35	12
sIgE			
Milk	+	+	+
Egg	+	+	+
Wheat	+	-	+
Peanut	+	+	+
Soy	-	-	+
Fish	-	-	+
Others	rice	crab	rice
Treatment	Dietary allergen exclusion	Elemental formula	Dietary allergen exclusion
Follow-up duration (months)	14	12	26
Resolution of esophageal stricture	Yes	Yes	Yes

2.2. Exome Capture and Illumina Sequencing

Genomic DNA from each patient's blood was isolated using DNeasy Blood & Tissue Kit (Cat. No. 69504, Qiagen, Valencia, CA, USA) following the manufacturer's protocol. The libraries for exome sequencing were created using the Nextera Rapid Capture Exome and Expanded Exome Kit (Illumina, San Diego, CA, USA). TruSeq SBS v3 whole-exome, 2×101 paired end sequencing was performed on the Illumina Hiseq1500 platform according to the manufacturer's instructions.

2.3. Read Mapping and Variant Calling

The paired-end reads were aligned to the hg19 human reference genome using BWA (Burrows-Wheeler Aligner) [6]. Picard Sort Sam was used to convert the SAM (sequence alignment map) file into a BAM (binary sequence alignment map) file, and to sort the BAM file order by starting positions [7]. Picard Mark Duplicates was used to remove PCR duplicates (7). The read group information was very important for downstream GATK (genome analysis toolkit) functionality. Picard Add Or Replace Read Groups replaced all read groups in the input file with a single new read group and assigned all reads to this read group in the output BAM [7]. Samtools indexed the BAM file for fast random access to the human reference genome [8]. The Genome Analysis Toolkit (GATK) pipeline was used for recalibration, local realignment around indels and variation calling [9]. SNPs with a quality score less than 20, a depth of coverage less than 4, call ratios below 0.85 and HWE (Hardy-Weinberg equilibrium) below 10^{-6} were removed. SNP & Variation Suite™ software (Golden Helix, Inc., Bozeman, MT, USA) was used for variation annotation and genotype association tests. Predictions of protein functional effect changes with those variants were performed by Sift and Polyphen 2 [10,11]. DAVID was utilized to perform Gene Ontology to identify the cellular biological processes of genes with pediatric refractory esophageal stricture with food allergy SNPs [12]. PubMatrix analysis [13], a multiplex literature mining tool, was used as described previously [14] to build the relationship between genes with milk-protein allergy variations and allergy-associated diseases in PubMed.

3. Results

For the discovery phase, 91,024 variants were detected by whole-exome sequencing in three patients. After filtering lower quality alleles, 62,971 high quality variants were kept for the subsequent analysis. 12,741 variants of 1370 genes were kept after filtering out 'healthy' wildtype or SNPs from the 1000 genome phase 3 population [15] found in the three patients, and 90.57% of the variants were SNPs (Figure 1). The majority of variants were located in non-coding intronic and intergenic regions (82.53%) (Figure 2A). Further analysis of variants within the coding regions revealed that 55.13% of variants identified in the three patients were nonsynonymous SNPs (Figure 2B). Interestingly, phenotypic damage analysis of these variants by SIFT and Polyphen 2 HVAR showed that 204 and 89 variants existing in the three patients were predicted as damaging variants, respectively.

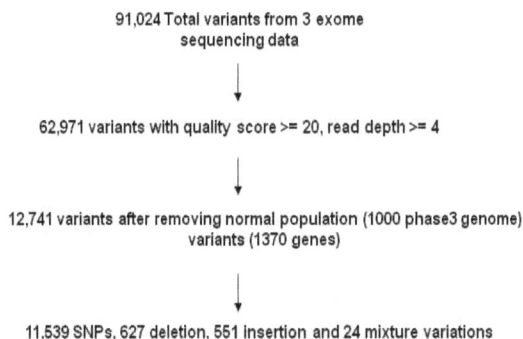

91,024 Total variants from 3 exome sequencing data

↓

62,971 variants with quality score >= 20, read depth >= 4

↓

12,741 variants after removing normal population (1000 phase3 genome) variants (1370 genes)

↓

11,539 SNPs, 627 deletion, 551 insertion and 24 mixture variations

Figure 1. Workflow of identifying new genetic variants in three children with RES plus food allergy. Identified total variants were first subjected to the quality control and then filtered against 'normal variants' of the 1000 Genomes Project exome sequences (quality score ≥ 20, read depth ≥ 4). The remaining variants were applied for the further analyses.

The 12,741 variants identified in the three patients were located in 1370 genes. Among them, 182 genes were enzymes, 48 genes were transporters and 27 genes were ion channels. The 30 significant biological processes were enriched for genes with these variants ($p < 0.05$). Figure 3 shows the top 20 biological processes' enrichment. Sixty-two genes with 177 variants were enriched in cell adhesion, 15 genes with 169 variants were enriched in digestion, seven genes with 10 variants were enriched in receptor metabolic process, four genes with five variants were enriched in bile acid and bile salt transport, and 82 genes with 483 variants were enriched in neurological system process, all of which are important biological processes for pediatric refractory esophageal stricture combined with food allergy (Figure 4). The majority of these variants in digestion (66.27%) and neurological system process (68.12%) were located in coding regions (Figure 4).

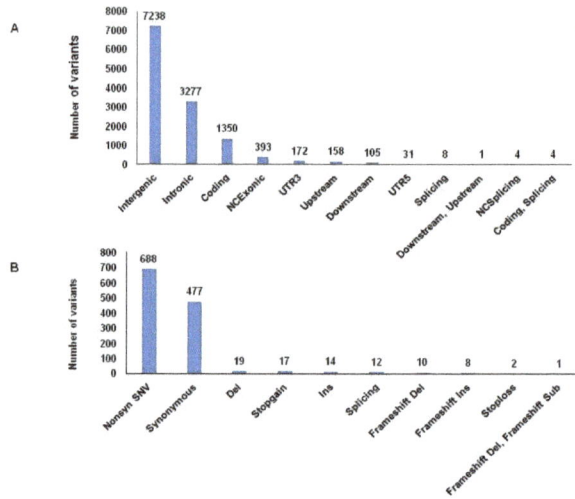

Figure 2. Variant location and type analyses. (**A**) Variant locations. Variant distribution in each of 12 regions are displayed in bar graphs. UTR, untranslated region; NC, noncoding region. (**B**) Variant types. Distribution of 10 different variant types are presented in bar graphs. Del, deletion; Sub, substitution.

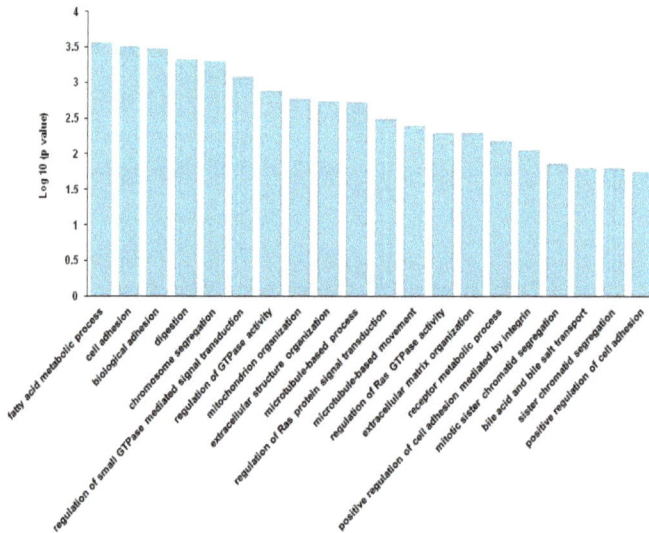

Figure 3. Top 20 biological processes' enrichment of genes with variants found in all three patients. All disease-associated genes with variants found in all three patients were supplied for biological process analysis using the software program DAVID, as described in Methods. Only the top 20 biological processes are presented.

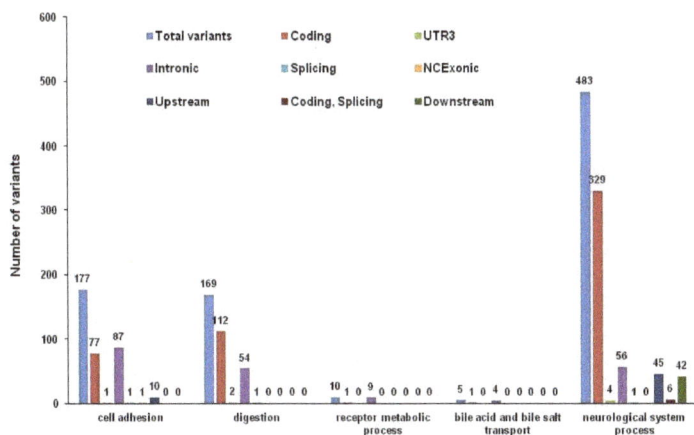

Figure 4. Variant type distribution in five relevant pathways or biological processes. Variant type (eight) distributions in five relevant pathways or biological processes are displayed in bar graphs.

To identify potential etiologic genes, we ranked variant counts by genes. Three hundred and fifty-six genes had splicing and coding region variations, and the genes MUC6, OR8U1, OR8U8, PDE4DIP and KCNJ12 ranked in the top five. To further mine relationships between genes with RES with food allergy variations and allergy-associated diseases in PubMed, we submit the top 100 genes and 17 allergy-associated diseases into PubMatrix. This approach identified the genes MUC5B, FANCD2, MUC6, TPSAB1, MUC16, MAP2K3, NCOR1, PRSS1 and KRT18 as being linked to the most allergy terms (Figure 5).

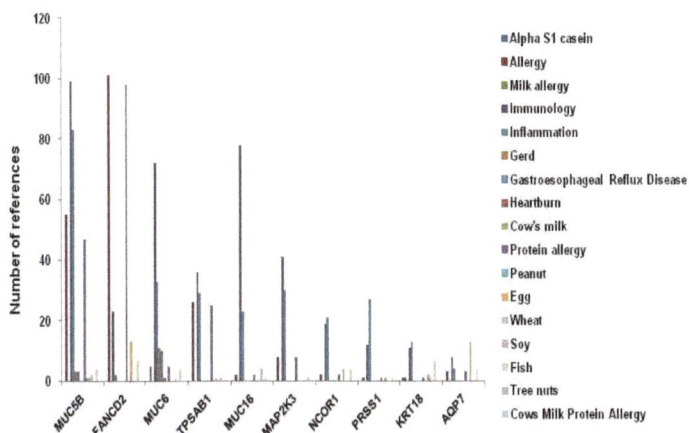

Figure 5. Top 10 PubMatrix genes with variants in splicing and coding regions found in all three patients. Top genes were applied to PubMatrix analysis to probe whether they have been previously associated with any of the 17 allergy-related diseases or conditions. The top 10 genes with the most previous association reports in literature are presented.

4. Discussion

We identified three children with refractory esophageal stricture who were found to have food allergies to milk, eggs and peanuts. One patient had an esophageal mucosal eosinophil count of 35/hpf, and most likely has eosinophilic esophagitis. Two other patients had esophageal mucosal eosinophil counts of 9/hpf and 12/hpf, respectively, and did not meet histological criteria ($\geq$15 eos/hpf) for eosinophilic esophagitis [16]. All patients responded well to dietary allergen exclusion, with resolution of esophageal strictures. To our knowledge, this is the first report associating food allergies with complicated refractory esophageal stricture in children who subsequently responded well to dietary allergen exclusion. Based on our report, it is important to consider cow's milk protein allergy or multiple food allergies in children with refractory esophageal stricture.

This study applied whole-exome sequencing analysis to systematically identify genome-wide coding variants which may underlie genetic susceptibility to pediatric refractory esophageal stricture with food allergy from three children. Our analyses identified 12,741 variants of 1370 genes in these patients after filtering the 1000 Genome Project Phase 3 controls [15]. Three hundred and fifty-six genes with 1350 variants had splicing and coding region variations, among them 688 variants were nonsynonymous SNPs. The potential candidate genes in pediatric refractory esophageal stricture with food allergy are involved in ion channel, transporter, cell adhesion, digestion, receptor metabolic process, bile acid and bile salt transport and neurological system processes. These biological functions and pathways have a major impact on esophageal function, which is consistent with the pathogenesis of pediatric refractory esophageal stricture with food allergy.

Through searching the literature for the top 100 found genes in the three patients with refractory esophageal stricture with food allergy variations, 50 genes were previously linked to 17 allergy-associated diseases, 21 genes were previously associated with allergy, and 19 genes were linked specifically to protein allergy. This finding lends a strong support that WES (whole exome sequencing) is a promising approach to identify genetically susceptible genes linked with both refractory esophageal stricture and food allergy. However, none of these top genes are linked to cow's milk and milk allergy, and 50 genes have not been previously associated with any of the 17 allergy-associated diseases. These 50 genes represent newly identified allergy-associated genes, opening new avenues to investigate new genetic risk factors in refractory esophageal stricture combined with food allergy.

Among top candidate genes, the MUC6 gene encodes a secreted glycoprotein that plays an important role in the cytoprotection of epithelial surfaces and mechanical trauma in the gastrointestinal tract [17,18]. Eighty-six variations were found in MUC6 splicing and coding regions in the three patients with RES and food allergies. Ten gastroesophageal reflux diseases and five protein allergy studies in the literature were reported to link to MUC6.

The majority of SNPs (82.53%) identified in this study map to non-coding regions of the genome, which complicates the analysis of these variations. However, this is a common finding in GWAS (genome-wide association study) studies and suggests that non-coding SNPs are located in functional regulatory regions, such as splicing regulatory elements, enhancer elements, DNase hypersensitivity regions and chromatin marks [19]. Thus, these non-coding SNPs may regulate the expression of nearby genes.

5. Conclusions

This study has demonstrated the power of WES to identify new genetic risk factors within the whole-exome scale in children with refractory esophageal stricture as well as food allergies. It should be mentioned that our study is limited to only three patients, and thus no solid conclusion can be drawn without a proper control and a large sample size. Replication of our findings in larger and different populations, in addition to experimental delineation of the underlying molecular mechanisms, is warranted to validate the candidate variants identified here as true genetic biomarkers and to develop them into potential therapeutic targets in refractory esophageal stricture presenting with food allergy.

Acknowledgments: We thank Craig Friesen from Children's Mercy Hospital for critical reading of the manuscript.

Author Contributions: Min Yang participated in acquisition, analysis and interpretation of data, statistical analysis, and drafting of the initial manuscript; Min Xiong, Huan Chen, Lanlan Geng and Peiyu Chen all participated in acquisition, analysis and interpretation of data; Shui Qing Ye participated in critical revision of the manuscript for important intellectual content; Sitang Gong and Ding-You Li conceptualized the study, revised the manuscript for important intellectual content, obtained funding and supervised the project.

Conflicts of Interest: The authors declare no conflict of interest.

References

1. Ball, W.S.; Strife, J.L.; Rosenkrantz, J.; Towbin, R.B.; Noseworthy, J. Esophageal strictures in children. Treatment by balloon dilatation. *Radiology* **1984**, *150*, 263e4. [CrossRef] [PubMed]
2. Alshammari, J.; Quesnel, S.; Pierrot, S.; Couloigner, V. Endoscopic balloon dilatation of esophageal strictures in children. *Int. J. Ped. Otorhinolaryngol.* **2011**, *75*, 1376–1379. [CrossRef] [PubMed]
3. El Hassani, A.; Michaud, L.; Chartier, A.; Penel-Capelle, D.; Sfeir, R.; Besson, R.; Turck, D.; Gottrand, F. Cow's milk protein allergy after neonatal intestinal surgery. *Arch. Pediatr.* **2005**, *12*, 134–139. [CrossRef] [PubMed]
4. Ikeda, K.; Ida, S.; Kawahara, H.; Kawamoto, K.; Etani, Y.; Kubota, A. Importance of evaluating for cow's milk allergy in pediatric surgical patients with functional bowel symptoms. *J. Pediatr. Surg.* **2011**, *46*, 2332–2335. [CrossRef] [PubMed]
5. Matsuki, T.; Kaga, A.; Kanda, S.; Suzuki, Y.; Tanabu, M.; Sawa, N. Intestinal malrotation with suspected cow's milk allergy: A case report. *BMC Res. Notes* **2012**, *5*, 481. [CrossRef] [PubMed]
6. Li, H.; Durbin, R. Fast and accurate long read alignment with Burrows-Wheeler transform. *Bioinformatics* **2009**, *25*, 1754–1760. [CrossRef] [PubMed]
7. Van der Auwera, G.A.; Carneiro, M.O.; Hartl, C.; Poplin, R.; Del Angel, G.; Levy-Moonshine, A.; Jordan, T.; Shakir, K.; Roazen, D.; Thibault, J.; et al. From FastQ data to high confidence variant calls: The Genome Analysis Toolkit best practices pipeline. *Curr. Protoc. Bioinform.* **2013**, *43*, 11.10.1–11.10.33.
8. Li, H.; Handsaker, B.; Wysoker, A.; Fennell, T.; Ruan, J.; Homer, N.; Marth, G.; Abecasis, G.; Durbin, R.; 1000 Genome Project Data Processing Subgroup. The Sequence Alignment/Map format and SAMtools. *Bioinformatics* **2009**, *25*, 2078–2079. [PubMed]
9. McKenna, A.; Hanna, M.; Banks, E.; Sivachenko, A.; Cibulskis, K.; Kernytsky, A.; Garimella, K.; Altshuler, D.; Gabriel, S.; Daly, M.; et al. The Genome Analysis Toolkit: A MapReduce framework for analyzing next-generation DNA sequencing data. *Genome Res.* **2010**, *20*, 1297–1303. [CrossRef] [PubMed]
10. Adzhubei, I.A.; Schmidt, S.; Peshkin, L.; Ramensky, V.E.; Gerasimova, A.; Bork, P.; Kondrashov, A.S.; Sunyaev, S.R. A method and server for predicting damaging missense mutations. *Nat. Methods.* **2010**, *7*, 248–249. [CrossRef] [PubMed]
11. Kumar, P.; Henikoff, S.; Ng, P.C. Predicting the effects of coding non-synonymous variants on protein function using the SIFT algorithm. *Nat. Protoc.* **2009**, *4*, 1073–1081. [CrossRef] [PubMed]
12. Huang da, W.; Sherman, B.T.; Lempicki, R.A. Systematic and integrative analysis of large gene lists using DAVID bioinformatics resources. *Nat. Protoc.* **2009**, *4*, 44–57. [CrossRef] [PubMed]
13. Becker, K.G.; Hosack, D.A.; Dennis, G., Jr.; Lempicki, R.A.; Bright, T.J.; Cheadle, C.; Engel, J. PubMatrix: A tool for multiplex literature mining. *BMC Bioinform.* **2003**, *4*, 61. [CrossRef] [PubMed]
14. Xiong, M.; Heruth, D.P.; Zhang, L.Q.; Ye, S.Q. Identification of lung-specific genes by meta-analysis of multiple tissue RNA-seq data. *FEBS Open Bio* **2016**, *6*, 774–781. [CrossRef] [PubMed]
15. 1000 Genomes Project Consortium. A global reference for human genetic variation. *Nature* **2015**, *526*, 68–74.
16. Dellon, E.S. Eosinophilic esophagitis: Diagnostic testsandcriteria. *Curr. Opin. Gastroenterol.* **2012**, *28*, 382–388. [CrossRef] [PubMed]
17. Reis, C.A.; David, L.; Correa, P.; Carneiro, F.; de Bolós, C.; Garcia, E.; Mandel, U.; Clausen, H.; Sobrinho-Simões, M. Intestinal metaplasia of human stomach displays distinct patterns of mucin (MUC1, MUC2, MUC5AC, and MUC6) expression. *Cancer Res.* **1999**, *59*, 1003–1007. [PubMed]
18. Corfield, A.P.; Carroll, D.; Myerscough, N.; Probert, C.S. Mucins in the gastrointestinal tract in health and disease. *Front. Biosci.* **2001**, *6*, D1321–D1357. [CrossRef] [PubMed]
19. Zhang, F.; Lupski, J.R. Non-coding genetic variants in human disease. *Hum. Mol. Genet.* **2015**, *24*, R102–R110. [CrossRef] [PubMed]

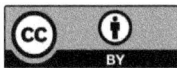

![nutrients logo] *nutrients*

Article

Genetic Variants Involved in One-Carbon Metabolism: Polymorphism Frequencies and Differences in Homocysteine Concentrations in the Folic Acid Fortification Era

Josiane Steluti [1,*], Aline M. Carvalho [1], Antonio A. F. Carioca [1], Andreia Miranda [1], Gilka J. F. Gattás [2], Regina M. Fisberg [1] and Dirce M. Marchioni [1]

[1] Department of Nutrition, School of Public Health, Sao Paulo University, Avenida Doutor Arnaldo, 715-Cerqueira César, São Paulo—SP, São Paulo 01246-904, Brazil; aline.carvalho.usp@gmail.com (A.M.C.); nutriaugusto@gmail.com (A.A.F.C.); andreia.am.miranda@gmail.com (A.M.); rfisberg@usp.br (R.M.F.); marchioni@usp.br (D.M.M.)
[2] Department of Legal Medicine, Bioethics and Occupational Health, School of Medicine, University of São Paulo, Avenida Doutor Arnaldo, 455-Cerqueira César, São Paulo—SP, São Paulo 01246-903, Brazil; gfgattas@usp.br
* Correspondence: jsteluti@usp.br; Tel.: +55-11-3061-7856

Received: 24 March 2017; Accepted: 18 May 2017; Published: 25 May 2017

Abstract: Folate and other B vitamins are essential co-factors of one-carbon metabolism, and genetic variants, such as polymorphisms, can alter the metabolism. Furthermore, the adoption of food fortification with folic acid showed a decrease of homocysteine concentration. The aim of this study was to investigate the frequencies of the polymorphisms of enzymes and carrier proteins involved in one-carbon metabolism, and to evaluate homocysteine concentrations in the presence of these genetic variants in a population exposed to mandatory food fortification with folic acid. Using data from a population-based cross-sectional study in São Paulo, Brazil, the study population comprised 750 participants above 12 years of age of both genders. A linear regression model was used to evaluate the homocysteine concentrations according to genetic variants and folate level. The results showed that the minor allelic frequencies were 0.33 for MTHFR (rs1801133), 0.24 for MTHFR (rs1801131), 0.19 for MTR (rs1805087), 0.42 for MTRR (rs1801394), 0.46 for RFC1 (rs1051266), and 0.47 for DHFR (19-bp deletion). The genetic variants of MTHFR 677C>T, MTRR 66A>G and RFC-1 80G>A were different according to race. The homocysteine concentrations increased in the CT and TT compared to CC genotypes of polymorphism *MTHFR* 677C>T in all populations, and differences between the homocysteine concentrations according to the genotypes of *MTHFR* 677C>T were observed regardless of folate level.

Keywords: one-carbon metabolism; folic acid fortification; genetic variants; homocysteine; polymorphisms

---

1. Introduction

One-carbon metabolism plays an important role in complex and essential metabolic pathways, as hundreds of intracellular transmethylation reactions, including DNA methylation and DNA synthesis, have been implicated in carcinogenesis [1] and processes closely associated with homocysteine (Hcy) metabolism [2]. Vitamins, particularly folate (B9) and other B vitamins, such as B6 and B12, are essential co-factors of one-carbon metabolism (Figure 1) [3].

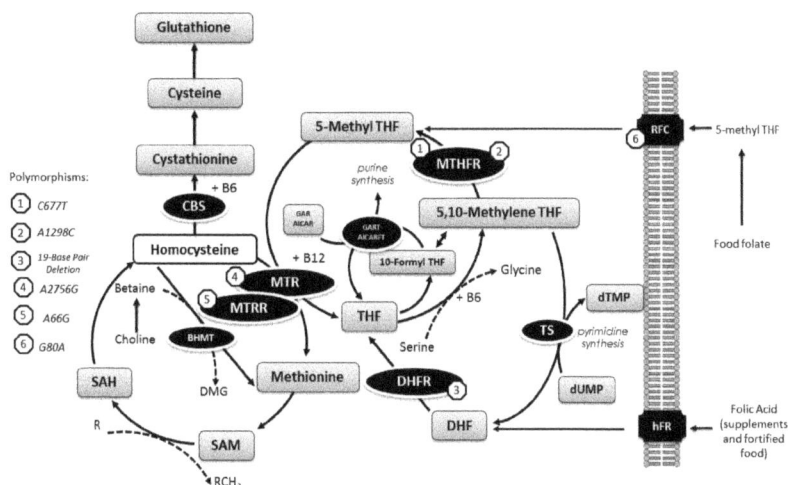

Figure 1. Overview of one-carbon metabolism considering metabolites, enzymes, coenzymes, and genetic variants. Abbreviations: methylenetetrahydrofolate reductase (MTHFR), methionine synthase (MTR), methionine synthase reductase (MTRR), reduced folate carrier (RFC), dihydrofolate reductase (DHFR), tetrahydrofolate (THF), cystathionine β-synthase (CBS), dihydrofolate (DHF), human folate receptor (hFR), *S*-adenosylmethionine (SAM), *S*-adenosylhomocysteine (SAH), thymidylate synthase (TS), deoxyuridine monophosphate (dUMP), deoxythymidine monophosphate (dTMP), Betaine–Homocysteine *S*-Methyltransferase (BHMT), dimethyglycine (DMG), glycinamide ribonucleotide (GAR), 5-aminoimidazole-4-carboxamide ribonucleotide (AICAR), glycinamide ribonucleotide transformylase (GART), 5-aminoimidazole-4-carboxamide ribonucleotide formyltransferase (AICARFT).

Studies have shown that the elevation of homocysteine levels is an important risk marker for the occurrence of adverse events, such as dementia, Alzheimer's disease, bone fractures, cancers, and particularly cardiovascular diseases [4,5]. Environmental and genetic factors modify homocysteine concentrations, for example, polymorphisms can alter metabolism, generating homocysteine accumulation [6]. However, increases in the levels of some vitamins, particularly folate and other vitamins, such as B6 and B12, modulates metabolic functions [5], consequently facilitating the remethylation of homocysteine, thereby hindering increases in the concentrations of this metabolite [6]. As a result, an important reduction of homocysteine concentration in some populations was observed after the adoption of food fortification with folic acid (synthetic form of folate) in several countries [7,8].

This observation highlights the importance of adequate nutrient intake, knowledge concerning genetic variant frequencies, and evaluation of country conditions in which the mandatory policy is to fortify foods with folic acid, as has occurred in Brazil since 2002. Furthermore, despite the accumulated evidence, there are gaps in the knowledge of the frequencies of genetic variants in several primarily healthy populations, and the impact of individual responses to diseases remains unknown. The objective of the present study was to investigate the frequency of the genetic variants involved in one-carbon metabolism and to evaluate homocysteine concentrations in accordance with the presence of these genetic variants considering the folate plasma level.

2. Materials and Methods

2.1. Study and Sample Population

We used the data from 'Health Survey of Sao Paulo' (ISA-Capital), a population-based and cross-sectional household health survey conducted in 2008 [9]. The study population comprised residents of private households in the urban area of São Paulo, Brazil. This complex probabilistic sample was obtained using conglomerates in two stages: census and household sectors (data from National Survey of Households 2005, IBGE). Six sample domains, comprising adolescents (12 to 19 years of age), adults (20 to 59 years of age), and elderly (60 years of age and older) individuals of both genders, were considered, and a total of 2691 participants were included to facilitate general data collection. Among these participants, blood samples and blood pressure and anthropometric measurements were obtained from 750 individuals. Other details of the sampling have been previously published [10].

In the present study, we considered all participants aged 12 years or older at the time of collection. A total of 750 individuals (158 adolescents, 303 adults, and 289 elderly) responded to a social-economic survey and underwent anthropometric measurement, and subsequently, blood samples were collected for genotyping.

The Ethical and Research Committee of the School of Public Health University of São Paulo (Protocol number 2001) approved this study, and informed consent was obtained from all participants.

2.2. Data Collection and Processing

In 2008, household information was obtained from randomly selected residents using structured questionnaires applied by previously trained interviewers. Demographic, social-economic, lifestyle, referred morbidity, family-history diseases, supplementation, medicine, and diet information were collected. In a subsequent home visit, blood samples were collected and anthropometric measurements were recorded.

2.3. Diet

Two 24-h recalls (24hR) were performed as a dietary survey. Food consumption described in both recalls was converted into energy and nutrient values using the Nutrition Data System for Research (NDSR, version 2007, Nutrition Coordinating Center (NCC), University of Minnesota, Minneapolis, MN, USA). This software is used to calculate the folate quantity in three different ways: (1) natural folate—the vitamin naturally present in food; (2) synthetic folate (folic acid)—vitamin added to fortified food and dietary supplements; and (3) dietary folate equivalents (DFE)—sum of the dietary quantity of natural folate and synthetic folate, considering the difference in the bioavailability of both forms. Additionally, synthetic folate values and, consequently, the DFE values were corrected, considering the mandatory fortification of wheat and corn flour in Brazil since 2004. Moreover, the Multiple Source Method (MSM) was used to measure folate intake to estimate the usual consumption distribution of nutrients, mitigating the effects of intra-individual variation when at least two dietary measurements per individual are available [11].

2.4. Anthropometric Measures

Weight and height were measured and the anthropometric data were used to calculate Body Mass Index (BMI), and the individuals were classified, according to the BMI cut-off points of the World Health Organization (WHO) [12], as underweight—BMI < 18.5 kg/m^2; eutrophic—BMI 18.5–24.9 kg/m^2, and overweight—BMI ≥ 25 kg/m^2. A previously trained nurse technician performed all measurements.

2.5. Blood Collection

A trained nurse technician performed blood collection at home using disposable needles and syringes according to the standardized procedures described in the Guidelines for the Assessment of Food Consumption in population studies which reported an experience of the Health Survey in São Paulo [9]. The blood samples were collected through venipuncture after 12-h fasting.

Approximately 20 mL of blood were collected in tubes containing EDTA (ethylenediaminetetraacetic acid) and plastic serum tubes which had spray-coated silica through venipuncture. The tubes were stored in Styrofoam packages with recyclable ice packs and were transported to the Laboratory of Human Nutrition at School of Public Health, followed by centrifugation and processing into aliquots of serum and plasma, and storage at −80 °C.

2.6. Biochemical Analysis

The folate dosage was determined through High-Performance Liquid Chromatography (HPLC) with electrochemical detection [13]. The B6 concentrations were analyzed by HPLC with fluorometric detection using the ImmunDiagnostik AG® HPLC-Analytik system [14]. Vitamin B12 concentrations were determined by a chemiluminescence immunoassay with paramagnetic particles for the quantitative determination of vitamin levels in human serum and plasma using the Access Immunoassay System® (Beckman Coulter, Inc., Galway, Ireland). The immunoassay method of chemiluminescence microparticles using the ARCHITECT Homocysteine Reagent Kit (Abbott Diagnostics Division, Abbott Park, IL, USA) was used to analyze the plasma concentrations of homocysteine. All tests were performed according to the manufacturer's instructions.

Mean intra-assay coefficients of variation (CVs) for B6, B12, folate, and homocysteine, respectively, were 7.2%, 7.0%, 2.0%, and 2.3%, and mean inter-assay CVs were 5.9%, 8.5%, 3.4%, and 4.0%, respectively.

2.7. DNA Extraction and Genotyping

The DNA was extracted using the DNA salt extraction method [15]. Subsequently, the DNA was quantified using a Nanodrop® 1000 Spectrophotometer (Wilmington, DE, USA).

The PCR-allele technique was used for genotyping in duplicates with 100% of concordance [16]. This assay facilitates the simultaneous amplification and detection of DNA using a common reverse primer in each reaction tube and two marked primers with two different fluorophores that recognize specific sequences corresponding to each allele. A fluorescence reader was used to capture the emitted fluorescence signal for clusterizing and identifying genotypes.

The following six polymorphisms in the genes involved in folate metabolism were analyzed: 677C>T (rs1801133) and 1298A>C (rs1801131) of methylenetetrahydrofolate reductase—MTHFR; 2756A>G (rs1805087) of methionine synthase—MTR; 66A>G (rs1801394) of methionine synthase reductase—MTRR; 80G>A (rs1051266) of reduced folate carrier 1-RFC-1; and a 19-bp deletion in dihydrofolate reductase—DHFR. In this study, the genotyping call rate was >97% for the polymorphisms.

2.8. Statistical Analysis

For each polymorphism in the population, the minimum allele frequency was calculated, and the Hardy-Weinberg equilibrium was verified. The frequencies of female and male, age group, and self-declared races, and median of folate and homocysteine concentrations were stratified according to genotypes for each of the gene encoding enzymes or carrier proteins. The chi-square test and Kruskal-Wallis test were performed to verify differences between frequencies and medians, respectively. The folate concentration was also considered to evaluate the differences in homocysteine concentrations in the presence of genetic variants. Therefore, the population was divided into tertiles of the folate plasma concentration with mean, respectively: first (14.9 nmol/L), second (27.5 nmol/L), and third (50.7 nmol/L). A linear regression model was used to evaluate differences in the homocysteine concentrations in accordance with genetic variants by total population and folate concentration tertiles. The model considered the log-transformed homocysteine concentration as a dependent variable and the genetic variants as independent variables, divided into three categories: (1) homozygous wild-type, (2) heterozygous mutation, and (3) homozygous mutation for enzyme or carrier genotypes. The models were adjusted according to race, sex, age, estimated consumption of total folate (mcg of DFE/day), body mass index, serum concentrations of vitamins, folate, B6, and B12. In addition, we used the interaction terms of genotypes and folate plasma concentration in these linear regression models.

All statistical analyses were done using the STATA® software (version 10.0, 2007; College Station, TX, USA). A significance level of 5% was considered in all analyses.

3. Results

The present study involved a total of 750 participants as a representative sample of the population of São Paulo, Brazil, of which 58.1% of the participants were women and 41.9% of the participants were men, averaging 46.7 years of age (95% CI: 45.0–48.4 years). In relation to the nutritional status of the population according to the BMI classification, 46.1% of the population was overweight (BMI > 25 kg/m^2). Moreover, in terms of race, most of the participants were self-declared Whites (59.2%), followed by Mixed (white/black) (30.7%), Blacks (8.3%), and Asians/Indigenous (1.9%). Non-smokers represented 85.2% of the population. The median of homocysteine and folate concentrations in the studied population were 8.8 μmol/L and 27.4 nmol/L, respectively.

The primary information concerning the polymorphisms studied in this population, such as gene location, change of DNA molecule bases and consequent amino acid alterations, Hardy-Weinberg equilibrium, and minor allele frequencies, are listed in Table 1. The chi-square test ($p > 0.05$) revealed that the population was in Hardy-Weinberg equilibrium for all of the alleles studied. The genotype frequencies of the genetic variants in the studied population according to sex, age group, and self-declared race, and the respective homocysteine and folate concentrations according to genotypes are listed in Table 2. Individuals presenting genotypes CT and TT for the MTHFR 677C>T polymorphism presented higher homocysteine levels than individuals with genotype CC ($p = 0.026$), whereas individuals presenting genotypes GA and GG for the MTR 2756A>G polymorphism presented lower folate concentrations than individuals with genotype AA ($p = 0.015$). Race was observed to show statistically significant differences in the genotypes of MTHFR 677>T ($p = 0.035$), MTRR 66A>G ($p = 0.000$), and RFC-1 80G>A ($p = 0.003$).

Table 1. Panel of genetic variants, minimum allele frequency, and Hardy-Weinberg equilibrium of the six polymorphisms involved in one-carbon metabolism.

Polymorphisms	Location	Gene	Changes		p [a]	MAF
			DNA	Amino acids		
rs1801131	1p36.3	MTHFR	A→C	Glu→Ala	0.392	0.24
rs1801133	1p36.3	MTHFR	C→T	Ala→Val	0.428	0.33
rs1805087	1q43	MTR	A→G	Asp→Gly	0.333	0.19
rs1801394	5p15.31	MTRR	A→G	-	0.154	0.42
rs1051266	21q22.3	RFC1	G→A	His→Arg	0.141	0.46
19-bp deletion	5q11.2–q13.2	DHFR	-	-	0.807	0.47

[a] *p*-value for Hardy-Weinberg equilibrium. MAF, minor allele frequency; RFC-1, reduced folate carrier 1; DHFR, dihydrofolate reductase; MTHFR, 5,10-methylenetetrahydrofolate reductase; MTR, methionine synthase; MTRR, methionine synthase reductase.

The association between genetic variants involved in one-carbon metabolism and homocysteine concentration was assessed (Table 3). Only MTHFR 677C>T was significantly associated with Hcy concentration in the total population ($p = 0.000$). The increasing risk allele (T) was related to the increase in Hcy concentration. In the presence of genetic variants stratified by folate level tertiles, the same effect was observed in MTHFR 677C>T. The individuals carrying the risk allele had higher Hcy concentrations than those of non-carriers in the first tertile ($p = 0.006$) and third tertile ($p = 0.038$) of folate concentration. However, no interaction was observed between genotypes and folate concentration on homocysteine concentration ($p > 0.05$).

Table 2. Genotype frequencies of the enzymes MTHFR, MTR, MTRR, and DHFR and the carrier protein RFC-1 according to sex, age group, and race; and the medians of homocysteine and folate concentrations according to genotypes.

SNP	MTHFR 677C>T				MTHFR 1298A>C				MTR 2756A>G				MTRR 66A>G				RFC1 80G>A				DHFR Deletion			
Genotypes	C:C	C:T	T:T	p-Value	A:A	A:C	C:C	p-Value	A:A	A:G	G:G	p-Value	A:A	A:G	G:G	p-Value	G:G	G:A	A:A	p-Value	WT:WT	WT:del	del:del	p-Value
Total (%) [1]	46.0	42.7	11.3		58.6	34.2	6.2		66.0	29.8	4.2		35.6	44.8	19.6		30.5	47.0	22.5		28.4	50.2	21.4	
Sex (%) [1]																								
male	43.4	44.3	12.3	0.462	60.6	34.5	4.9	0.376	67.8	27.7	4.6	0.548	35.0	45.2	19.8	0.961	31.6	45.1	23.4	0.682	20.1	52.9	27.0	0.455
female	47.8	41.6	10.6		57.2	35.6	7.21		64.7	31.3	3.9		36.0	44.5	19.5		29.7	48.4	21.9		22.4	48.2	29.4	
Age group (%) [1]																								
12–19 years	42.0	44.0	14.0	0.662	61.9	33.6	4.5	0.593	69.5	26.6	3.9	0.139	33.3	44.4	22.2	0.193	28.5	45.7	25.8	0.763	24.4	48.1	27.6	0.801
20–59 years	48.2	41.2	10.6		56.0	36.3	7.7		69.5	26.2	4.4		36.9	47.8	15.4		32.1	45.7	22.2		19.4	52.0	28.6	
60+ years	45.8	43.7	10.6		59.6	34.8	5.7		60.5	35.3	4.2		35.5	41.8	22.7		29.9	48.9	21.1		21.9	49.5	28.6	
Race (%) [1]																								
White	42.4	44.4	13.2	0.035 *	54.9	37.5	7.6	0.056	68.4	28.9	2.8	0.183	28.7	46.2	25.2	0.000 *	32.4	47.3	20.3	0.003 *	30.3	51.3	18.5	0.120
Black	59.7	38.7	1.6		69.4	27.4	3.2		65.6	29.5	4.9		54.8	38.7	6.5		29.5	57.4	13.1		16.1	51.6	32.3	
Mixed (white/black)	49.3	41.0	9.7		63.7	32.3	4.0		61.2	31.7	7.1		43.1	43.5	13.5		28.4	44.4	27.1		28.1	47.8	24.1	
Asian/Indigenous	42.9	35.7	21.4		41.7	41.7	16.7		71.4	28.6	0.0		42.9	50.0	7.1		7.7	30.8	61.5		28.6	50.0	21.4	
Hcy, μmol/L (median) [2]	8.3	9.0	9.3	0.026 *	8.7	8.9	7.5	0.180	8.6	8.9	8.7	0.569	9.0	8.2	9.4	0.097	8.9	8.8	8.5	0.401	8.4	8.9	8.8	0.355
Folate, nmol/L (median) [2]	27.9	27.9	24.1	0.088	26.5	28.5	22.8	0.565	28.0	25.1	21.0	0.015 *	26.6	27.0	28.1	0.423	29.0	27.4	25.4	0.396	27.5	28.0	25.6	0.935

[1] p-value for the chi-square test; [2] p-value for the Kruskal-Wallis test; * A p-value < 0.05 was considered statistically significant.

Table 3. Associations between the genotypes involved in one-carbon metabolism and homocysteine concentration by total population and folate concentration tertiles.

Homocysteine [1]	Total		Folate Concentration						*p*-Interaction [3]
			First Tertile		Second Tertile		Third Tertile		
	Mean	SEM	Mean	SEM	Mean	SEM	Mean	SEM	
MTHFR 677C>T									
C:C	9.3	0.2	9.7	0.4	9.6	0.4	8.9	0.3	0.208
C:T	10.3	0.4	10.5	0.8	10.0	0.4	10.5	1.0	
T:T	12.6	1.3	12.6	1.3	10.2	1.7	13.9	3.9	
p-value [2]	0.000 *		0.006 *		0.162		0.038 *		
MTHFR 1298A>C									
A:A	10.5	0.4	11.0	0.6	9.5	0.4	10.9	1.0	0.327
A:C	9.7	0.2	10.3	0.5	10.0	0.5	9.0	0.3	
C:C	9.2	0.7	7.1	0.6	12.1	1.6	8.4	1.3	
p-value [2]	0.304		0.121		0.190		0.187		
MTR 2756A>G									
A:A	10.0	0.3	10.1	0.4	9.5	0.3	10.4	0.8	0.397
A:G	10.4	0.5	11.5	1.2	10.5	0.7	9.2	0.4	
G:G	9.1	0.5	9.6	0.7	8.5	1.0	9.8	1.5	
p-value [2]	0.439		0.583		0.859		0.374		
MTRR 66A>G									
A:A	10.2	0.4	10.4	0.5	10.0	0.6	10.6	1.1	0.825
A:G	10.0	0.4	10.6	0.8	9.5	0.5	9.6	0.9	
G:G	10.1	0.4	9.8	0.9	10.1	0.6	10.4	0.7	
p-value [2]	0.576		0.59		0.612		0.388		
RFC1 80G>A									
G:G	10.7	0.5	11.7	1.2	11.0	0.8	9.2	0.5	0.214
G:A	10.1	0.4	9.6	0.4	9.7	0.4	11.2	1.2	
A:A	9.4	0.3	10.5	0.7	8.5	0.5	9.2	0.5	
p-value [2]	0.281		0.920		0.001 *		0.396		
deletion DHFR									
WT:WT	10.4	0.6	10.5	1.3	9.7	0.8	10.8	1.3	0.535
WT:del	10.1	0.3	10.2	0.4	9.8	0.4	10.1	0.8	
del:del	10.1	0.4	11.2	0.8	10.3	0.6	8.9	0.5	
p-value [2]	0.312		0.071		0.667		0.836		

[1] Hcy concentration data are mean and SEM. Hcy concentration values were Log transformed before analysis. [2] Linear regression model adjusted by race, sex, age, estimated consumption of total folate (mcg of DFE/day), body mass index, serum concentrations of vitamins folate, B6, and B12. [3] *p*-value of genotypes-folate concentration interaction term at the linear regression model. * *p*-values were considered significant ($p < 0.05$).

4. Discussion

Herein, we conducted a population-based study of individuals in the city of São Paulo, Brazil, to evaluate the frequencies of the primary polymorphisms associated with one-carbon metabolism, the associations between these genotypes and sex, age, and self-declared race, and the differences in metabolic responses considering genetic variants. The results showed that (1) the allele frequencies in the population were in equilibrium and similar to those in other populations; (2) the genotype frequencies of MTHFR 677C>T, MTRR 66A>G, and RFC-1 80G>A were significantly different according to race; and (3) statistically significant differences between the mean homocysteine concentrations according to the genotypes of MTHFR 677C>T were observed independently of folate level.

Among the described polymorphisms of the enzyme MTHFR, the variants 677C>T and 1298A>C are the most well studied. Americans of Hispanic origin presented a higher prevalence of homozygotes TT for MTHFR 677C>T, which was found in 25% of the population. The prevalence of this genotype among white Americans was between 10% and 15%, and a lower prevalence of this genotype was observed for African and African-Americans, with 0% and 1%, respectively [4,17,18]. The results from case-control studies showed that the homozygote prevalence (TT) for this variant (677C>T) was 9.5% in control Brazilian individuals who were considered to be healthy [19], while the homozygote prevalence was 1.9% in individuals of African origin and 11.8% in individuals of Caucasian origin [20]. Herein, we observed that 11.3% of the population presented as being homozygous (TT) for the variant

677C>T, considering a homozygote prevalence of 13.2% and 1.6% among White and Black races, respectively. In a study concerning the polymorphism 1298A>C, 40% heterozygotes (AC) and 6% mutant homozygotes CC were observed in a healthy Brazilian population [21], consistent with the results of the present study (34.2% AC and 6.2% CC). In the United Kingdom, 44.8% heterozygotes AC and 9.3% mutant homozygotes CC were observed in an elderly population (*n* = 1041) [22].

The prevalence of 3.7% homozygotes GG and 19.7% heterozygotes AG for the MTR variant 2756A>G was observed in the control individuals from a Brazilian population [23], whereas in the present study, we observed a prevalence of 4.2% homozygotes and 29.8% heterozygotes. The homozygotes GG were detected at a frequency of 2–3% in Japanese, Chinese, Korean, and European individuals and at approximately 1–5% in Americans [24]. However, the MTRR polymorphism is extremely common. The prevalence of this genotype among the individuals examined in the present study was 44.8% heterozygotes AG and 19.6% homozygotes GG. However, in a previous study, the prevalence of the MTRR polymorphism among Brazilians was 54.3% and 17.6%, respectively [23].

The RFC-1 genetic variant is a mutation with high prevalence among the studied populations. Homozygotes AA showed a prevalence of 22.3% and heterozygotes AG showed a prevalence of 48.4% among a Brazilian population that attended a public health care center [25]. In contrast, in the present study, we detected a 22.5% prevalence of homozygotes AA and 47% prevalence of homozygotes AG, whereas in a British elderly population, the observed prevalence was 18.6% for AA and 50% for AG [22]. A 19-base pair deletion in the DHFR gene was also prevalent among these populations. The homozygote and heterozygote variants for this deletion accounted for 17.2% and 51.3%, respectively, of the population in the United States [26]. However, in the Brazilian population, the DHFR polymorphism has only been reported in studies of individuals with DS, presenting a frequency of genotype Del:Del in 20.9% of these individuals [27]. In the present study, the observed genotype frequency of Del:Del was 21.4%.

In relation to the homocysteine concentration, several studies have shown that an increase in folate consumption, particularly folic acid via fortification or supplementation, consequently increases folate intake and serum vitamin concentrations, and decreases homocysteine concentrations [28]. Additional studies have shown no alterations in the homocysteine concentration when folate is adequate. However, with low folate concentrations, there is a significant increase in the homocysteine concentration in individuals presenting genetic variants as methylenetetrahydrofolate reductase C677T mutation [29]. In contrast, the results of the present study showed that the mean homocysteine concentration was significantly lower ($p < 0.05$) in individuals with wild-type compared to the increasing risk allele (T) for the MTHFR 677C>T polymorphism regardless of folate concentrations tertiles. Similar results were found in other studies of folic acid supplementation. The mutation MTHFR TT was associated with lower folate concentrations and higher homocysteine concentration, and the trend of TT compared to CC was maintained even at different folic acid doses [30]. Indeed, for the remethylation of Hcy into methionine, the enzyme MTHFR is responsible for converting 5.10-methyltetrahydrofolate into 5-methyltetrahydrofolate, the circulating and physiologically active form of folate and primary methyl group donor for remethylation [3]. The results of a previous study showed that homozygotes (TT) for the MTHFR 677C>T mutation presented one-third of the expected activity for this enzyme [31]. It has been suggested that folic acid from fortified food primarily increases the intake and serum concentration of folate [32]. The synthetic form of folate, folic acid, needs to be converted into 5-methyltetrahydrofolate (5MeTHF) through the enzyme MTHFR. However, the presence of the MTHFR 677C>T polymorphism would restrict this conversion, thereby decreasing homocysteine remethylation and consequently increasing homocysteine concentrations in the blood [3,30]. On the other hand, the effect of natural sources of folate on plasma homocysteine has not been assessed in studies. It is known that common folate form in food without fortification, i.e., naturally occurring folate, is 5MeTHF after absorption, and this form does not require conversion by enzyme MTHFR in the metabolism [33]. Thus, we emphasized the need for further research studies to elucidate this gap.

Another important finding is related to differences in genetic variations according to race. In the present study, race was differently presented ($p < 0.05$) among MTHFR 677>T, MTRR 66A>G, and RFC-1 80G>A genotypes. Some researchers criticize the use and limitations of self-declared race and consider the use of individual genetic ancestry to be the best measure of racial differences in genetic variations [34]. Nevertheless, significant differences in the prevalence of polymorphisms among self-declared races were observed, suggesting the importance of population miscegenation [35]. Therefore, the race variable must be considered in future population studies evaluating potential differences in serum concentrations of folate, homocysteine, B vitamins, and other molecules, consistent with previous studies [36,37].

Accordingly, the knowledge of genetic variability in epidemiological studies remains scarce in Brazil, primarily in representative samples of healthy populations. However, several studies have attempted to associate disease outcomes with genetic variability among individual populations. In the last two decades, several studies have reported that MTHFR polymorphisms, particularly 677C>T and 1298A>C, are associated with an increased risk for neural tube defects [38], cardiovascular diseases [39], schizophrenia [40], neoplasia [41–43], and hyperhomocysteinemia [44]. In contrast with other diseases related to folate metabolism, the MTR variant has not been associated with hyperhomocysteinemia, an increased risk of neural tube defects, or vascular diseases [4,45]. Several studies have investigated the association of the MTR variant with the development of neoplasia; however, the results are conflicting. The results of a meta-analysis of the MTRR 66A>G polymorphism showed that the genotype GG is associated with an increase in risk of carcinomas [46]. With respect to RFC-1, several studies have related the genetic variants for RFC-1 with an increased risk for neural tube defects [47]. The 19-base pair deletion in the DHFR gene has only been reported in studies concerning individuals with Down syndrome [27,48].

Despite these findings, a potential limitation of the present study was the use of self-declared race, as this variable reflects the influence of social-economic and cultural status, although, until recently, genetic ancestry analysis was not performed in population-based studies in the city of São Paulo. Accordingly, even self-declared race is not an adequate genetic indicator, but rather this variable could represent an exposition indicator of social factors [49]. Therefore, epidemiological studies with representative samples are important to promote these results for further discussions concerning this issue.

5. Conclusions

In conclusion, adequate folate levels are an important point in this discussion, as Brazil is a country that has a public health policy of mandatory folic acid fortification. Folic acid fortification considerably reduces the inadequacy of folate prevalence within levels considered to be safe in the inhabitant population of São Paulo [32]; however, the profile of genetic variability among this population remains unknown. Indeed, the presence of these polymorphisms modifies the metabolism and alters the concentrations of these metabolites, as differences in homocysteine concentrations were observed in individuals with genetic variants of MTHFR 677C>T. These effects in health and disease are inconclusive; therefore, the evaluation of such variants must be considered in future epidemiological studies. Consequently, studies concerning the frequencies and factors associated with genetic variants in the enzymes involved in metabolic processes are becoming increasingly important.

Acknowledgments: This work was supported by Municipal Health Secretariat of São Paulo; National Counsel of Technological-CNPq; and Scientific Development and São Paulo Research Foundation–FAPESP (Grant Numbers: 2010/19899-5, 2011/19788-1, and 2012/05505-0).

Author Contributions: J.S., R.M.F. and D.M.M. conceived and designed the research. G.J.F.G. performed the experiments. J.S., A.M.C., A.A.F.C. and A.M. analyzed the data. J.S., A.M.C., A.A.F.C., A.M. and D.M.M. drafted the manuscript.

Conflicts of Interest: The authors declare no conflict of interest.

References

1. Ulrich, C.M. Nutrigenetics in cancer research—Folate metabolism and colorectal cancer. *J. Nutr.* **2005**, *135*, 2698–2702. [PubMed]
2. Stover, P.J. Polymorphisms in 1-carbon metabolism, epigenetics and folate-related pathologies. *J. Nutr. Nutr.* **2011**, *4*, 293–305. [CrossRef] [PubMed]
3. Williams, K.T.; Schalinske, K.L. New insights into the regulation of methyl group and homocysteine metabolism. *J. Nutr.* **2007**, *137*, 311–314. [PubMed]
4. Eldibany, M.M.; Caprini, J.A. Hyperhomocysteinemia and thrombosis: An overview. *Arch. Pathol. Lab. Med.* **2007**, *131*, 872–884. [PubMed]
5. Clarke, R.; Halsey, J.; Lewington, S.; Lonn, E.; Armitage, J.; Manson, J.E.; Bønaa, K.H.; Spence, J.D.; Nygård, O.; Jamison, R.; et al. Effects of lowering homocysteine levels with B vitamins on cardiovascular disease, cancer, and cause-specific mortality: Meta-analysis of 8 randomized trials involving 37 485 individuals. *Arch. Intern. Med.* **2010**, *170*, 1622–1631. [PubMed]
6. DeVos, L.; Chanson, A.; Liu, Z.; Ciappio, E.D.; Parnell, L.D.; Mason, J.B.; Tucker, K.L.; Crott, J.W. Associations between single nucleotide polymorphisms in folate uptake and metabolizing genes with blood folate, homocysteine, and DNA uracil concentrations. *Am. J. Clin. Nutr.* **2008**, *88*, 1149–1158. [PubMed]
7. Jacques, P.F.; Selhub, J.; Bostom, A.G.; Wilson, P.W.F.; Rosenberg, I.H. The effect of folic acid fortification on plasma folate and total homocysteine concentrations. *N. Engl. J. Med.* **1999**, *340*, 1449–1454. [CrossRef] [PubMed]
8. Ganji, V.; Kafai, M.R. Trends in serum folate, RBC folate, and circulating total homocysteine concentrations in the United States: Analysis of data from National Health and Nutrition Examination Surveys, 1988–1994, 1999–2000, and 2001–2002. *J. Nutr.* **2006**, *136*, 153–158. [PubMed]
9. Marchioni, D.M.L.; Fisberg, R.M. *Manual de Avaliação do Consumo Alimentar em Estudos Populacionais: A Experiência do Inquérito de Saúde em São Paulo (ISA)*; Faculdade de Saúde Pública da USP: São Paulo, Brazil, 2012.
10. Verly, E., Jr.; Steluti, J.; Fisberg, R.M.; Marchioni, D.M. A quantile regression approach can reveal the effect of fruit and vegetable consumption on plasma homocysteine levels. *PLoS ONE* **2014**, *9*, e111619. [CrossRef]
11. Haubrock, J.; Noethlings, U.; Volatier, J.L.; Dekkers, A.; Ocke, M.; Harttig, U.; Illner, A.K.; Knüppel, S.; Andersen, L.F.; Boeing, H.; et al. Estimating Usual Food Intake Distributions by Using the Multiple Source Method in the EPIC-Potsdam Calibration Study. *J. Nutr.* **2011**, *141*, 914–920.
12. WHO—World Health Organization. *Obesity: Preventing and Managing the Global Epidemic Report of a World Health Organization Consultation*; World Health Organization: Geneva, Switzerland, 2000; p. 256.
13. Bagley, P.J.; Selhub, J. Analysis of folate from distribution by affinity followed by reversed-phase chromatography with electrical detection. *Clin. Chem.* **2000**, *46*, 404–411. [PubMed]
14. Rybak, M.E.; Jain, R.B.; Pfeiffer, C.M. Clinical vitamin B6 analysis: An interlaboratory comparison of pyridoxal 5′-phosphate measurements in serum. *Clin. Chem.* **2005**, *51*, 1223–1231. [CrossRef] [PubMed]
15. Miller, S.; Dykes, D.; Polesky, H. A simple salting out procedure for extracting DNA from human nucleated cells. *Nucleic Acids Res.* **1988**, *16*, 1215. [CrossRef] [PubMed]
16. Myakishev, M.V.; Khripin, Y.; Hu, S.; Hamer, D.H. High-throughput SNP genotyping by allele-specific PCR with universal energy-transfer-labeled primers. *Genome Res.* **2001**, *11*, 163–169. [CrossRef] [PubMed]
17. Schneider, J.A.; Rees, D.C.; Liu, Y.T.; Clegg, J.B. Worldwide distribution of a common methylenetetrahydrofolate reductase mutation. *Am. J. Hum. Genet.* **1998**, *62*, 1258–1260. [CrossRef] [PubMed]
18. Botto, L.D.; Yang, Q. 5,10-Methylenetetrahydrofolate reductase gene variants and congenital anomalies: A HuGE review. *Am. J. Epidemiol.* **2000**, *151*, 862–877. [CrossRef] [PubMed]
19. Shinjo, S.K.; Oba-Shinjo, S.M.; da Silva, R.; Barbosa, K.C.; Yamamoto, F.; Scaff, M. Methylenetetrahydrofolate reductase gene polymorphism is not related to the risk of ischemic cerebrovascular disease in a Brazilian population. *Clinics* **2007**, *63*, 295–300. [CrossRef]
20. Voetsch, B.; Damasceno, B.P.; Camargo, E.C.; Massaro, A.; Bacheschi, L.A.; Scaff, M.; Annichino-Bizzacchi, J.M.; Arruda, V.R. Inherited thrombophilia as a risk factor for the development of ischaemic stroke in young adults. *Thromb. Haemost.* **2000**, *83*, 229–233. [PubMed]

21. Oliveira, K.C.; Bianco, B.; Verreschi, I.T.N.; Guedes, A.D.; Galera, B.B.; Galera, M.F.; Barbosa, C.P.; Lipay, M.V. Prevalence of the Polymorphism MTHFR A1298C and not MTHFR C677T Is Related to Chromosomal Aneuploidy in Brazilian Turner Syndrome Patients. *Arq. Bras. Endocrinol. Metabol.* **2008**, *52*, 1374–1381. [CrossRef] [PubMed]

22. Devlin, A.M.; Clarke, R.; Birks, J.; Evans, J.G.; Halsted, C.H. Interactions among polymorphisms in folate-metabolizing genes and serum total homocysteine concentrations in a healthy elderly population. *Am. J. Clin. Nutr.* **2006**, *3*, 708–713.

23. Lima, C.S.; Ortega, M.M.; Ozelo, M.C.; Araujo, R.C.; De Souza, C.A.; Lorand-Metze, I.; Annichino-Bizzacchi, J.M.; Costa, F.F. Polymorphisms of methylenetetrahydrofolate reductase (MTHFR), methionine synthase (MTR), methionine synthase reductase (MTRR), and thymidylate synthase (TYMS) in multiple myeloma risk. *Leuk. Res.* **2008**, *32*, 401–405. [CrossRef] [PubMed]

24. Sharp, L.; Little, J. Polymorphisms in genes involved in folate metabolism and colorectal neoplasia: A HuGE review. *Am. J. Epidemiol.* **2004**, *159*, 423–443. [CrossRef] [PubMed]

25. Barnabé, A.; Aléssio, A.C.; Bittar, L.F.; de MoraesMazetto, B.; Bicudo, A.M.; de Paula, E.V.; Höehr, N.F.; Annichino-Bizzacchi, J.M. Folate, vitamin B12 and Homocysteine status in the post-folic acid fortification era in different subgroups of the Brazilian population attended to at a public health care center. *Nutr. J.* **2015**, *14*, 19. [CrossRef] [PubMed]

26. Kalmbach, R.D.; Choumenkovitch, S.F.; Troen, A.P.; Jacques, P.F.; D'Agostino, R.; Selhub, J. A 19-base pair deletion polymorphism in dihydrofolate reductase is associated with increased unmetabolized folic acid in plasma and decreased red blood cell folate. *J. Nutr.* **2008**, *138*, 2323–2327. [CrossRef] [PubMed]

27. Mendes, C.C.; Raimundo, A.M.; Oliveira, L.D.; Zampieri, B.L.; Marucci, G.H.; Biselli, J.M.; Goloni-Bertollo, E.M.; Eberlin, M.N.; Haddad, R.; Riccio, M.F.; et al. DHFR 19-bp Deletion and SHMT C1420T Polymorphisms and Metabolite Concentrations of the Folate Pathway in Individuals with Down Syndrome. *Genet. Test. Mol. Biomark.* **2013**, *17*, 274–277. [CrossRef] [PubMed]

28. Hoey, L.; McNulty, H.; Askin, N.; Dunne, A.; Ward, M.; Pentieva, K.; Strain, J.; Molloy, A.M.; Flynn, C.A.; Scott, J.M. Effect of a voluntary food fortification policy on folate, related B vitamin status, and homocysteine in healthy adults. *Am. J. Clin. Nutr.* **2007**, *86*, 1405–1413. [PubMed]

29. Girelli, D.; Friso, S.; Trabetti, E.; Olivieri, O.; Russo, C.; Pessotto, R.; Faccini, G.; Pignatti, P.F.; Mazzucco, A.; Corrocher, R. Methylenetetrahydrofolate reductase C677T mutation plasma homocysteine, and folate in subjects from northern Italy with or without angiographically documented severe coronary atherosclerotic disease: Evidence for an important genetic-environmental interaction. *Blood* **1998**, *9*, 4158–4163.

30. Crider, K.S.; Zhu, J.H.; Hao, L.; Yang, Q.H.; Yang, T.P.; Gindler, J.; Maneval, D.R.; Quinlivan, E.P.; Li, Z.; Bailey, L.B.; et al. MTHFR 677C→T genotype is associated with folate and homocysteine concentrations in a large, population-based, double-blind trial of folic acid supplementation. *Am. J. Clin. Nutr.* **2011**, *93*, 1365–1372. [CrossRef] [PubMed]

31. Rozen, R. Genetic predisposition to hyperhomocysteinemia: Deficiency of methylenetetrahydrofolate reductase (MTHFR). *Thromb. Haemost.* **1997**, *78*, 523–526. [PubMed]

32. Marchioni, D.M.L.; Verly, E., Jr.; Steluti, J.; Cesar, C.L.G.; Fisberg, R.M. Ingestão de folato nos períodos pré e pós-fortificação mandatória: Estudo de base populacional em São Paulo, Brasil Folic acid intake before and after mandatory fortification: A population-based study in Sao Paulo, Brazil. *Cad. Saúde Pública* **2013**, *29*, 2083–2092. [CrossRef] [PubMed]

33. FAO/WHO—Food and Agriculture Organization/World Health Organization. Folate and Folic Acid. In *FAO/WHO Expert Consultation on Human Vitamin and Mineral Requirements*; FAO: Rome, Italy, 2001; pp. 53–63.

34. Parra, F.C.; Amado, R.C.; Lambertucci, J.R.; Rocha, J.; Antunes, C.M.; Pena, S.D. Color and genomic ancestry in Brazilians. *Proc. Natl. Acad. Sci. USA* **2003**, *100*, 177–182. [CrossRef] [PubMed]

35. Suarez-Kurtz, G. Pharmacogenomics and the genetic diversity of the Brazilian population. *Cad. Saude Publica* **2009**, *25*, 1650–1651. [CrossRef] [PubMed]

36. Rady, P.L.; Szucs, S.; Grady, J.; Hudnall, S.D.; Kellner, L.H.; Nitowsky, H.; Tyring, S.K.; Matalon, R.K. Genetic polymorphisms of methylenetetrahydrofolate reductase (MTHFR) and methionine synthase reductase (MTRR) in ethnic populations in Texas; a report of a novel MTHFR polymorphic site, G1793A. *Am. J. Med. Genet.* **2002**, *107*, 162–168. [CrossRef] [PubMed]

37. Yang, Q.-H.; Botto, L.D.; Gallagher, M.; Friedman, J.; Sanders, C.L.; Koontz, D.; Nikolova, S.; Erickson, J.D.; Steinberg, K. Prevalence and effects of gene-gene and gene-nutrient interactions on serum folate and serum total homocysteine concentrations in the United States: Findings from the third National Health and Nutrition Examination Survey DNA Bank. *Am. J. Clin. Nutr.* **2008**, *88*, 232–246. [PubMed]

38. Pangilinan, F.; Molloy, A.M.; Mills, J.L.; Troendle, J.F.; Parle-McDermott, A.; Signore, C.; O'Leary, V.B.; Chines, P.; Seay, J.M.; Geiler-Samerotte, K.; et al. Evaluation of common genetic variants in 82 candidate genes as risk factors for neural tube defects. *BMC Med. Genet.* **2012**, *13*, 62. [CrossRef] [PubMed]

39. Mehlig, K.; Leander, K.; De Faire, U.; Nyberg, F.; Berg, C.; Rosengren, A.; Björck, L.; Zetterberg, H.; Blennow, K.; Tognon, G.; et al. The association between plasma homocysteine and coronary heart disease is modified by the MTHFR 677C>T polymorphism. *Heart* **2013**, *99*, 1761–1765. [CrossRef] [PubMed]

40. Muntjewerff, J.W.; Kahn, R.S.; Blom, H.J.; Heijer, M. Homocysteine, methylenetetrahydrofolate reductase and risk of schizophrenia: A meta-analysis. *Mol. Psychiatry* **2006**, *11*, 143–149. [CrossRef] [PubMed]

41. Safarinejad, M.R.; Shafiei, N.; Safarinejad, N. Relationship between three polymorphisms of Methylenetetrahydrofolate reductase (MTHFR C677T, A1298C, and G1793A) gene and risk of Prostate cancer: A case control study. *Prostate* **2010**, *70*, 1645–1657. [CrossRef] [PubMed]

42. Arslan, S.; Karadayi, S.; Yildirim, M.E.; Ozdemir, O.; Akkurt, I. The association between methylene-tetrahydrofolate reductase gene polymorphism and lung cancer risk. *Mol. Biol. Rep.* **2011**, *38*, 991–996. [CrossRef] [PubMed]

43. Yu, L.; Chen, J. Association of MHTFR Ala222Val (rs1801133) polymorphism and breast cancer susceptibility: An update meta-analysis based on 51 research studies. *Diagn. Pathol.* **2012**, *7*, 171. [CrossRef] [PubMed]

44. Husemoen, L.L.N.; Skaaby, T.; Jørgensen, T.; Thuesen, B.H.; Fenger, M.; Grarup, N.; Sandholt, C.H.; Hansen, T.; Pedersen, O.; Linneberg, A. MTHFR C677T genotype and cardiovascular risk in a general population without mandatory folic acid fortification. *Eur. J. Nutr.* **2014**, *53*, 1549–1559. [CrossRef] [PubMed]

45. Wilson, A.; Platt, R.; Wu, Q.; Leclerc, D.; Christensen, B.; Yang, H.; Gravel, R.A.; Rozen, R. A Common Variant in Methionine Synthase Reductase Combined with Low Cobalamin (Vitamin B12) Increases Risk for Spina Bifida. *Mol. Genet. Metab.* **1999**, *67*, 317–323. [CrossRef] [PubMed]

46. Hu, J.; Zhou, G.W.; Wang, N.; Wang, Y.J. MTRR A66G polymorphism and breast cancer risk: A meta-analysis. *Breast Cancer Res. Treat.* **2010**, *124*, 779–784. [CrossRef] [PubMed]

47. Wang, H.G.; Wang, J.L.; Zhang, J.; Zhao, L.X.; Zhai, G.X.; Xiang, Y.Z.; Chang, P. Reduced folate carrier A80G polymorphism and susceptibility to neural tube defects: A meta-analysis. *Gene* **2012**, *510*, 180–184. [CrossRef] [PubMed]

48. Biselli, J.M.; Zampieri, B.L.; Goloni-Bertollo, E.M.; Haddad., R.; Fonseca, M.F.; Eberlin, M.N.; Vannucchi, H.; Carvalho, V.M.; Pavarino, E.C. Genetic polymorphisms modulate the folate metabolism of Brazilian individuals with Down syndrome. *Mol. Biol. Rep.* **2012**, *39*, 9277–9284. [CrossRef] [PubMed]

49. Laguardia, J. O uso da variável "raça" na pesquisa em saúde. *Physis* **2004**, *4*, 197–234. [CrossRef]

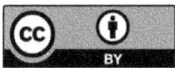

nutrients

MDPI

Brief Report

The *IL6* Gene Promoter SNP and Plasma IL-6 in Response to Diet Intervention

Brinda K. Rana [1,*], Shirley W. Flatt [2], Dennis D. Health [2], Bilge Pakiz [2], Elizabeth L. Quintana [2], Loki Natarajan [2] and Cheryl L. Rock [2]

[1] Department of Psychiatry, School of Medicine, University of California, San Diego, La Jolla, CA 92093-0738, USA

[2] Department of Family Medicine and Public Health, School of Medicine, University of California, San Diego, La Jolla, CA 92093-0901, USA; sflatt@ucsd.edu (S.W.F.); dheath@ucsd.edu (D.D.H.); bpakiz@ucsd.edu (B.P.); Elquintana@ucsd.edu (E.L.Q.); lnatarajan@ucsd.edu (L.N.); clrock@ucsd.edu (C.L.R.)

* Correspondence: bkrana@ucsd.edu; Tel.: +1-858-822-4010

Received: 16 March 2017; Accepted: 22 May 2017; Published: 27 May 2017

Abstract: We recently reported that interleukin-6 (IL-6), an inflammatory marker associated with breast pathology and the development of breast cancer, decreases with diet intervention and weight loss in both insulin-sensitive and insulin-resistant obese women. Here, we tested whether an individual's genotype at an *IL6* SNP, rs1800795, which has previously been associated with circulating IL-6 levels, contributes to changes in IL-6 levels or modifies the effect of diet composition on IL-6 in these women. We genotyped rs1800795 in overweight/obese women (N = 242) who were randomly assigned to a lower fat (20% energy), higher carbohydrate (65% energy) diet; a lower carbohydrate (45% energy), higher fat (35% energy) diet; or a walnut-rich (18% energy), higher fat (35% energy), lower carbohydrate (45% energy) diet in a 1-year weight loss intervention study of obesity-related biomarkers for breast cancer incidence and mortality. Plasma IL-6 levels were measured at baseline, 6 and 12 months. At baseline, individuals with a CC genotype had significantly lower IL-6 levels than individuals with either a GC or GG genotype (p < 0.03; 2.72 pg/mL vs. 2.04 pg/mL), but this result was not significant when body mass index (BMI) was accounted for; the CC genotype group had lower BMI (p = 0.03; 32.5 kg/m^2 vs. 33.6 kg/m^2). We did not observe a 2-way interaction of time*rs1800795 genotype or diet*rs1800795 genotype. Our findings provide evidence that rs1800795 is associated with IL-6 levels, but do not support a differential interaction effect of rs1800795 and diet composition or time on changes in circulating IL-6 levels. Diet intervention and weight loss are an important strategy for reducing plasma IL-6, a risk factor of breast cancer in women, regardless of their rs1800795 genotype.

Keywords: IL-6; rs1800795; diet intervention; BMI; walnut

1. Introduction

Elevated interleukin-6 (IL-6) has been consistently associated with breast pathology and the development of breast cancer [1]. The *IL6* rs1800795 SNP (-174G>C) is a focus of genetic studies on breast cancer risk because of its association with circulating IL-6 levels [2]. A study of 624 primary breast cancer patients in Sweden revealed that C carriers had a higher risk of early events than GG carriers [3]. However, the body of genetic studies have been inconclusive. A recent meta-analysis (12 studies; 10,137 breast cancer cases, 15,566 controls) was unable to establish an association between *IL6* genotypes and breast cancer risk [4].

We recently reported that diet intervention and weight loss are associated with decreased IL-6 in both insulin-sensitive and insulin-resistant obese women [5]. We follow-up with the question: does the rs1800795 genotype interact with the type of diet composition or time to affect IL-6? If so, rs1800795 may be used to personalize a weight reduction regimen to reduce breast cancer risk.

2. Materials and Methods

2.1. Subjects

Participants (N = 242) were from a behavioral weight loss intervention trial in San Diego, CA [5] which randomized 245 overweight and obese women from a screened sample of 1559 women. Inclusion criteria were: female, $\geq$21 years old; body mass index (BMI) between 27 and 40 kg/m^2; willing and able to participate in clinic visits, group sessions, and telephone and internet communications; able to provide data through questionnaires and telephone; willing to maintain contact with investigators for 12 months; willing to allow blood collections; no known allergy to tree nuts; and capable of performing a simple test for assessing cardiopulmonary fitness. Exclusion criteria were any of the following: inability to participate in physical activity due to severe disability; history or presence of a comorbid diseases where diet modification and increased physical activity may be contraindicated; self-reported pregnancy or breastfeeding or planning a pregnancy within the next year; currently involved in another diet intervention study or weight loss program; and having a history or presence of a significant psychiatric disorder or any condition that would interfere with participation in trial. The University of California, San Diego institutional review board approved the study protocol, and all participants provided written informed consent (Clinical Trial Registration: NCT01424007 [6]. Prior to enrollment, women were screened for diabetes and considered ineligible with a fasting blood glucose $\geq$125 mg/dL.

Enrolled participants were randomly assigned to one of the three study arms: lower fat (20% energy), higher carbohydrate (65% energy) diet; higher fat (35% energy), lower carbohydrate (45% energy) diet; or walnut-rich (18% energy), higher fat (35% energy), lower carbohydrate (45% energy) diet. All diet prescriptions limited saturated fat, so guidance for the higher fat diet emphasized lean meats and reduced-fat dairy foods, while encouraging monounsaturated fat as a major, but not sole source of fat in the diet. In all diets, prescribed protein intake exceeded recommended levels although lower fat diet had slightly lower levels compared to the other two diets. The randomization was stratified by menopausal status (older/younger than 55 years as a proxy) and by insulin resistance status (insulin sensitive or insulin resistant) with a homeostasis model assessment (HOMA) value of >3.0 indicative of insulin resistance. Fasting glucose and insulin were measured at the screening clinic visit to calculate HOMA for the baseline characterization of insulin resistance status. Data collection, anthropometric measurements and blood sample collection were conducted at clinic visits at baseline and 6 and 12 months.

Following randomization, participants were provided a detailed diet prescription and sample meal plans in an individual counseling session with a dietitian, with follow-up at regular intervals by telephone or email to provide additional support and reinforce adherence. The overall goal of the dietary guidance was to promote a reduction in energy intake, aiming for a 500–1000 kcal/day deficit relative to expenditure, according to the individualized prescribed diet plan (1200, 1500 or 1800 kcal/day). Specific instructions for the lower fat diet were to choose lean protein sources and reduced-fat dairy foods and to emphasize vegetables, fruit, and whole grains as healthy high-carbohydrate choices. Participants assigned to the lower carbohydrate diet were educated about higher vs. lower carbohydrate choices, as well as lean protein sources, and were instructed to achieve a high monounsaturated fat intake, and examples and recipes were discussed.

Participants assigned to the walnut-rich study group were also educated about higher vs. lower carbohydrate choices and lean protein sources. They were also instructed to consume an average of 42 g (1.5 oz) walnuts per day, within their energy-reduced diet plan, and were provided meal and snack suggestions and recipes to facilitate adherence. Walnuts were distributed to participants assigned to that group approximately every two weeks and they were instructed to record walnut consumption on a simple form. Diet prescriptions for participants assigned to the other two study groups excluded nuts.

All participants also were encouraged to use Web-based tracking programs that guide dietary intake toward the prescribed macronutrient distribution, conduct self-monitoring, and were provided both group-based behavioral weight loss intervention and one-on-one counseling on diet and activity as previously described [7].

2.2. Assays

We measured plasma IL-6 at baseline, 6 and 12 months using solid phase quantitative sandwich ELISA (R & D Systems, Inc., Minneapolis, MN, USA) with inter-assay Coefficients of Variability of 9%.

DNA was extracted from blood using the QIAamp DNA Blood Mini Kit (Qiagen, Hilden, Germany). Rs1800795 was genotyped using iPLEX Gold chemistry on a MassARRAY® System (Agena Bioscience, San Diego, CA, USA) at the Roswell Park Cancer Institute Genomics Shared Resource.

2.3. Statistical Analysis

Of the 242 participants genotyped, 192 completed the study, and one with IL-6 values higher than 100 pg/mL was excluded from the analysis. Two-sample chi-square and *t*-tests were used to compare demographics, baseline IL-6 and BMI between genotype groups. Mixed effect models (MEM) were used to model associations between genotype and longitudinal IL-6 levels, and likelihood ratio tests were used to test interaction effects of genotype with diet or time.

With a total sample size of 234 subjects, our study had 80% power to detect a weight loss difference of 3.8 kg and a between group biomarker (e.g., IL-6) effect-size of 0.89 between two diet arms in the insulin-sensitive or insulin-resistant subjects. As secondary analysis, our study explored whether biomarker changes between diet arms differed according to *IL6* genotype. We also conducted post-hoc power calculations for the main genotype effect on baseline IL-6 levels and the genotype*diet interaction on changes in IL-6, based on 2-sided tests with significance level set to 0.05. With 242 participants (18% CC genotype), we have 80% power to detect a mean difference of 0.68 pg/mL in the CC versus (GG or GC) groups assuming distributions similar to those observed in our study based on a 2-sided 2-sample *t*-test. For the interaction, we have 15% power to detect the observed 0.07 effect-size for changes in IL6 changes based on a F-test. Conversely, with the study sample size of 242, we have 80% power to detect a 0.2 interaction effect-size. Thus, for this exploratory analysis, our study had sufficient power to detect the observed differences in baseline IL6 levels by genotype, but not for genotype*diet effects on IL-6 changes.

3. Results

Rs1800795 genotypes are summarized in Table 1: 42% GG, 40% GC, and 18% CC. The CC genotype was not present in the 13 African American (AA) women (seven GC, six GG). The SNP was in Hardy–Weinberg equilibrium (χ^2 = 3.15) in the non-AA population. IL-6 and BMI at baseline were lower in participants with the CC genotype compared to carriers of the G allele.

In the mixed model, the CC group had lower IL6 compared to the GC/GG groups across time-points (p = 0.06, Model 1, Table 2), but this effect was attenuated with adjustment for BMI (Model 2, Table 2). Excluding AAs did not change results, so we report analyses with AAs included. The genotype*time interaction added to Model 1 was not significant, indicating that changes in marker levels were not different by genotype. Specifically, mean (95% CI) change in IL-6 levels between baseline and at 6 months for G allele carriers was −0.44 (−0.68, −0.20) compared to −0.44 (−0.96, +0.08) pg/mL for the CC group, and at 12 months, −0.99 (−1.24, −0.74) for G carriers versus −0.65 (−1.19, −0.11) for the CC group. Genotype did not modify the diet effect on longitudinal IL-6 levels (genotype and diet model vs. genotype, diet, genotype*diet model, likelihood ratio test p = 0.71).

Table 1. Baseline characteristics in 242 participants.

Characteristics	rs1800795 Genotype		
	GG or GC *N* (%)	CC *N* (%)	*p* [b]
Race/Ethnicity			0.17
White	142(80.2)	35 (19.8)	
African American	13 (100)	0	
Asian American	4 (100)	0	
Hispanic	33 (82.5)	7 (17.5)	
Mixed/Other	7 (87.5)	1 (12.5)	
IL-6 pg/mL [a]	2.72 (0.15)	2.04 (0.21)	0.01
IL-6 pg/mL non-African Americans [a]	2.61 (0.15)	2.04 (0.21)	0.03
BMI (kg/m^2) [a]	33.6 (0.2)	32.5 (0.4)	0.03
BMI (kg/m^2) non-African Americans [a]	33.5 (0.2)	32.5 (0.4) [c]	0.06

[a] Mean (S.E.M); [b] *p* value from Chi-square or 2-sample *t*-tests; [c] There were no African Americans in the CC group. IL-6, Interleukin-6; BMI, Body Mass Index.

Table 2. Associations between IL-6 level and genotype.

		Model 1		Model 2	
		Coefficient (95% CI)	*p* [a]	Coefficient (95% CI)	*p* [a]
GENOTYPE	GG or GC (Reference)				
	CC genotype	-0.55 ± 0.57	0.06	-0.42 ± 0.55	0.14
TIME POINT	Baseline (Reference)				
	6 months	-0.44 ± 0.22	<001	-0.19 ± 0.25	0.13
	12 months	-0.93 ± 0.23	<001	-0.66 ± 0.26	<001
	Body Mass Index			0.10 ± 0.05	<001

[a] Mixed effect model on *N* = 241 excluding one participant with plasma IL-6 >100 pg/mL. Coefficients were derived from Type III Sum of Squares. Model 1: IL-6 Level = Genotype + Time point + Random Intercept. Model 2: IL-6 Level = Genotype + Time point + BMI+ Random Intercept.

4. Discussion and Conclusions

We did not observe a significant effect of the rs1800795 genotype on longitudinal plasma IL-6 levels or an interaction effect with time or diet composition in obese women undergoing a 12-month dietary intervention to promote weight loss. Our results are consistent with a dietary intervention study (314 men, 407 women) in which the C allele was associated with higher serum IL-6 in men, but not in women, and no genotype*diet interaction was found [8]. In our study, BMI was lower in the CC group at baseline and remained lower at 6 and 12 months, possibly confounding the results. Consistent with our previous report, BMI as well as time is driving IL-6 levels, not rs1800795 genotype [5].

A limitation to our study is that our cohort was not underpowered to identify genotype*diet interaction effects on IL-6 changes. However, with a sample size of 242, we were powered to detect changes in baseline IL-6 levels by genotype. The relationship between IL-6, breast cancer risk factors, obesity measures, and rs1800795 is complex and previous genetic studies have been conflicting [2,9]. These conflicts may be due to the role of other *IL6* SNPs and resolved by applying haplotype-based strategies which include other *IL6* SNPs, but such studies require larger cohorts that are difficult to obtain for a longitudinal intervention study such as ours.

We conclude that, as shown in our previous report, diet intervention and weight loss is an important strategy for reducing plasma IL-6, a risk factor of breast cancer in women, but the *IL6* rs1800795 genotype does not interact with the diet type or time to affect IL-6 levels in our cohort.

Acknowledgments: The authors thank the Data and Safety Monitoring Committee (Richard Schwab, Jeanne Nichols and Sonia Jain). We thank Elaine Cornell, University of Vermont, for conducting the IL-6 analysis. SNP genotyping was performed by the Genomics Shared Resource supported by Roswell Park Cancer Institute and

Nutrients **2017**, *9*, 552

National Cancer Institute (NCI) grant P30CA016056. We also thank Hava-Shoshana Barkai and Lea Jacinto for operational support. This study was supported by the National Cancer Institute (NIH) grant, CA155435, and the California Walnut Commission.

Author Contributions: C.L.R. designed and led the trial effort with major contributions from E.L.Q and L.N.; B.K.R. and D.H. performed the assays; B.K.R, L.N. and S.F. conducted the data analysis; B.K.R., L.N. and C.L.R. wrote the paper and all authors revised the manuscript.

Conflicts of Interest: The authors declare no conflict of interest.

References

1. Lithgow, D.; Covington, C. Chronic inflammation and breast pathology: A theoretical model. *Biol. Res. Nurs.* **2005**, *7*, 118–129. [CrossRef] [PubMed]
2. Joffe, Y.T.; Collins, M.; Goedecke, J.H. The relationship between dietary fatty acids and inflammatory genes on the obese phenotype and serum lipids. *Nutrients* **2013**, *5*, 1672–1705. [CrossRef] [PubMed]
3. Markkula, A.; Simonsson, M.; Ingvar, C.; Rose, C.; Jernstrom, H. IL6 genotype, tumour ER-status, and treatment predicted disease-free survival in a prospective breast cancer cohort. *BMC Cancer* **2014**, *14*, 759. [CrossRef] [PubMed]
4. Yu, K.D.; Di, G.H.; Fan, L.; Chen, A.X.; Yang, C.; Shao, Z.M. Lack of an association between a functional polymorphism in the interleukin-6 gene promoter and breast cancer risk: A meta-analysis involving 25,703 subjects. *Breast Cancer Res. Treat.* **2010**, *122*, 483–488. [CrossRef] [PubMed]
5. Le, T.; Flatt, S.W.; Natarajan, L.; Pakiz, B.; Quintana, E.L.; Heath, D.D.; Rana, B.K.; Rock, C.L. Effects of Diet Composition and Insulin Resistance Status on Plasma Lipid Levels in a Weight Loss Intervention in Women. *J. Am. Heart Assoc.* **2016**, *5*, e002771. [CrossRef] [PubMed]
6. Clinical Trials.gov. Available online: https://clinicaltrials.gov/ct2/show/NCT01424007 (accessed on 26 May 2017).
7. Rock, C.L.; Flatt, S.W.; Pakiz, B.; Quintana, E.L.; Heath, D.D.; Rana, B.K.; Natarajan, L. Effects of diet composition on weight loss, metabolic factors and biomarkers in a 1-year weight loss intervention in obese women examined by baseline insulin resistance status. *Metabolism* **2016**, *65*, 1605–1613. [CrossRef] [PubMed]
8. Corella, D.; Gonzalez, J.I.; Bullo, M.; Carrasco, P.; Portoles, O.; Diez-Espino, J.; Covas, M.I.; Ruiz-Gutierrez, V.; Gomez-Gracia, E.; Aros, F.; et al. Polymorphisms cyclooxygenase-2-765G>C and interleukin-6-174G>C are associated with serum inflammation markers in a high cardiovascular risk population and do not modify the response to a Mediterranean diet supplemented with virgin olive oil or nuts. *J. Nutr.* **2009**, *139*, 128–134. [CrossRef] [PubMed]
9. Yu, Z.; Han, S.; Cao, X.; Zhu, C.; Wang, X.; Guo, X. Genetic polymorphisms in adipokine genes and the risk of obesity: A systematic review and meta-analysis. *Obesity* **2012**, *20*, 396–406. [CrossRef] [PubMed]

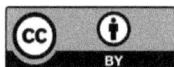

nutrients

MDPI

Article

Genome-Wide Association Study of Dietary Pattern Scores

Frédéric Guénard [1], Annie Bouchard-Mercier [1], Iwona Rudkowska [2], Simone Lemieux [1], Patrick Couture [3] and Marie-Claude Vohl [1,*]

[1] Institute of Nutrition and Functional Foods (INAF), School of Nutrition, Laval University, Québec, QC G1V 0A6, Canada; frederic.guenard@fsaa.ulaval.ca (F.G.); Annie.Bouchard-Mercier@fsaa.ulaval.ca (A.B.-M.); Simone.Lemieux@fsaa.ulaval.ca (S.L.)

[2] Endocrinology and Nephrology Unit, Centre de recherche du CHU de Québec, Laval University, Québec, QC G1V 4G2, Canada; Iwona.Rudkowska@crchudequebec.ulaval.ca

[3] Institute of Nutrition and Functional Foods (INAF), Endocrinology and Nephrology Unit, Centre de recherche du CHU de Québec, Laval University, Québec, QC G1V 4G2, Canada; patrick.couture@crchudequebec.ulaval.ca

* Correspondence: Marie-Claude.Vohl@fsaa.ulaval.ca; Tel.: +1-418-656-2131 (ext. 4676)

Received: 13 April 2017; Accepted: 21 June 2017; Published: 23 June 2017

Abstract: Dietary patterns, representing global food supplies rather than specific nutrients or food intakes, have been associated with cardiovascular disease (CVD) incidence and mortality. The contribution of genetic factors in the determination of food intakes, preferences and dietary patterns has been previously established. The current study aimed to identify novel genetic factors associated with reported dietary pattern scores. Reported dietary patterns scores were derived from reported dietary intakes for the preceding month and were obtained through a food frequency questionnaire and genome-wide association study (GWAS) conducted in a study sample of 141 individuals. Reported Prudent and Western dietary patterns demonstrated nominal associations ($p < 1 \times 10^{-5}$) with 78 and 27 single nucleotide polymorphisms (SNPs), respectively. Among these, SNPs annotated to genes previously associated with neurological disorders, CVD risk factors and obesity were identified. Further assessment of SNPs demonstrated an impact on gene expression levels in blood for SNPs located within/near *BCKDHB* ($p = 0.02$) and the hypothalamic glucosensor *PFKFB3* ($p = 0.0004$) genes, potentially mediated through an impact on the binding of transcription factors (TFs). Overrepresentations of glucose/energy homeostasis and hormone response TFs were also observed from SNP-surrounding sequences. Results from the current GWAS study suggest an interplay of genes involved in the metabolic response to dietary patterns on obesity, glucose metabolism and food-induced response in the brain in the adoption of dietary patterns.

Keywords: association study; dietary patterns; food preferences; Prudent; Western

1. Introduction

Millions of people in both developed and developing countries are affected by cardiovascular diseases (CVDs), one of the world's leading causes of morbidity and mortality [1]. Obesity is known to increase the risk of CVD [2] and a combination of decreased levels of physical activity and an increase in adverse eating behaviors contributes to the obesity pandemic [3]. There is also clear evidence of individual variability in response, suggesting that genetic susceptibility may have an important contribution to individual risk [4].

Single nutrients or food components have been studied to understand their impact on the development of chronic diseases [5,6]. Accordingly, individual dietary components have been associated with increased or decreased risk of diseases without consideration of the cumulative or synergistic effects of the consumption of multiple nutrients within a diet, a concept extensively discussed [5–7]. An alternative method for estimating diet may be to measure global food supply, thus taking into account the potential synergistic effects of multiple components within the diet [5]. One of the methods used to regroup foods that are consumed together involves factor analysis. This 'a posteriori' hypothesis-free derivation method uses observed/reported dietary data in order to extract dietary patterns [8]. Despite an ongoing debate on the validity of memory-based dietary assessment methods (M-BMs; e.g., 24-h dietary recalls and food frequency questionnaires (FFQs)), especially concerning their use in the formulation of national dietary guidelines [9,10], dietary patterns have been demonstrated to be concurrently valid and reproducible in comparison to other M-BMs [11], and are associated with CVD mortality [12] and risk factors such as diabetes, blood pressure, obesity and dyslipidemia [13–15]. Multiple studies summarized in a meta-analysis and in systematic reviews [16,17] identified the Prudent dietary pattern as a protective factor for CVD and reported an opposite relationship for the Western dietary pattern. The Prudent dietary pattern is mostly characterized by the consumption of vegetables, fruits, whole-grain products, fish and non-hydrogenated fats, whereas the Western dietary pattern is characterized by higher intakes of red meats, processed meats, refined grains, French fries and sweets/desserts [14,18].

Genetic variations in several genes were associated with macronutrient intakes such as protein, fat and carbohydrate [19,20]. Expanding single nutrients or food components, food preferences and dietary patterns were shown to be influenced by genetic variations [19,20]. Greater desirability for "unhealthy" food items was associated with gene variation in the dopamine-related *COMT* gene [21] and the rare allele of the rs9939609 single nucleotide polymorphism (SNP) in the fat mass and obesity-associated (*FTO*) gene has been associated with food preference; carriers of the rare allele consumed more biscuits and pastry and less soft drinks compared with TT carriers [20].

In line with abovementioned association of Prudent and Western dietary patterns with CVD and CVD risk factors, potential contribution of genetic susceptibility to CVD risk, and taking into account the debate on the validity of M-BM [9,10] combined with the lack of error-free, practical, and affordable method to assess whole dietary pattern data [22–24], our group previously demonstrated that gene expression profiles differed in individuals with high vs. low scores for both Prudent and Western dietary patterns [25], and that expression profiles may potentially modulate the risk of chronic diseases including CVD [25]. The current study aimed to assess the association of SNPs with the reported Prudent and Western dietary patterns scores. We conducted unbiased genome-wide approach and identified reported dietary pattern-related genetic variations. Further assessment of SNPs from associations identified was carried out through gene expression level and *in silico* analyses, and suggested interplay of genes involved in the metabolic response to dietary patterns in the adoption of dietary patterns.

2. Materials and Methods

2.1. Subjects

One hundred and forty-one individuals were selected among the 210 participants who completed the Fatty Acid Sensor (FAS) study, primarily aiming to understand how genes and environment act together to define CVD risk profile [26]. Individuals recruited in the FAS study had to be non-smokers and be free of any thyroid or metabolic disorders requiring treatment such as diabetes, hypertension, severe dyslipidemia, and coronary heart disease. A concurrently validated FFQ was administered by a registered dietician before omega-3 fatty acid supplementation [27]. Dietary patterns were derived by factor analysis from dietary intakes reported in FFQ. Further details on FAS study participants and recruitment criteria were published elsewhere [26]. This trial was registered at clinicaltrials.gov as NCT01343342. The subset of 141 individuals was originally selected among the FAS study participants based on DNA material availability and response to an *n*-3 polyunsaturated fatty acid supplementation [28]. The experimental protocol was approved by the Ethics Committees of Laval University Hospital Research Center and Laval University. The study was conducted in accordance with the Declaration of Helsinki and all participants provided written informed consent before their inclusion.

2.2. Anthropometric Measurements and Biochemical Profiling

Body weight (kg), height (m) and waist circumference (cm) were measured according to standardized methods [29]. Resting blood pressure (mm Hg) was measured in triplicate after a 10-min rest in a sitting position, phases I and V of Korotkoff sounds being respectively used for systolic (SBP) and diastolic (DBP) blood pressures [30]. Blood samples were collected prior the supplementation period from an antecubital vein into Vacutainer tubes (Becton, Dickinson and Company, Franklin Lakes, NJ, USA) containing ethylenediaminetetraacetic acid after a 12-h overnight fast and 48-h alcohol abstinence. Blood buffy coat and plasma were separated by centrifugation. Plasma total cholesterol (total-C, mmol/L) and triglyceride (TG, mmol/L) concentrations were measured using enzymatic assays [31] on an Olympus AU400e analyzer (Olympus America Inc., Melville, NY, USA). The high-density lipoprotein cholesterol (HDL-C; mmol/L) fraction was obtained after precipitation of very low-density lipoprotein cholesterol and low-density lipoprotein cholesterol (LDL-C) particles. LDL-C (mmol/L) was calculated with the Friedewald formula [32]. Fasting insulinemia (pmol/L) was measured by radioimmunoassay with polyethylene glycol separation [33] and fasting glucose concentrations (mmol/L) were enzymatically measured [34].

2.3. Dietary Assessment and Food Pattern Derivation

Habitual dietary intake for the month preceding the study was determined by a 91-item FFQ including 27 items with 1 to 3 sub-questions [27] and specifically based on food habits of Quebecers. This FFQ was previously shown to be reproducible and concurrently valid based on comparisons with a 3-day dietary record [27]. Participants had to answer to each question during a face-to-face interview with a registered dietician and were asked to report how often they consumed each type of food: daily, weekly, monthly or none at all during the last month. Examples of portion size were provided to ensure that each participant estimated correctly the proportion eaten. Information was compiled and the Nutrition Data System for Research software version 4.03 with Nutrient Database v2011 (Nutrition Coordination Center, University of Minnesota, Minneapolis, MN, USA) was used to analyze FFQ data. This database includes more than 16,000 food items with complete nutritional values for 112 nutrients. Similar food items from the FFQ were grouped, as previously described [14], and based on similarity of nutrient profiles, culinary usage and groups used in other studies [8]. Twenty-seven food groups were then formed and used for factor analyses to generate reported dietary patterns. The FACTOR procedure from Statistical Analysis Software (SAS) was used to derive factors from all participants considering eigenvalue >1, values at Scree test and interpretability to determine the number of factors to retain. Briefly, two main reported dietary patterns were derived. These patterns were similar to Prudent and Western dietary patterns from the literature [18]. Each individual was given a score for both reported dietary patterns. The SCORE procedure of SAS was used to calculate scores from the sum of food groups multiplied by their respective factor loading. These scores reflect the degree of each participant's reported dietary intake conformance to a dietary pattern. Further details on reported dietary assessment, food grouping, food pattern derivation and factor loadings were provided elsewhere [25].

2.4. Genome-Wide Genotyping and Quality Control

DNA was isolated from blood buffy coats using the GenElute™ Blood Genomic DNA kit (Sigma, St. Louis, MO, USA). Quantification and verification of DNA quality were conducted via NanoDrop spectrophotometer (Thermo Scientific, Wilmington, DE, USA) and PicoGreen DNA methods. Illumina HumanOmni-5-Quad BeadChip® (Illumina Inc., San Diego, CA, USA) were used to genotype more than 4,300,000 SNPs at the genome-wide level in the 141 individuals. Samples were tested for call rate (>95%) and gender mismatch based on genotyping data. All 141 samples were used in further analysis. Genotyping arrays were processed at the McGill University/Génome Québec Innovation Center (Montreal, QC, Canada) according to manufacturer's recommendations. SNP allele frequencies and tests for Hardy–Weinberg equilibrium (HWE) were performed using PLINK [35] (version 1.07). SNP quality control was conducted and SNPs failing one of the criteria were excluded from analyses. Specifically, SNPs with insufficient call rate (<95%) or genotype distribution deviating from Hardy–Weinberg equilibrium (p values < 1.87×10^{-8}) were excluded. In addition, monomorphic (non-variable) SNPs or with a minor allele frequency (MAF) < 0.01 were removed from analyses. Thus, a total of 1,632,526 SNPs were excluded, leaving 2,668,805 SNPs for statistical analyses.

2.5. Gene Expression Analyses

Pre-supplementation gene expression data were retrieved from previously published data [36] for 30 of the 141 individuals. Briefly, gene expression profiling was performed on RNA extracted from peripheral blood mononuclear cells using the Illumina Human-6 v3 Expression BeadChip and carried out at the McGill University/Génome Québec Innovation Center (Montreal, QC, Canada). The microarray data re-analysis was performed using the FlexArray software [37] and the Lumi algorithm. Robust multiarray average background adjustment was applied followed by log2 variance stabilization and quartile normalization. Transcripts were considered as expressed if they were detected in 25% of the samples.

2.6. Functional Analyses

Potential impacts of reported dietary patterns associated-SNPs herein identified on amino acid (aa) sequence and at protein level were analyzed using Variant Effect Predictor (VEP) [38]. Potential impacts of these SNPs on transcription factor (TF) binding sites and prediction of TF binding affinities based on DNA sequences were conducted using TRAP [39] an online tool comparing SNP surrounding sequences with known TF recognition sequences. TRAP has the capacity to identify TF binding sites among a SNP-surrounding sequence and to estimate TF affinity to the common and rare alleles. It also offers the possibility to identify overrepresented/enriched TFs among a group of sequences submitted, thus highlighting potential disruption of global regulators of biological mechanisms and providing biological insights for the associations identified. Sequences overlapping SNPs of interest (30 bp upstream and downstream) were submitted for analysis as input sequences. The Transfac vertebrates 2010.1 database was used as TF matrix file and human promoter sequences were introduced as background model.

2.7. Statistical Analysis

Clinical data were expressed as mean ± standard deviation for the full cohort and according to sex. Differences in clinical data between men and women were tested using Student's *t*-test for continuous variables and Chi-square test for categorical variables. The general linear model (type III sum of squares) with adjustments for the effects of age, sex and body mass index (BMI) was used to test the associations of SNPs with CVD risk factors (fasting plasma lipids, glucose, insulin, SBP and DBP) as well as the associations of prudent and Western reported dietary pattern scores with these CVD risk factors. Transformations were applied for TG (logarithmic transformation; log10) and insulin levels (negative inverse transformation; $1/(-1*X)$) to meet the criteria for normality. Partial Pearson correlations were computed to assess the relation between reported dietary pattern scores and associated CVD risk factors. Associations between SNPs and scores for prudent and Western reported dietary patterns were tested under linear regression using PLINK including age, sex and BMI as covariates. Nominal genome-wide association threshold of $p < 1.0 \times 10^{-5}$ was used to identify SNPs associated to reported dietary patterns. This significance threshold was used in order to avoid discounting true positive association based on the fact that statistical tests in genome-wide association studies (GWASs) are not independent due to linkage disequilibrium (LD) between SNPs and therefore the traditional method to adjust significance thresholds for multiple testing overcorrects when used in GWASs [40,41]. To evaluate the contribution of SNPs to the variance of reported dietary pattern scores, stepwise regression analysis was conducted. Differences in gene expression levels between genotype groups for reported dietary pattern-associated SNPs were tested using analysis of variance (general linear model, type III sum of squares) with adjustments for the effects of age, sex and BMI. LD (r^2) between SNPs demonstrating significant associations was calculated from our data and from the 1000 Genomes Project phase 1v3 data [42] using Haploview [43] and LD calculator (https://caprica.genetics.kcl.ac.uk/~ilori/ld_calculator.php), respectively. SAS software version 9.3 (SAS Institute Inc., Cary, NC, USA) was used to test for differences in clinical data, associations and correlation of reported dietary pattern scores with CVD risk factors, and differences in gene expression levels according to genotype groups.

3. Results

3.1. Subjects' Description

The current study included 141 individuals from a previously described supplementation study aimed at assessing gene–environment interactions on CVD risk profile [26]. Individuals included here were overweight, middle-aged men and women (68 men and 73 women; Table 1). Men and women had similar BMI, while men had higher SBP ($p < 0.0001$) and lower HDL-C levels than women ($p < 0.0001$). Comparing reported dietary pattern scores derived from dietary intakes reported for the month preceding the study, women were characterized by higher Prudent and lower Western scores than men ($p = 0.04$ and 0.01, respectively). When categorizing individuals with high (>0) vs. low (<0) scores for both reported dietary patterns, men were more prone to showing a high score for Western reported dietary pattern ($p = 0.0006$) while no difference between sex was identified for the Prudent reported dietary pattern score ($p = 0.11$).

Table 1. Description of the genotyping cohort.

Characteristics	All	Men	Women
Number	141	68	73
Age (years)	31.6 ± 8.8	31.1 ± 8.0	32.0 ± 9.6
BMI (kg/m^2)	28.4 ± 3.8	28.1 ± 3.7	28.7 ± 3.8
Waist girth (cm)	94.5 ± 11.0	96.3 ± 11.2	92.9 ± 10.7
Lipid profile			
Total-C (mmol/L)	4.90 ± 0.97	4.88 ± 1.03	4.92 ± 0.92
LDL-C (mmol/L)	2.88 ± 0.88	3.01 ± 0.95	2.75 ± 0.80
HDL-C (mmol/L)	1.42 ± 0.38 [b]	1.25 ± 0.29	1.58 ± 0.39
TG (mmol/L)	1.32 ± 0.68	1.37 ± 0.72	1.27 ± 0.65
Total-C/HDL-C	3.66 ± 1.10 [b]	4.10 ± 1.16	3.25 ± 0.88
Blood pressure (mm Hg)			
SBP	113.0 ± 12.3 [b]	118.5 ± 12.9	107.8 ± 9.1
DBP	68.5 ± 8.4	68.7 ± 8.6	68.3 ± 8.3
Fasting glucose (mmol/L)	5.00 ± 0.46	5.06 ± 0.47	4.94 ± 0.44
Insulin (pmol/L)	93.2 ± 87.5	100.6 ± 119.2	86.4 ± 39.6
Self-reported diet scores			
Prudent	-0.022 ± 1.012 [a]	-0.207 ± 1.041	0.150 ± 0.960
High/low scores (>0)	70/71	29/39	41/32
Western	-0.009 ± 0.980 [a]	0.202 ± 1.087	-0.207 ± 0.829
High/low score (>0)	70/71^2	44/24	26/47

Values presented (means $\pm$ standard deviation) are untransformed and unadjusted. Sex differences are identified. [a] p value < 0.05. [b] p value < 0.0001 Abbreviations: BMI, body mass index; Total-C, total cholesterol; LDL-C, low-density lipoprotein cholesterol; HDL-C, high-density lipoprotein cholesterol; TG, triglycerides; SBP, systolic blood pressure; DBP, diastolic blood pressure.

3.2. Dietary Scores and CVD Risk Factors

Reported dietary pattern, characterized by high intakes of vegetables, fruits, whole grain products, non-hydrogenated fats for the Prudent and by high intakes of refined grain products, desserts, sweets and processed meats for the Western were tested for associations with CVD risk factors. Although limited by our sample size, the respective SNP frequency and their potential effect size, assessment of associations of Prudent score with CVD risk factors using correlation analysis revealed that DBP ($r = -0.259$, $p = 0.002$) and fasting insulin levels ($r = -0.282$, $p = 0.0008$), both showed inverse correlation with the Prudent score following adjustments for age, sex and BMI.

3.3. Association between SNPs and Reported Dietary Patterns

Associations were tested between 2,668,805 SNPs and each reported dietary pattern including age, sex and BMI as covariates. A total of 78 and 27 SNPs was associated with the Prudent and Western reported dietary pattern scores, respectively ($p < 1 \times 10^{-5}$; Figure 1, Tables S1 and S2). Associations identified were unique; none of the SNPs showed an association with both Prudent and Western scores. Low LD was generally observed in our study sample between Prudent-associated SNPs considering SNPs on the same chromosome, with few exceptions of large regions on chromosomes 2 (5 SNPs; 250 kb), 19 (3 SNPs; 118 kb) and 20 (12 SNPs; 476 kb) demonstrating strong LD ($r^2 \geq 0.8$). LD calculation from the 1000 Genomes Project data revealed moderate LD ($r^2 \geq 0.6$) between SNPs located within these regions. No such large region with strong LD was observed between SNPs associated with Western score with a mean LD of 0.23 in the present study sample.

SNPs associated with Prudent reported dietary pattern score were mainly located in gene regions, with 44 of the 78 Prudent score-associated-SNPs being located in gene regions. Most of these SNPs were intronic, while 5 were exonic, one was located in promoter and another in the 3'near gene region. Prudent-associated intergenic SNP rs13042507 is located near the *CTCFL* gene previously associated with type 2 diabetes (T2D) [44]. SNPs annotated to genes previously associated to obesity traits (*LINGO2* [45], *NELL1* [46]) and neurological disorders (schizophrenia (*ACSM1* [47], *KIF26B* [48], *NALCN* [49])), and alcohol and nicotine dependence (*LINGO* [50], *SH3BP5* [51]) were found among Prudent reported dietary pattern score associated-SNPs. SNPs associated to Western reported dietary pattern score were mostly intergenic; 19 of the 27 significant SNPs being intergenic while 7 were intronic and another was located in 3' near gene region. SNPs from genes associated with alcohol dependence (*ESR1*) and obesity traits (*RGS7*, *NRG3* and *ESR1*) were observed among Western reported dietary pattern score-associated SNPs.

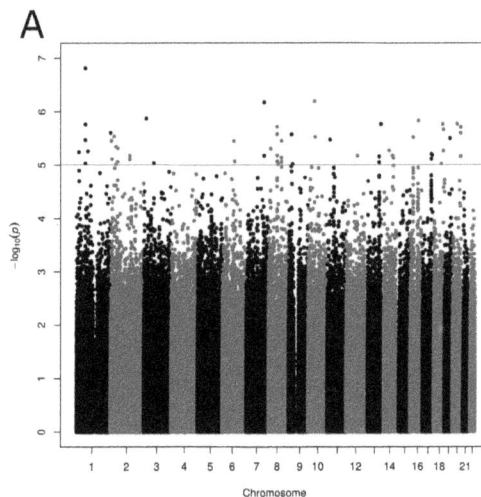

Figure 1. *Cont.*

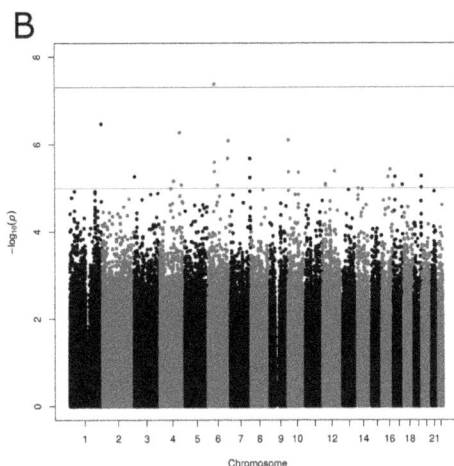

Figure 1. Manhattan plot showing *p* values obtained from genome-wide association studies between single nucleotide polymorphisms and reported dietary pattern scores: (**A**) Prudent; (**B**) Western reported dietary patterns. *p* values obtained using linear regression model with age, sex and BMI as covariates. Suggestive ($p < 1.0 \times 10^{-5}$) and conventional ($p < 5.0 \times 10^{-8}$) genome-wide association thresholds are represented by blue and red lines, respectively.

To get further insights on the contribution of SNPs in variability of reported dietary patterns, and to identify potential leading SNPs for regions demonstrating multiple significant associations, stepwise regression was performed from Prudent- and Western-associated SNPs. Among Prudent-associated SNPs, 14 SNPs contributed to explaining 76.2% of the Prudent reported dietary pattern score variability, while sex and BMI explained 2.0% and 1.0% of variability, respectively. From the 27 Western-associated SNPs, 9 explained 63.6% of variability in the Western reported dietary pattern score while confounding factors (age, sex, BMI) did not seem to contribute to variability. Potential leading SNPs revealed by stepwise regression analysis are highlighted in Tables S1 and S2.

3.4. Impact of SNPs on CVD Risk Factors

In order to test the potential implication of reported dietary pattern-associated SNPs in the associations between reported dietary patterns and CVD risk factors, we further tested reported dietary pattern-associated SNPs for associations with CVD risk factors. In line with associations identified here between Prudent reported dietary pattern scores and CVD risk factors (DBP and insulin), a total of three significant associations were identified with insulin levels (Table 2). Among these, the rs6499924 SNP located within *CNGB1*, showed the most significant association with insulin levels ($p = 0.0005$). Significant associations between SNPs located in the gluconeogenesis-regulating *PCK1* gene region and fasting glucose levels were also found although the Prudent reported dietary pattern score was not associated with fasting glucose levels in our previous analysis. Regarding Western-associated SNPs, five significant associations were identified between Western reported dietary pattern score-associated SNPs and total-C, including SNPs located within or near *RGS7*, *TET2*, *ARID1B* and *PFKFB3*.

Table 2. Significant associations identified between reported dietary pattern-associated SNPs and cardiometabolic risk factors.

SNP ID [a]	rs Number	Gene	Associated Pattern	Total-C	LDL-C	HDL-C	Total-C/HDL-C	SBP	Fasting Glucose	Insulin
kgp4289407	rs114123656	LINC01246 [b]	Prudent	—	—	—	—	—	—	0.02
kgp6444538	rs115510004	LOC645949 [b]	Prudent	—	—	0.008	—	—	—	—
rs10097298	rs10097298	LOC100130298 [b]	Prudent	—	—	—	—	—	0.03	—
kgp2826446	rs76838052	C10orf142 [b]	Prudent	—	0.02	—	—	0.03	—	—
kgp9480099	rs74842138	GDF10 [b]	Prudent	0.04	—	—	—	—	—	—
rs714547	rs714547	STON2	Prudent	—	—	0.004	0.03	—	—	0.02
rs163269	rs163269	ACSM1	Prudent	—	—	—	—	—	—	0.0005
rs649924	rs649924	CNGB1	Prudent	—	—	—	—	0.04	—	—
kgp5504930	rs13042507	CTCFL [b]	Prudent	—	—	0.02	—	—	0.02	—
kgp6972810	rs73180793	PCK1 [b]	Prudent	—	—	0.02	—	—	0.02	—
kgp12008054	rs6070157	PCK1	Prudent	—	—	0.04	—	—	0.02	—
kgp10614850	rs11552145	PCK1	Prudent	—	—	—	—	—	0.01	—
kgp9374426	rs116812750	RGS7	Western	0.02	0.009	—	—	0.01	—	—
kgp8978882	rs112040989	LOC101929468 [b]	Western	0.03	—	—	—	0.02	—	—
kgp9399667	rs112764838	TET2 [b]	Western	0.03	—	—	—	0.02	—	—
kgp9469075	rs72736220	LOC100996286 [b]	Western	—	—	—	—	0.03	—	—
kgp29240591	rs148696004	TLL1 [b]	Western	—	—	—	—	—	0.01	—
rs200247	rs200247	TFAP2D [b]	Western	—	—	—	—	0.04	—	—
kgp9033598	rs79041188	ESR1	Western	—	—	—	—	0.05	—	—
kgp26148321	rs141382233	ARID1B [b]	Western	0.02	0.01	—	—	—	—	—
kgp4441528	rs2535974	ACTR3B [b]	Western	—	—	—	—	0.008	—	—
kgp1054774	rs113152482	PFKFB3	Western	0.03	—	—	—	—	—	—
rs1348307	rs1348307	LINC00706 [b]	Western	—	—	—	—	—	0.006	0.0008
rs7911681	rs7911681	NRG3	Western	—	—	—	—	—	0.03	—
kgp6498073	rs112633616	LOC101928441 [b]	Western	—	0.03	—	—	—	—	—
kgp27660318	rs140957346	EEA1	Western	—	—	—	—	—	0.03	—
kgp25610618	rs140552175	LOC101928880	Western	—	0.05	—	—	0.02	0.002	—

[a] SNP ID and annotated genes according to Illumina® HumanOmni5-Quad BeadChip. [b] Nearest gene according to Illumina® HumanOmni5-Quad BeadChip annotations. Significant p values are shown while non-significant ones are represented by dashes (—). No significant associations between SNPs and BMI, triglyceride levels or DBP were found. Abbreviations: SNP, single nucleotide polymorphism; Total-C, total cholesterol; HDL-C, high-density lipoprotein cholesterol; LDL-C, low-density lipoprotein cholesterol; SBP, systolic blood pressure; DBP, diastolic blood pressure.

3.5. Impact of SNPs on Gene Expression Level

To assess the physiological impact of reported dietary pattern-associated SNPs and to provide potential molecular mechanisms underlying associations identified, we tested the association of SNPs with gene expression levels using gene expression data retrieved from a previous study [36] conducted on 30 individuals from our study sample (Table S3). Corresponding gene expression data were obtained for SNPs located in the gene region while expression levels of the nearest gene were retrieved for intergenic SNPs. Among genes annotated to diet associated-SNPs, 55 were found on gene expression array and 21 were detected in peripheral blood mononuclear cells. Despite few of the SNPs tested being associated with gene expression levels in this small study sample of 30 individuals, two intergenic SNPs associated with the Prudent reported dietary pattern (rs1454469, rs976145) were associated with expression levels ($p = 0.02$ for both) of *BCKDHB* (NM_183050). Rare allele carriers of these SNPs had higher expression levels (Figure 2A,B). These two SNPs demonstrated strong LD ($r^2 = 1.0$) in our sample as well as in data from the 1000 Genomes Project. Testing Western reported dietary pattern-associated SNPs for association with expression levels, rs113152482 rare allele carriers showed higher *PFKFB3* (NM_004566) expression levels following adjustments for the effect of age, sex and BMI ($p = 0.0004$; Figure 2C). It is interesting to note that this SNP was highlighted by stepwise regression analysis as it contributed to 1.3% of the variability of the Western reported dietary pattern score.

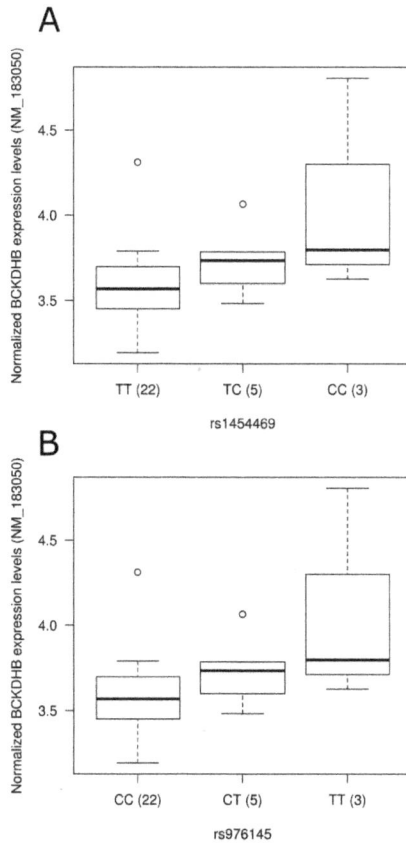

Figure 2. *Cont.*

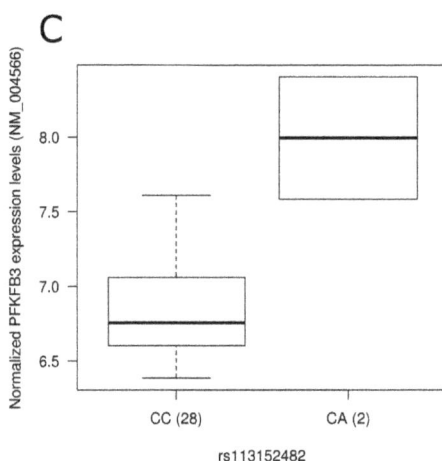

Figure 2. Representation of expression levels according to genotype groups for transcripts showing significant association with the presence of single nucleotide polymorphisms in blood. Expression levels of the *BCKDHB* gene (NM_183050) according to (**A**) rs1454469 and (**B**) rs976145 genotype groups; (**C**) Expression level of *PFKFB3* (NM_004566) according to rs113152482 genotype groups. Normalized expression levels are shown. The line in the middle of the rectangle represents the median while first and third quartiles are represented by box borders. Whiskers represent first and third quartiles ±1.5 interquartile ranges.

3.6. Functional Analysis of SNPs

To provide further mechanistic insights for associations identified between SNPs, Prudent and Western reported dietary pattern scores, CVD risk factors and expression levels, we conducted TF analysis from SNP-surrounding sequences. Considering all Prudent-associated SNPs, FOXM1, glucocorticoid receptor (GR), CEBP and CEBPB were found among the most overrepresented TF binding sites. STAT family members and HMGA1 TFs were overrepresented from SNP-surrounding sequences for SNP associated with either Prudent or Western reported dietary patterns (Tables S4 and S5). IRF8 and PDX1 TFs were also overrepresented among surrounding sequences from SNPs associated with either the Prudent or the Western reported dietary pattern. Focusing on SNPs associated to CVD risk factors identified here, SNP rs6499924 associated with fasting insulin levels showed creation of potential GABP-alpha and ATF5 binding sites in the presence of the rare allele. Among glucose level-associated SNPs located in the *PCK1* gene region, rs6070157 resulted in aa change that was predicted to be tolerated or benign. For SNPs associated with gene expression, the rs976145 SNP associated to *BCKDHB* gene expression levels showed creation of HIF2A binding site while the presence of the rare allele of rs1454469 SNP, also located within the *BCKDHB* gene region, was predicted to disrupt IRX2 and IRX3 binding sites and to create a MEF2 binding site. Western reported dietary pattern-associated rs113152482 SNP, found to be associated with *PFKFB3* gene expression, showed the creation of a potential NFAT1 binding site.

4. Discussion

Using factor analysis from reported dietary intakes obtained from a concurrently validated FFQ [27], we first derived dietary patterns corresponding to Prudent and Western dietary patterns [14,18] previously reported to be associated respectively with protective and deleterious effects on CVD [16,17]. We thereafter tested associations between SNPs and reported dietary pattern scores using a nominal threshold of $p < 1.0 \times 10^{-5}$. This genome-wide association threshold was used to account the non-independency of statistical tests conducted [40,41] and combined with functional analyses to provide potential mechanistic insights for the associations identified. Although not reaching the conventional $p < 5.0 \times 10^{-8}$ GWAS significance threshold or Bonferroni corrected threshold, it provides clues for the discovery of biologically relevant associations. Identification of associations between reported dietary pattern-associated SNPs, CVD risk factors and gene expression levels argued for such biological importance of SNPs identified. Nonetheless, the most significant association observed here, between rs13212846 and the Western score ($p = 4.16 \times 10^{-8}$), reached a conventional $p < 5.0 \times 10^{-8}$ GWAS significance threshold. This SNP is located ~285 kb upstream the *DEFB112* gene encoding an antimicrobial and cytotoxic peptides made by neutrophils [52]. Another SNP located upstream of the *DEFB112* gene (~259 kb) was previously associated with BMI [53]. However, very low LD is observed between the BMI-associated rs17665162 SNP and the Western score-associated rs13212846 SNP herein identified. Globally, low LD observed between reported dietary pattern-associated SNPs and subsequent regression analysis demonstrated that a limited number of SNPs explains a large proportion of the variability in reported dietary pattern scores. These results suggest that: (1) some of the SNPs identified herein may act under an additive model; and (2) some other SNPs may act through common functional mechanisms with major SNPs potentially alleviating the impact of certain SNPs in common biological mechanism.

In line with the relationship between dietary patterns and CVD risk factors, the current study identified the rs13042507 SNP, near the *CTCFL* gene previously associated with T2D [44]. This SNP, herein associated with the Prudent reported dietary pattern, shows very low LD (0.008; 1000 Genomes Project data) with the rs328506 SNP associated with decreased risk of T2D [44], thus not allowing a potential biological link between Prudent dietary pattern and T2D-associated risk previously reported [54]. Nonetheless, association of reported dietary pattern-associated SNPs with CVD risk factors were also identified in the current study. Three SNPs (rs73180793, rs11552145, rs6070157) located within the gluconeogenesis-regulating *PCK1* gene region were found to be associated with fasting glucose levels. Although subjects recruited had to be non-diabetics, these associations are coherent with a potential association between *PCK1* SNPs and T2D [44], and between Prudent-like dietary patterns and decreased risk of T2D [54]. Testing Western reported dietary pattern -associated SNPs with CVD risk factors, the most significant association found involved the rs1348307 SNP located within the long intergenic non-protein coding RNA 706 (*LINC00706*) and fasting insulin levels ($p = 0.0008$). Although association between Western reported dietary pattern score and insulin levels was not observed in our cohort of overweight/obese men and women, such association of Western reported dietary pattern-associated SNPs with insulin level is coherent with a correlation of the Western score with insulin levels, as previously reported in men [55].

Mechanistic insights for the associations identified are provided herein through analysis of gene expression levels in blood and TF analysis. Increased expression levels of the *BCKDHB* gene (NM_183050) were observed in the presence of rare allele of Prudent reported dietary pattern-associated SNPs rs1454469 and rs976145, both SNPs demonstrating perfect LD in our study sample. Mutations in the *BCKDHB* gene are known to be responsible for the maple syrup urine disease (Online Mendelian Inheritance in Man #248600) characterized by mental and physical retardation, feeding problems, and a maple syrup odor of the urine. Specifically, the presence of SNP rs1454469 was predicted to create an MEF2 binding site. In *Caenorhabditis elegans* chemosensory neurons, MEF2 TF was recently found to be involved in sensory neuron–gut interaction, linking feeding state conditions to the regulation of chemoreceptor genes via insulin signaling [56]. An association between the Western diet associated-SNP rs113152482 and gene expression of *PFKFB3* in blood was also identified. *PFKFB3* encodes inducible 6-phosphofructo-2-kinase and is expressed in the brain [57]. It was shown to act as an essential glucosensor in hypothalamic neurons, linking glycolysis, AMP-activated protein kinase signaling and neuropeptide expression in mouse [58]. The rs113152482 SNP, highlighted by stepwise regression and explaining 1.3% of Western score variability, was predicted to disrupt the NFAT1 binding site. NFAT signaling plays critical roles in the development of multiple organ systems, including pancreas [59] and nervous system [60], and was reported to play a role in glucose homeostasis in pancreatic β-cells cellular models [61].

Having a global look at TF overrepresentation from surrounding sequences of reported dietary pattern-associated SNPs, overrepresentation of FOXM1 and GR TF were observed from Prudent reported dietary pattern-associated SNPs. FOXM1 is involved in cell proliferation, is necessary for the maintenance of adult beta-cell mass, beta-cell proliferation and glucose homeostasis, and was shown to be up-regulated in obesity [62]. Glucocorticoids (GCs) are known to mobilize the endocannabinoid system which is essential for negative feedback regulation of the hypothalamic–pituitary–adrenal axis [63]. In addition, a recent study using Cushing's syndrome patients as a unique model of chronic GCs exposure demonstrated a negative correlation of urine cortisone with food-related choice thus implying a potential role of GR in food-choice behavior [64]. STAT family members and PDX1 TF were found to be overrepresented from SNP-surrounding sequences from both Prudent and Western reported dietary pattern-associated SNPs (Tables S5 and S6). STAT TFs were shown to be involved in energy homeostasis through an activation of the JAK-STAT pathway by leptin and their role in leptin-mediated satiety [65]. Specifically, STAT5 TF herein overrepresented is recruited by many hormones and cytokines that regulate food intake [66] whereas the PDX1 TF is involved in pancreatic development and glucose metabolism [67].

Results presented here tend to highlight a potential involvement of obesity-related and glucose metabolism genes in the adoption of dietary patterns concordant with a potential involvement of obesity genes in nutrient-specific food preference proposed following the analysis of obesity-associated loci revealed through genome-wide association study [19]. Notably, variants associated with body weight and BMI were previously reported to be associated with appetite, energy intake and eating behaviors [20,68], and several obesity genes were reported to be expressed in the hypothalamus, a center for energy balance and regulation of food intake. Specifically, interplay exists between food-induced brain responses and eating behaviour [69], and hypothalamus is a brain area specifically involved in food reward [70] thus potentially influencing food choice and the adoption of dietary patterns.

The current study used unbiased genome-wide approach to assess the genetics of the adoption of Prudent and Western reported dietary pattern scores. Results from the 91-items FFQ administered in the current study are based on reported data known to be biased by omissions, false memories, intentional misreporting and gross misestimation [9], and face-to-face interviews may have affected participants' responses due to social desirability bias [71]. While these biases cannot be measured in the current study, the use of a population-specific FFQ [27] combined with an extensive database of food items with nutritional values available for 112 nutrients may partially alleviate the impact of self-reported nutritional assessment method on the derivation of reported dietary patterns. Despite subject to the imperfection of self-reported data and the ongoing debate on the validity of the memory-based dietary assessment methods [9,10], the concurrent validity and reproducibility of the FFQ used here were previously reported using a home- and self-completed 3-day food record [27], a dietary assessment method subject to recall bias, thus arguing for concurrent validity of the FFQ administered although validation was not performed in the current study and actual dietary intakes were not measured. Interactions between genetic and dietary factors as well as the impact of developmental processes on CVD risk factors were not analyzed, the main objective of the study being to identify associations between SNPs and reported dietary patterns to provide novel potential targets and biological mechanisms for CVD prevention. Since differences in reported dietary pattern scores between men and women have been identified herein from reported dietary intakes, sex has been included as a covariate in genome-wide analyses. However, analyses have not been conducted separately in men and women. BMI was also included as a covariate in our analysis, suggesting that association identified are BMI independent. However, we acknowledge that other CVD risk-associated confounding factors, e.g., developmental programming [72,73] and physical activity [74], were not taken into account for testing associations between reported dietary pattern-associated SNPs and CVD risk factors. Further generalization of conclusions at the population level merits further validation in general population, our cohort being composed of overweight individuals. An impact of SNPs on blood cell expression levels was observed here for a limited number SNPs. Nonetheless, we cannot rule out the possibility that they may exert their effect in other tissues.

Collectively, the association of SNPs with reported dietary pattern scores, CVD risk factors and expression levels argues for an impact of genetic variations on the determination of the adoption of Prudent and Western dietary patterns. Integration of association, expression and transcription factor data tends to reveal the involvement of obesity, glucose metabolism and neurological genes in the adoption of dietary patterns. As proposed herein, reported dietary pattern-associated SNPs may potentially act through an impact on glucose metabolism and food- and energy-sensing pathways.

Supplementary Materials: The following are available online at www.mdpi.com/2072-6643/9/7/649/s1, Table S1: Associations identified between SNPs and Prudent dietary pattern, Table S2: Associations identified between SNPs and Western dietary pattern, Table S3: Description of gene expression cohort, Table S4: Transcription factors overrepresented in surrounding regions (60 bp) of Prudent dietary pattern-associated SNPs, Table S5: Transcription factors overrepresented in surrounding regions (60 bp) of Western dietary pattern-associated SNPs.

Acknowledgments: The authors thank participants in the study for their excellent collaboration. We would like to thank Hubert Cormier, Véronique Garneau, Alain Houde, Catherine Ouellette, Catherine Raymond and Élisabeth Thifault for their participation in the recruitment of the participants, the study coordination and the data collection. We acknowledge the contribution of the McGill University and Génome Quebec Innovation Centre for processing of Illumina HumanOmni-5-Quad arrays. I.R. holds a Junior 1 Research Scholar from the Fonds de Recherche du Québec-Santé (FRQ-S). M.C.V. is a Canada Research Chair in Genomics Applied to Nutrition and Health. This study was supported by a grant from the Canadian Institutes of Health Research (CIHR MOP-110975).

Author Contributions: I.R., S.L., P.C. and M.C.V. conceived and designed the experiments; F.G., A.B.M. and I.R. performed the experiments; F.G. and A.B.M. analyzed the data or performed statistical analysis; F.G. wrote the paper; and M.C.V. has primary responsibility for final content.

Conflicts of Interest: The authors declare no conflict of interest.

References

1. Mendis, S.; Davis, S.; Norrving, B. Organizational update: The world health organization global status report on noncommunicable diseases 2014; one more landmark step in the combat against stroke and vascular disease. *Stroke* **2015**, *46*, e121–e122. [CrossRef] [PubMed]

2. Mokdad, A.H.; Ford, E.S.; Bowman, B.A.; Dietz, W.H.; Vinicor, F.; Bales, V.S.; Marks, J.S. Prevalence of obesity, diabetes, and obesity-related health risk factors, 2001. *JAMA* **2003**, *289*, 76–79. [CrossRef] [PubMed]

3. Livingstone, M.B.; McCaffrey, T.A.; Rennie, K.L. Childhood obesity prevention studies: Lessons learned and to be learned. *Public Health Nutr.* **2006**, *9*, 1121–1129. [CrossRef] [PubMed]

4. Miller, W.C.; Lindeman, A.K.; Wallace, J.; Niederpruem, M. Diet composition, energy intake, and exercise in relation to body fat in men and women. *Am. J. Clin. Nutr.* **1990**, *52*, 426–430. [PubMed]

5. Jacobs, D.R.; Tapsell, L.C. Food synergy: The key to a healthy diet. *Proc. Nutr. Soc.* **2013**, *72*, 200–206. [CrossRef] [PubMed]

6. Zarraga, I.G.; Schwarz, E.R. Impact of dietary patterns and interventions on cardiovascular health. *Circulation* **2006**, *114*, 961–973. [CrossRef] [PubMed]

7. Hu, F.B. Dietary pattern analysis: A new direction in nutritional epidemiology. *Curr. Opin. Lipidol.* **2002**, *13*, 3–9. [CrossRef] [PubMed]

8. Newby, P.K.; Tucker, K.L. Empirically derived eating patterns using factor or cluster analysis: A review. *Nutr. Rev.* **2004**, *62*, 177–203. [CrossRef] [PubMed]

9. Archer, E.; Pavela, G.; Lavie, C.J. The Inadmissibility of What We Eat in America and NHANES Dietary Data in Nutrition and Obesity Research and the Scientific Formulation of National Dietary Guidelines. *Mayo Clin. Proc.* **2015**, *90*, 911–926. [CrossRef] [PubMed]

10. Davy, B.M.; Estabrooks, P.A. The Validity of Self-reported Dietary Intake Data: Focus on the "What We Eat In America" Component of the National Health and Nutrition Examination Survey Research Initiative. *Mayo Clin. Proc.* **2015**, *90*, 845–847. [CrossRef] [PubMed]

11. Nanri, A.; Shimazu, T.; Ishihara, J.; Takachi, R.; Mizoue, T.; Inoue, M.; Tsugane, S. Reproducibility and validity of dietary patterns assessed by a food frequency questionnaire used in the 5-year follow-up survey of the Japan Public Health Center-Based Prospective Study. *J. Epidemiol.* **2012**, *22*, 205–215. [CrossRef] [PubMed]

12. Heidemann, C.; Schulze, M.B.; Franco, O.H.; van Dam, R.M.; Mantzoros, C.S.; Hu, F.B. Dietary patterns and risk of mortality from cardiovascular disease, cancer, and all causes in a prospective cohort of women. *Circulation* **2008**, *118*, 230–237. [CrossRef] [PubMed]

13. Malik, V.S.; Fung, T.T.; van Dam, R.M.; Rimm, E.B.; Rosner, B.; Hu, F.B. Dietary patterns during adolescence and risk of type 2 diabetes in middle-aged women. *Diabetes Care* **2012**, *35*, 12–18. [CrossRef] [PubMed]

14. Paradis, A.M.; Godin, G.; Perusse, L.; Vohl, M.C. Associations between dietary patterns and obesity phenotypes. *Int. J. Obes. (Lond.)* **2009**, *33*, 1419–1426. [CrossRef] [PubMed]

15. Shen, J.; Wilmot, K.A.; Ghasemzadeh, N.; Molloy, D.L.; Burkman, G.; Mekonnen, G.; Gongora, M.C.; Quyyumi, A.A.; Sperling, L.S. Mediterranean Dietary Patterns and Cardiovascular Health. *Annu. Rev. Nutr.* **2015**, *35*, 425–449. [CrossRef] [PubMed]

16. Rodriguez-Monforte, M.; Flores-Mateo, G.; Sanchez, E. Dietary patterns and CVD: A systematic review and meta-analysis of observational studies. *Br. J. Nutr.* **2015**, *114*, 1341–1359. [CrossRef] [PubMed]

17. Sherzai, A.; Heim, L.T.; Boothby, C.; Sherzai, A.D. Stroke, food groups, and dietary patterns: A systematic review. *Nutr. Rev.* **2012**, *70*, 423–435. [CrossRef] [PubMed]

18. Hu, F.B.; Rimm, E.B.; Stampfer, M.J.; Ascherio, A.; Spiegelman, D.; Willett, W.C. Prospective study of major dietary patterns and risk of coronary heart disease in men. *Am. J. Clin. Nutr.* **2000**, *72*, 912–921. [PubMed]

19. Bauer, F.; Elbers, C.C.; Adan, R.A.; Loos, R.J.; Onland-Moret, N.C.; Grobbee, D.E.; van Vliet-Ostaptchouk, J.V.; Wijmenga, C.; van der Schouw, Y.T. Obesity genes identified in genome-wide association studies are associated with adiposity measures and potentially with nutrient-specific food preference. *Am. J. Clin. Nutr.* **2009**, *90*, 951–959. [CrossRef] [PubMed]

20. Brunkwall, L.; Ericson, U.; Hellstrand, S.; Gullberg, B.; Orho-Melander, M.; Sonestedt, E. Genetic variation in the fat mass and obesity-associated gene (FTO) in association with food preferences in healthy adults. *Food Nutr. Res.* **2013**, *57*. [CrossRef] [PubMed]

21. Wallace, D.L.; Aarts, E.; d'Oleire, U.F.; Dang, L.C.; Greer, S.M.; Jagust, W.J.; D'Esposito, M. Genotype status of the dopamine-related catechol-O-methyltransferase (COMT) gene corresponds with desirability of "unhealthy" foods. *Appetite* **2015**, *92*, 74–80. [CrossRef] [PubMed]

22. Bhupathiraju, S.N.; Hu, F.B. One (small) step towards precision nutrition by use of metabolomics. *Lancet Diabetes Endocrinol.* **2017**, *5*, 154–155. [CrossRef]

23. Dietary Guidelines Advisory Committee. *Scientific Report of the 2015 Dietary Guidelines Advisory Committee*; Departments of Agriculture and Health and Human Services: Washington, DC, USA, 2015.

24. Hebert, J.R.; Hurley, T.G.; Steck, S.E.; Miller, D.R.; Tabung, F.K.; Peterson, K.E.; Kushi, L.H.; Frongillo, E.A. Considering the value of dietary assessment data in informing nutrition-related health policy. *Adv. Nutr.* **2014**, *5*, 447–455. [CrossRef] [PubMed]

25. Bouchard-Mercier, A.; Paradis, A.M.; Rudkowska, I.; Lemieux, S.; Couture, P.; Vohl, M.C. Associations between dietary patterns and gene expression profiles of healthy men and women: A cross-sectional study. *Nutr. J.* **2013**, *12*, 24. [CrossRef] [PubMed]

26. Thifault, E.; Cormier, H.; Bouchard-Mercier, A.; Rudkowska, I.; Paradis, A.M.; Garneau, V.; Ouellette, C.; Lemieux, S.; Couture, P.; Vohl, M.C. Effects of age, sex, body mass index and APOE genotype on cardiovascular biomarker response to an *n*-3 polyunsaturated fatty acid supplementation. *J. Nutrigenet Nutrigenom.* **2013**, *6*, 73–82. [CrossRef] [PubMed]

27. Goulet, J.; Nadeau, G.; Lapointe, A.; Lamarche, B.; Lemieux, S. Validity and reproducibility of an interviewer-administered food frequency questionnaire for healthy French-Canadian men and women. *Nutr. J.* **2004**, *3*, 13. [CrossRef] [PubMed]

28. Rudkowska, I.; Guenard, F.; Julien, P.; Couture, P.; Lemieux, S.; Barbier, O.; Calder, P.C.; Minihane, A.M.; Vohl, M.C. Genome-wide association study of the plasma triglyceride response to an *n*-3 polyunsaturated fatty acid supplementation. *J. Lipid Res.* **2014**, *55*, 1245–1253. [CrossRef] [PubMed]

29. Lohman, T.; Roche, A.; Martorel, R. *The Airlie (VA) Consensus Conference*; Human Kinetics Publishers: Champaign, IL, USA, 1988; pp. 39–80.

30. Padwal, R.S.; Hemmelgarn, B.R.; Khan, N.A.; Grover, S.; McKay, D.W.; Wilson, T.; Penner, B.; Burgess, E.; McAlister, F.A.; Bolli, P.; et al. The 2009 Canadian Hypertension Education Program recommendations for the management of hypertension: Part 1—Blood pressure measurement, diagnosis and assessment of risk. *Can. J. Cardiol.* **2009**, *25*, 279–286. [CrossRef]

31. McNamara, J.R.; Schaefer, E.J. Automated enzymatic standardized lipid analyses for plasma and lipoprotein fractions. *Clin. Chim. Acta* **1987**, *166*, 1–8. [CrossRef]

32. Friedewald, W.T.; Levy, R.I.; Fredrickson, D.S. Estimation of the concentration of low-density lipoprotein cholesterol in plasma, without use of the preparative ultracentrifuge. *Clin. Chem.* **1972**, *18*, 499–502. [PubMed]

33. Desbuquois, B.; Aurbach, G.D. Use of polyethylene glycol to separate free and antibody-bound peptide hormones in radioimmunoassays. *J. Clin. Endocrinol. Metab.* **1971**, *33*, 732–738. [CrossRef] [PubMed]

34. Richterich, R.; Dauwalder, H. [Determination of plasma glucose by hexokinase-glucose-6-phosphate dehydrogenase method]. *Schweiz. Med. Wochenschr.* **1971**, *101*, 615–618. [PubMed]

35. Purcell, S.; Neale, B.; Todd-Brown, K.; Thomas, L.; Ferreira, M.A.; Bender, D.; Maller, J.; Sklar, P.; de Bakker, P.I.; Daly, M.J.; et al. PLINK: A tool set for whole-genome association and population-based linkage analyses. *Am. J. Hum. Genet.* **2007**, *81*, 559–575. [CrossRef] [PubMed]

36. Rudkowska, I.; Paradis, A.M.; Thifault, E.; Julien, P.; Tchernof, A.; Couture, P.; Lemieux, S.; Barbier, O.; Vohl, M.C. Transcriptomic and metabolomic signatures of an *n*-3 polyunsaturated fatty acids supplementation in a normolipidemic/normocholesterolemic Caucasian population. *J. Nutr. Biochem.* **2013**, *24*, 54–61. [CrossRef] [PubMed]

37. Blazejczyk, M.; Miron, M.; Nadon, R. *FlexArray: A Statistical Data Analysis Software for Gene Expression Microarrays*; Canadian Bioinformatics Help Desk (CBHD) Newsletter: Montreal, QC, Canada, 2007.

38. McLaren, W.; Pritchard, B.; Rios, D.; Chen, Y.; Flicek, P.; Cunningham, F. Deriving the consequences of genomic variants with the Ensembl API and SNP Effect Predictor. *Bioinformatics* **2010**, *26*, 2069–2070. [CrossRef] [PubMed]

39. Thomas-Chollier, M.; Hufton, A.; Heinig, M.; O'Keeffe, S.; Masri, N.E.; Roider, H.G.; Manke, T.; Vingron, M. Transcription factor binding predictions using TRAP for the analysis of ChIP-seq data and regulatory SNPs. *Nat. Protoc.* **2011**, *6*, 1860–1869. [CrossRef] [PubMed]

40. Duggal, P.; Gillanders, E.M.; Holmes, T.N.; Bailey-Wilson, J.E. Establishing an adjusted p-value threshold to control the family-wide type 1 error in genome wide association studies. *BMC Genom.* **2008**, *9*, 516. [CrossRef] [PubMed]

41. Nicodemus, K.K.; Liu, W.; Chase, G.A.; Tsai, Y.Y.; Fallin, M.D. Comparison of type I error for multiple test corrections in large single-nucleotide polymorphism studies using principal components versus haplotype blocking algorithms. *BMC Genet.* **2005**, *6* (Suppl. 1), S78. [CrossRef] [PubMed]

42. Sudmant, P.H.; Rausch, T.; Gardner, E.J.; Handsaker, R.E.; Abyzov, A.; Huddleston, J.; Zhang, Y.; Ye, K.; Jun, G.; Hsi-Yang, F.M.; et al. An integrated map of structural variation in 2,504 human genomes. *Nature* **2015**, *526*, 75–81. [CrossRef] [PubMed]

43. Barrett, J.C.; Fry, B.; Maller, J.; Daly, M.J. Haploview: Analysis and visualization of LD and haplotype maps. *Bioinformatics* **2005**, *21*, 263–265. [CrossRef] [PubMed]

44. Saxena, R.; Saleheen, D.; Been, L.F.; Garavito, M.L.; Braun, T.; Bjonnes, A.; Young, R.; Ho, W.K.; Rasheed, A.; Frossard, P.; et al. Genome-wide association study identifies a novel locus contributing to type 2 diabetes susceptibility in Sikhs of Punjabi origin from India. *Diabetes* **2013**, *62*, 1746–1755. [CrossRef] [PubMed]

45. Rask-Andersen, M.; Almen, M.S.; Lind, L.; Schioth, H.B. Association of the LINGO2-related SNP rs10968576 with body mass in a cohort of elderly Swedes. *Mol. Genet. Genom.* **2015**, *290*, 1485–1491. [CrossRef] [PubMed]

46. Comuzzie, A.G.; Cole, S.A.; Laston, S.L.; Voruganti, V.S.; Haack, K.; Gibbs, R.A.; Butte, N.F. Novel genetic loci identified for the pathophysiology of childhood obesity in the Hispanic population. *PLoS ONE* **2012**, *7*, e51954. [CrossRef] [PubMed]

47. Athanasiu, L.; Mattingsdal, M.; Kahler, A.K.; Brown, A.; Gustafsson, O.; Agartz, I.; Giegling, I.; Muglia, P.; Cichon, S.; Rietschel, M.; et al. Gene variants associated with schizophrenia in a Norwegian genome-wide study are replicated in a large European cohort. *J. Psychiatr. Res.* **2010**, *44*, 748–753. [CrossRef] [PubMed]

48. Fanous, A.H.; Zhou, B.; Aggen, S.H.; Bergen, S.E.; Amdur, R.L.; Duan, J.; Sanders, A.R.; Shi, J.; Mowry, B.J.; Olincy, A.; et al. Genome-wide association study of clinical dimensions of schizophrenia: Polygenic effect on disorganized symptoms. *Am. J. Psychiatry* **2012**, *169*, 1309–1317. [CrossRef] [PubMed]

49. Wang, K.S.; Liu, X.F.; Aragam, N. A genome-wide meta-analysis identifies novel loci associated with schizophrenia and bipolar disorder. *Schizophr. Res.* **2010**, *124*, 192–199. [CrossRef] [PubMed]

50. Kapoor, M.; Wang, J.C.; Wetherill, L.; Le, N.; Bertelsen, S.; Hinrichs, A.L.; Budde, J.; Agrawal, A.; Almasy, L.; Bucholz, K.; et al. Genome-wide survival analysis of age at onset of alcohol dependence in extended high-risk COGA families. *Drug Alcohol. Depend.* **2014**, *142*, 56–62. [CrossRef] [PubMed]

51. Zuo, L.; Zhang, F.; Zhang, H.; Zhang, X.Y.; Wang, F.; Li, C.S.; Lu, L.; Hong, J.; Lu, L.; Krystal, J.; et al. Genome-wide search for replicable risk gene regions in alcohol and nicotine co-dependence. *Am. J. Med. Genet. B Neuropsychiatr. Genet.* **2012**, *159B*, 437–444. [CrossRef] [PubMed]

52. Schutte, B.C.; Mitros, J.P.; Bartlett, J.A.; Walters, J.D.; Jia, H.P.; Welsh, M.J.; Casavant, T.L.; McCray, P.B., Jr. Discovery of five conserved beta -defensin gene clusters using a computational search strategy. *Proc. Natl. Acad. Sci. USA* **2002**, *99*, 2129–2133. [CrossRef] [PubMed]

53. Locke, A.E.; Kahali, B.; Berndt, S.I.; Justice, A.E.; Pers, T.H.; Day, F.R.; Powell, C.; Vedantam, S.; Buchkovich, M.L.; Yang, J.; et al. Genetic studies of body mass index yield new insights for obesity biology. *Nature* **2015**, *518*, 197–206. [CrossRef] [PubMed]

54. Heidemann, C.; Hoffmann, K.; Spranger, J.; Klipstein-Grobusch, K.; Mohlig, M.; Pfeiffer, A.F.; Boeing, H. A dietary pattern protective against type 2 diabetes in the European Prospective Investigation into Cancer and Nutrition (EPIC)—Potsdam Study cohort. *Diabetologia* **2005**, *48*, 1126–1134. [CrossRef] [PubMed]

55. Fung, T.T.; Rimm, E.B.; Spiegelman, D.; Rifai, N.; Tofler, G.H.; Willett, W.C.; Hu, F.B. Association between dietary patterns and plasma biomarkers of obesity and cardiovascular disease risk. *Am. J. Clin. Nutr.* **2001**, *73*, 61–67. [PubMed]

56. Gruner, M.; Grubbs, J.; McDonagh, A.; Valdes, D.; Winbush, A.; van der Linden, A.M. Cell-Autonomous and Non-Cell-Autonomous Regulation of a Feeding State-Dependent Chemoreceptor Gene via MEF-2 and bHLH Transcription Factors. *PLoS Genet.* **2016**, *12*, e1006237. [CrossRef] [PubMed]

57. Kessler, R.; Eschrich, K. Splice isoforms of ubiquitous 6-phosphofructo-2-kinase/fructose-2,6-bisphosphatase in human brain. *Brain Res. Mol. Brain Res.* **2001**, *87*, 190–195. [CrossRef]

58. Li, H.; Guo, X.; Xu, H.; Woo, S.L.; Halim, V.; Morgan, C.; Wu, C. A role for inducible 6-phosphofructo-2-kinase in the control of neuronal glycolysis. *J. Nutr. Biochem.* **2013**, *24*, 1153–1158. [CrossRef] [PubMed]

59. Goodyer, W.R.; Gu, X.; Liu, Y.; Bottino, R.; Crabtree, G.R.; Kim, S.K. Neonatal beta cell development in mice and humans is regulated by calcineurin/NFAT. *Dev. Cell* **2012**, *23*, 21–34. [CrossRef] [PubMed]

60. Kipanyula, M.J.; Kimaro, W.H.; Seke Etet, P.F. The Emerging Roles of the Calcineurin-Nuclear Factor of Activated T-Lymphocytes Pathway in Nervous System Functions and Diseases. *J. Aging Res.* **2016**, *2016*, 5081021. [CrossRef] [PubMed]

61. Lawrence, M.C.; Borenstein-Auerbach, N.; McGlynn, K.; Kunnathodi, F.; Shahbazov, R.; Syed, I.; Kanak, M.; Takita, M.; Levy, M.F.; Naziruddin, B. NFAT targets signaling molecules to gene promoters in pancreatic beta-cells. *Mol. Endocrinol.* **2015**, *29*, 274–288. [CrossRef] [PubMed]

62. Davis, D.B.; Lavine, J.A.; Suhonen, J.I.; Krautkramer, K.A.; Rabaglia, M.E.; Sperger, J.M.; Fernandez, L.A.; Yandell, B.S.; Keller, M.P.; Wang, I.M.; et al. FoxM1 is up-regulated by obesity and stimulates beta-cell proliferation. *Mol. Endocrinol.* **2010**, *24*, 1822–1834. [CrossRef] [PubMed]

63. Evanson, N.K.; Tasker, J.G.; Hill, M.N.; Hillard, C.J.; Herman, J.P. Fast feedback inhibition of the HPA axis by glucocorticoids is mediated by endocannabinoid signaling. *Endocrinology* **2010**, *151*, 4811–4819. [CrossRef] [PubMed]

64. Moeller, S.J.; Couto, L.; Cohen, V.; Lalazar, Y.; Makotkine, I.; Williams, N.; Yehuda, R.; Goldstein, R.Z.; Geer, E.B. Glucocorticoid Regulation of Food-Choice Behavior in Humans: Evidence from Cushing's Syndrome. *Front. Neurosci.* **2016**, *10*, 21. [CrossRef] [PubMed]

65. Ladyman, S.R.; Grattan, D.R. JAK-STAT and feeding. *JAKSTAT* **2013**, *2*, e23675. [CrossRef] [PubMed]

66. Furigo, I.C.; Ramos-Lobo, A.M.; Frazao, R.; Donato, J., Jr. Brain STAT5 signaling and behavioral control. *Mol. Cell. Endocrinol.* **2016**. [CrossRef] [PubMed]

67. Gao, T.; McKenna, B.; Li, C.; Reichert, M.; Nguyen, J.; Singh, T.; Yang, C.; Pannikar, A.; Doliba, N.; Zhang, T.; et al. Pdx1 maintains beta cell identity and function by repressing an alpha cell program. *Cell Metab.* **2014**, *19*, 259–271. [CrossRef] [PubMed]

68. Dougkas, A.; Yaqoob, P.; Givens, D.I.; Reynolds, C.K.; Minihane, A.M. The impact of obesity-related SNP on appetite and energy intake. *Br. J. Nutr.* **2013**, *110*, 1151–1156. [CrossRef] [PubMed]

69. Smeets, P.A.; Charbonnier, L.; van, M.F.; van der Laan, L.N.; Spetter, M.S. Food-induced brain responses and eating behaviour. *Proc. Nutr. Soc.* **2012**, *71*, 511–520. [CrossRef] [PubMed]

70. Levy, D.J.; Glimcher, P.W. Comparing apples and oranges: Using reward-specific and reward-general subjective value representation in the brain. *J. Neurosci.* **2011**, *31*, 14693–14707. [CrossRef] [PubMed]

71. Heitmann, B.L.; Lissner, L.; Osler, M. Do we eat less fat, or just report so? *Int. J. Obes. Relat. Metab. Disord.* **2000**, *24*, 435–442. [CrossRef] [PubMed]

72. Blackmore, H.L.; Ozanne, S.E. Programming of cardiovascular disease across the life-course. *J. Mol. Cell. Cardiol.* **2015**, *83*, 122–130. [CrossRef] [PubMed]

73. Guenard, F.; Deshaies, Y.; Cianflone, K.; Kral, J.G.; Marceau, P.; Vohl, M.C. Differential methylation in glucoregulatory genes of offspring born before vs. after maternal gastrointestinal bypass surgery. *Proc. Natl. Acad. Sci. USA* **2013**, *110*, 11439–11444. [CrossRef] [PubMed]

74. Despres, J.P. Physical Activity, Sedentary Behaviours, and Cardiovascular Health: When Will Cardiorespiratory Fitness Become a Vital Sign? *Can. J. Cardiol.* **2016**, *32*, 505–513. [CrossRef] [PubMed]

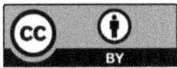

nutrients

MDPI

Review

Calcium Intake and the Risk of Ovarian Cancer: A Meta-Analysis

Xingxing Song [1], Zongyao Li [1], Xinqiang Ji [2] and Dongfeng Zhang [1,*]

[1] Department of Epidemiology and Health Statistics, the College of Public Health of Qingdao University, 38 Dengzhou Road, Qingdao 266021, Shandong, China; songxx1217@163.com (X.S.); lizy199002@163.com (Z.L.)

[2] Modern Educational Technology Center, Qingdao University, Qingdao 266021, Shandong, China; jixinqiang@qdu.edu.cn

[*] Correspondence: zhangdf1961@126.com or zhangdongfeng@qdu.edu.cn; Tel.: +86-532-8299-1712; Fax: +86-532-8380-1499

Received: 16 April 2017; Accepted: 24 June 2017; Published: 30 June 2017

Abstract: Several epidemiological studies have evaluated the association between calcium intake and the risk of ovarian cancer. However, the results of these studies remain controversial. Thus, we performed a meta-analysis to explore the association between calcium intake and the risk of ovarian cancer. Pubmed, Embase and Web of Science were searched for eligible publications up to April 2017. Pooled relative risks (RRs) with 95% confidence intervals (CIs) were calculated using the random-effects model. Small-study effect was estimated using Egger's test and the funnel plot. Among 15 epidemiological studies involving 493,415 participants and 7453 cases eligible for this meta-analysis, 13 studies were about dietary calcium intake, 4 studies about dairy calcium intake and 7 studies about dietary plus supplemental calcium intake. When comparing the highest with the lowest intake, the pooled RRs of ovarian cancer were 0.80 (95% CI 0.72–0.89) for dietary calcium, 0.80 (95% CI 0.66–0.98) for dairy calcium and 0.90 (95% CI 0.65–1.24) for dietary plus supplemental calcium, respectively. Dietary calcium was significantly associated with a reduced risk of ovarian cancer among cohort studies (RR = 0.86, 95% CI 0.74–0.99) and among case-control studies (RR = 0.75, 95% CI 0.64–0.89). In subgroup analysis by ovarian cancer subtypes, we found a statistically significant association between the dietary calcium (RR = 0.78, 95% CI 0.69–0.88) and the risk of epithelial ovarian cancer (EOC). This meta-analysis indicated that increased calcium intake might be inversely associated with the risk of ovarian cancer; this still needs to be confirmed by larger prospective cohort studies.

Keywords: calcium; intake; ovarian cancer; meta-analysis

1. Introduction

Ovarian cancers include three major histologic types: epithelial, sex cord/stromal and germ cell cancer. Approximately 90% of ovarian cancers are classified as epithelial ovarian cancer (EOC) [1,2]. There are more than 200,000 new ovarian cancer cases and 140,000 deaths of ovarian cancer per year, globally [3]. Ovarian cancer is the seventh most common cause of cancer death among women worldwide and the fifth leading cause of cancer death among women in the United States (US) [3,4].

The majority of cases are usually diagnosed at an advanced stage [5,6], contributing to poor survival. Given the suboptimal prognosis for this disease [7], it is necessary to explore modifiable risk factors to prevent ovarian cancer. Several factors have been confirmed to be associated with the risk of ovarian cancer, such as inheritance [8], anthropometric factors [9], hormonal and reproductive factors [10]. For dietary and nutritional factors, no specific dietary factors are consistently implicated in ovarian cancer [11]. Nonetheless, several meta-analyses have found that dairy products [12] and egg [13] may increase the risk of ovarian cancer, while fish [14], soy [15] and vegetables [16] may reduce the risk of ovarian cancer.

As an important component in foods, calcium has been identified as being associated with many diseases, for instance, cardiovascular disease [17], stroke [18] and breast cancer [19]. Some studies have found that calcium intake may play a role in the development of ovarian cancer [20–22]. Accordingly, numerous epidemiological studies have been carried out to evaluate the association between calcium intake and the risk of ovarian cancer. However, the results are inconsistent [23–35]. Four studies found that calcium intake was inversely related to ovarian cancer risk [27,30–32], while other studies found no evidence of an association [23–26,28,29,33–35]. Therefore, we systematically conducted a meta-analysis to (1) further investigate the associations between dietary calcium and dairy calcium intake and the risk of ovarian cancer; (2) further explore the effect of dietary plus supplemental calcium intake on the risk of ovarian cancer.

2. Materials and Methods

We followed the Preferred Reporting Items for Systematic reviews and Meta-Analyses (PRISMA) guidelines in this meta-analysis [36].

2.1. Literature Search Strategy

A literature search was performed up to April 2017 for relevant available articles from the PubMed, Embase and Web of Science databases. We used the search terms "nutrition" OR "diet" OR "dietary" OR "calcium" in combination with ("ovarian" OR "ovary") and ("neoplasm" OR "carcinoma" OR "cancer" OR "tumor"). We also reviewed the reference lists of the included studies for undetected relevant studies.

2.2. Inclusion Criteria

The inclusion criteria were as follows: (1) a case-control or cohort study published as an original study; (2) the exposure of interest was calcium intake; (3) the outcome of interest was ovarian cancer; (4) relative risk (RR) with 95% confidence interval (CI) were available (or data could be calculated). (5) the most recent and complete study was selected if data from the same population had been published more than once.

All studies were carefully searched and reviewed independently by two investigators. If the two investigators disagreed about the eligibility of an article, it was resolved by consensus with a third reviewer.

2.3. Quality Assessment

The Newcastle-Ottawa quality assessment scale was used to assess the quality of the original studies. Quality of selection, comparability, and exposure or outcome of study participants are three major parameters. And a higher score represents better methodological quality.

2.4. Data Extraction

The following data were extracted from each study by two investigators independently: the first author, publication year, country in which the study was conducted, study design, follow-up duration, age range or mean age at baseline, sample size, number of cases, dietary assessment method, the most adjusted RR with 95% CI for the highest versus lowest category of the intake of calcium, and the covariates that were adjusted for in each study.

2.5. Statistical Analysis

Pooled measure was calculated as the inverse variance-weighted mean of the logarithm of RR with 95% CI to assess the strength of association between calcium intake and the risk of ovarian cancer.

The random effect model was used to combine study-specific RRs (95% CIs) [37]. The I^2 was adopted to assess the heterogeneity between studies (I^2 values of 0%, 25%, 50% and 75% represented no, low, moderate and high heterogeneity, respectively) [38]. Meta-regression was performed to assess the potentially important covariates that might exert substantial impacts on between-study heterogeneity. We also conducted subgroup analyses stratified by study design, continent, whether the study adopted validated food frequency questionnaires (FFQs) as the exposure assessment method, and whether the results were adjusted for covariates of parity and tubal ligation. Influence analysis was performed with one study removed at a time to assess whether the results could have been affected markedly by a single study [39]. In the cumulative meta-analysis, studies were added one at a time according to the published year, and the results were summarized sequentially. Small-study effect was assessed with visual inspection of the funnel plot and Egger's test [40].

All statistical analyses were performed with STATA version 12.0 (Stata Corporation, College Station, TX, USA). All reported probabilities (*p*-values) were two-sided with $p \leq 0.05$ considered statistically significant.

3. Results

3.1. Literature Search and Study Characteristics

Initially, 3395 articles from Pubmed, 7486 from Web of Science and 5142 from Embase were identified. Two additional articles were also found from reference lists. After reviewing the titles and abstracts, 162 articles about the association of calcium intake with risk of ovarian cancer were identified. After reviewing the full texts, 148 articles were subsequently excluded: two were from the same population; three were systematic review; five were about the risk of ovarian cancer mortality and 138 did not provide RR concerning the association between calcium intake and the risk of ovarian cancer. Finally, a total of 14 published articles [23–27,29–35,41,42], including 15 studies were eligible for this meta-analysis. The detailed steps of our literature search are shown in Figure 1.

Among these included studies, 13 studies evaluated the relationship between dietary calcium and risk of ovarian cancer [24–27,29–35,42]. Seven studies evaluated the relationship between dietary plus supplemental calcium and risk of ovarian cancer [23,25,27,30,35,41,42]. Four studies evaluated the relationship between dairy calcium and risk of ovarian cancer [26,29,32]. With regard to the location, 11 studies were conducted in North America [23,25,27,29,30,32,34,35,41,42] and four studies in Europe [24,26,31,33]. As for study design, eight studies were case-control studies [24,26,27,30–34], and seven were cohort studies [23,25,29,35,41,42]. 11 studies used validated food frequency questionnaires (FFQs) for the assessment of calcium intake [23,25,27,29–32,34,35,42]. The basic characteristics of the included studies for calcium intake with risk of ovarian cancer are shown in Table 1. The quality assessment showed that the Newcastle-Ottawa score of each study was not less than 7, indicating that the methodological quality was generally good. The quality assessment result is showed in Supplementary Material Table S1.

3.2. Quantitative Synthesis

The main results are summarized in Table 2.

3.2.1. Dietary Calcium and the Risk of Ovarian Cancer

A total of 13 studies, with eight case-control studies and five cohort studies were included, involving 367,057 participants and 7034 cases. Four studies revealed a significant association between dietary calcium intake and the risk of ovarian cancer, while the other nine studies found no association. For the highest vs. lowest category of dietary calcium intake, the pooled RR of ovarian cancer was 0.80 (95% CI 0.72–0.89, $I^2 = 32.8\%$, $P_{\text{heterogeneity}} = 0.120$, Figure 2). In further analysis by ovarian cancer subtypes, dietary calcium intake was also significantly associated with a reduced risk of EOC (RR = 0.78, 95% CI: 0.69–0.88).

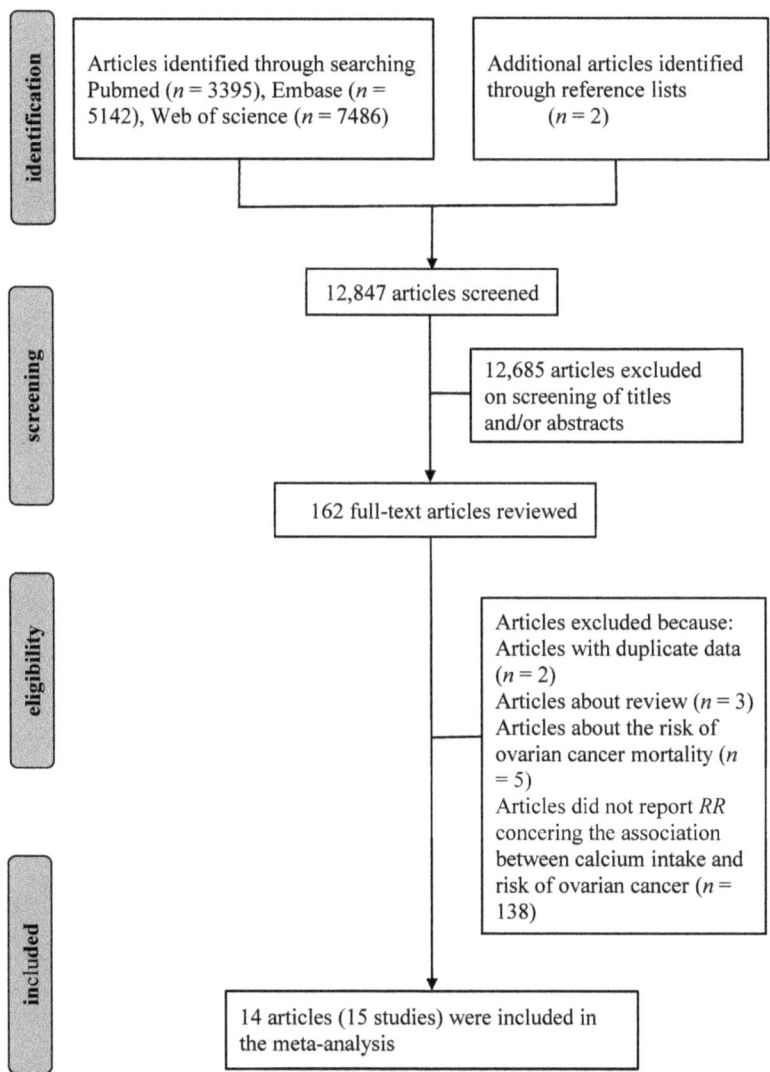

Figure 1. Flowchart of the selection of studies included in the meta-analysis.

Table 1. Characteristics of the studies included on the intake of calcium and the risk of ovarian cancer.

Author [Ref.]	Year	Country	Age Range/Mean Age (Case/Control)	Follow Years (Median)	Study Design	Dietary Assessment	Sample Size (Case)	Range of Calcium (Highest/Lowest) (mg/Day)	Exposure	Outcome	RR (95% CI)	Adjustment for Covariates
Goodman, M.T. [32]	2002	US	54.8	NA	CC	Validated FFQ	1165 (558)	Highest: >1107.9 Lowest: <528.1	Dietary calcium	EOC	0.46 (0.27, 0.76)	Age, ethnicity, study center, education, energy intake, parity, oral contraceptive use, tubal ligation
								Highest: >631.4 Lowest: <182.9	Dairy calcium	EOC	0.55 (0.36, 0.84)	
Merritt, M.A. [29]	2014	US	25–55	28	Cohort	Validated FFQ	76243 (609)	Highest: >1018 Lowest: <433	Dairy calcium	EOC	0.80 (0.59, 1.09)	Total caloric intake, menopausal status, number of pregnancies and parity, oral contraceptive use, tubal ligation and family history of ovarian cancer
Merritt, M.A. [29]	2014	US	25–55	28	Cohort	Validated FFQ	88356 (155)	Highest: >675.4 Lowest: <277.7	Dairy calcium	EOC	0.86 (0.68, 1.10)	
Merritt, M.A. [27]	2013	US	52.5/52.4	NA	CC	Validated FFQ	3898 (1909)	Highest: >859.3 Lowest: <543.7	Dietary calcium	EOC	0.74 (0.62, 0.89)	Age, number of pregnancies, oral contraceptive use, tubal ligation, family history of ovarian cancer in a first degree relative, study center, study phase and total calories
								Highest: >1318.8 Lowest: <654.9	Total calcium	EOC	0.62 (0.49, 0.79)	Age, number of pregnancies, oral contraceptive use, tubal ligation, family history of ovarian cancer in a first degree relative, study center, study phase, total calories, total vitamin D and lactose
Qin, B. [30]	2016	US	57.3/54.9	NA	CC	Validated FFQ	1146 (490)	Highest: >819.6 Lowest: <362.4	Dietary calcium	EOC	0.52 (0.28, 0.98)	Age, region, and total energy intake, education, parity, oral contraceptive use, menopausal status, tubal ligation, family history of breast/ovarian cancer, daylight hours spent outdoors in summer months, pigmentation, recreational physical activity, BMI, other sugar intake excluding lactose, plus quartiles of total vitamin D, and lactose, supplemental intake of calcium
								Highest: >1233.7 Lowest: <478.6	Total calcium	EOC	0.51 (0.30, 0.86)	Age, region, and total energy intake, education, parity, oral contraceptive use, menopausal status, tubal ligation, family history of breast/ovarian cancer, daylight hours spent outdoors in summer months, pigmentation, recreational physical activity, BMI, other sugar intake excluding lactose, plus quartiles of total vitamin D, and lactose
Tzonou, A. [33]	1993	Greece	<75	NA	CC	FFQ	389 (189)	Highest: >1500 Lowest: <500	Dietary calcium	EOC	0.93 (0.38, 2.29)	Total calories

Table 1. *Cont.*

Author [Ref.]	Year	Country	Age Range/Mean Age (Case/Control)	Follow Years (Median)	Study Design	Dietary Assessment	Sample Size (Case)	Range of Calcium (Highest/Lowest) (mg/Day)	Exposure	Outcome	RR (95% CI)	Adjustment for Covariates
Chang, E.T. [23]	2007	US	50	8.1	Cohort	Validated FFQ	97275 (280)	Highest: >1127 Lowest: <461	Total calcium	EOC	0.90 (0.57, 1.43)	Race, total energy intake, parity, oral contraceptive use, strenuous exercise, wine consumption, and menopausal status/hormone therapy use; use of dietary supplements, excluded short-term supplement users
Bidoli, E. [31]	2001	Italy	56/57	NA	CC	Validated FFQ	3442 (1031)	NA	Dietary calcium	EOC	0.70 (0.60, 1.00)	Age, study center, year of interview, education, BMI, parity, oral contraceptive use, occupational physical activity, and energy intake
Salazar, M.E. [34]	2002	Mexico	53/54	NA	CC	Validated FFQ	713 (84)	Highest: ≥1205 Lowest: <800	Dietary calcium	EOC	0.59 (0.32, 1.10)	Age, total energy intake, number of live births, recent changes in weight, physical activity and diabetes
Kushi, L.H. [41]	1999	US	55-69	10	Cohort	FFQ	29083 (139)	Highest: >1372 Lowest: <731	Total calcium	EOC	1.66 (0.96, 2.88)	Age, total energy intake, number of live births, age at menopause, family history of ovarian cancer in a first-degree relative, hysterectomy/unilateral oophorectomy status, waist-to-hip ratio, level of physical activity, cigarette smoking, and educational level
Fairfield, K.M. [42]	2004	US	30-55	16	Cohort	Validated FFQ	80326 (301)	NA	Dietary calcium	OC	0.85 (0.36, 2.00)	Age, BMI, caffeine intake, duration of oral contraceptive use, parity, tubal ligation and smoking, energy
								NA	Total calcium	OC	1.47 (0.88, 2.47)	
Koralek, D.O. [35]	2006	US	61	NA	Cohort	Validated FFQ	31925 (146)	NA	Dietary calcium	OC	0.67 (0.43, 1.04)	Age, menopause type, parity, oral contraceptive use, and postmenopausal hormone use at baseline, energy
								NA	Total calcium	OC	0.65 (0.36, 1.16)	Total vitamin D, lactose, age, menopause type, parity, age at menarche, oral contraceptive use, and postmenopausal hormone use at baseline, energy
Chiaffarino, F. [24]	2007	Italy	56/57	NA	CC	FFQ	2904 (493)	NA	Dietary calcium	EOC	0.90 (0.89, 1.10)	Age, study center, year of interview, education, parity, oral contraceptive use, family history of ovarian and/or breast cancer in first degree relatives and energy intake

Table 1. *Cont.*

Author [Ref.]	Year	Country	Age Range/Mean Age (Case/Control)	Follow Years (Median)	Study Design	Dietary Assessment	Sample Size (Case)	Range of Calcium (Highest/Lowest) (mg/Day)	Exposure	Outcome	RR (95% CI)	Adjustment for Covariates
Faber, M.T. [26]	2012	Denmark	58.9/57.1	NA	CC	FFQ	2208 (554)	Highest: ≥1200 Lowest: <400	Dairy calcium	EOC	1.00 (0.68, 1.48)	Age, pregnancy, number of pregnancies, oral contraceptive use, duration of oral contraceptive use, hormone replacement therapy use, and family history of breast and/or ovarian cancer, lactose intake
								Highest: >1101 Lowest: <409	Dietary calcium	OC	1.02 (0.75, 1.37)	Energy, race/ethnicity, education, marital status, BMI, family history of cancer, vigorous physical activity, menopausal hormone therapy use, alcohol consumption, and intakes of red meat and total energy smoking, parity, oral contraceptive use, and duration of hormone replacement use, supplement calcium, and additional variables race/ethnicity, education, marital status, BMI, family history of cancer, vigorous physical activity
Park, Y. [25]	2009	US	50–71	7	Cohort	Validated FFQ	74342 (515)	Highest: >1881 Lowest: <494	Total calcium	OC	1.14 (0.85, 1.52)	Race/ethnicity, education, marital status, BMI, family history of cancer, vigorous physical activity, menopausal hormone therapy use, alcohol consumption, and intakes of red meat and total energy smoking, parity, oral contraceptive use, and duration of hormone replacement use, and additional variables race/ethnicity, education, marital status, BMI, family history of cancer, vigorous physical activity

Abbreviations: RR, relative risk; CI, confidence interval; US, United States; Total calcium, dietary plus supplemental calcium; CC, case-control study; Cohort, cohort study; EOC, epithelial ovarian cancer; OC, ovarian cancer; BMI, body mass index; FFQ, food frequency questionnaire; NA, not available.

Table 2. Summary risk estimates of the association between the intake of calcium and the risk of ovarian cancer.

Exposure	Outcome	Subgroup	No. of Studies	Pooled RR (95% CI)	I^2 (%)	$P_{\text{heterogeneity}}$
Dietary calcium	OC	All studies	13	0.80 (0.72, 0.89)	32.8	0.12
		Cohort	5	0.86 (0.74, 0.99)	0	0.614
		Case-control	8	0.75 (0.64, 0.89)	53.3	0.036
		North America	9	0.76 (0.66, 0.87)	26.4	0.209
		Europe	4	0.86 (0.75, 0.99)	18.9	0.296
		Validated FFQ	10	0.75 (0.67, 0.85)	20.5	0.254
		FFQ	3	0.91 (0.82, 1.00)	0	0.875
		Adjustment for parity				
		Yes	9	0.79 (0.69, 0.91)	42.5	0.084
		No	4	0.77 (0.66, 0.90)	0	0.424
		Adjustment for tubal ligation				
		Yes	6	0.74 (0.64, 0.86)	20.1	0.282
		No	7	0.85 (0.75, 0.97)	21.7	0.264
Dietary calcium	EOC	All studies	10	0.78 (0.69, 0.88)	40.5	0.087
Total calcium	OC	All studies	7	0.90 (0.65, 1.24)	76.1	0.000
Dairy calcium	OC	All studies	4	0.80 (0.66, 0.98)	34.5	0.205

Abbreviations: RR, relative risk; CI, confidence interval; Total calcium, dietary plus supplemental calcium; EOC, epithelial ovarian cancer; OC, ovarian cancer.

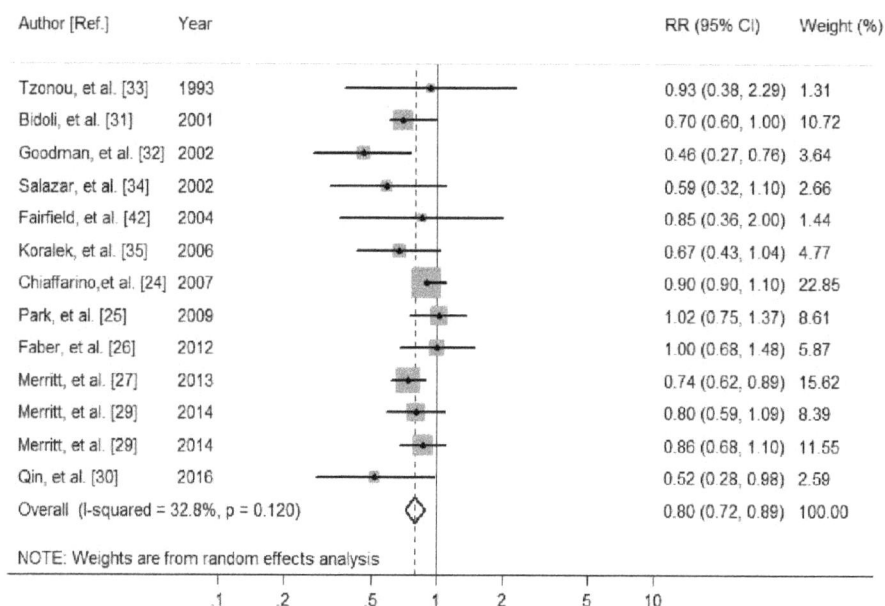

Author [Ref.]	Year		RR (95% CI)	Weight (%)
Tzonou, et al. [33]	1993		0.93 (0.38, 2.29)	1.31
Bidoli, et al. [31]	2001		0.70 (0.60, 1.00)	10.72
Goodman, et al. [32]	2002		0.46 (0.27, 0.76)	3.64
Salazar, et al. [34]	2002		0.59 (0.32, 1.10)	2.66
Fairfield, et al. [42]	2004		0.85 (0.36, 2.00)	1.44
Koralek, et al. [35]	2006		0.67 (0.43, 1.04)	4.77
Chiaffarino,et al. [24]	2007		0.90 (0.90, 1.10)	22.85
Park, et al. [25]	2009		1.02 (0.75, 1.37)	8.61
Faber, et al. [26]	2012		1.00 (0.68, 1.48)	5.87
Merritt, et al. [27]	2013		0.74 (0.62, 0.89)	15.62
Merritt, et al. [29]	2014		0.80 (0.59, 1.09)	8.39
Merritt, et al. [29]	2014		0.86 (0.68, 1.10)	11.55
Qin, et al. [30]	2016		0.52 (0.28, 0.98)	2.59
Overall (I-squared = 32.8%, p = 0.120)			0.80 (0.72, 0.89)	100.00

NOTE: Weights are from random effects analysis

Figure 2. Meta-analysis of the association between dietary calcium intake and ovarian cancer risk. The size of the gray box is positively proportional to the weight assigned to each study, which is inversely proportional to the standard error of the relative risks, and horizontal lines represent the 95% confidence intervals.

In subgroup analysis stratified by continent in which the studies were conducted, dietary calcium was significantly associated with decreased ovarian cancer risk among studies conducted in North America (*RR* = 0.76, 95% CI 0.66–0.87) and Europe (RR = 0.86, 95% CI 0.75–0.99). When stratified by study design subtype, a statistically significant effect of dietary calcium on ovarian cancer risk was observed both among case-control studies (RR = 0.75, 95% CI 0.64–0.89) and cohort studies (RR = 0.86, 95% CI 0.74–0.99). For subgroup analysis stratified by dietary assessment method, the inverse association was also statistically significant in validated FFQs group (RR = 0.75, 95% CI 0.67–0.85) and in no-validated FFQs group (RR = 0.91, 95% CI 0.82–1.00). The remaining results of subgroup analyses are shown in Table 2.

3.2.2. Dietary Plus Supplemental Calcium Intake and the Risk of Ovarian Cancer

For dietary plus supplemental calcium intake, seven studies (two case-control studies and five cohort studies) involving 317,995 participants and 3780 cases were included. Two studies revealed a significant association between dietary plus supplemental calcium intake and the risk of ovarian cancer, while the other five studies found no association. The pooled RR of ovarian cancer was 0.90 (95% CI 0.65–1.24, I^2 = 76.1%, $P_{heterogeneity}$ = 0.0001, Supplementary Material Figure S1) for the highest vs. lowest category of dietary plus supplemental calcium intake.

3.2.3. Dairy Calcium Intake and the Risk of Ovarian Cancer

For dairy calcium intake, four studies (two case-control studies and two cohort studies) involving 155,859 participants and 2330 cases were included, and the pooled RR of ovarian cancer was 0.80 (95% CI 0.66–0.98, I^2 = 34.5%, $P_{heterogeneity}$ = 0.205, Supplementary Material Figure S2) for the highest vs. lowest category of dairy calcium intake.

3.3. Cumulative Meta-Analysis

Cumulative meta-analysis for the association between dietary calcium and the risk of ovarian cancer was conducted to indicate the dynamic trend of results and assess the influence of an individual study on the overall results (Figure 3). The results indicated that there was not an association between dietary calcium and the risk of ovarian cancer until adding the study conducted in 2001 [31] (cumulative RR: 0.71 (95% CI: 0.56–0.91)). Since 2012, the significant association remained stable thereafter (cumulative RR: 0.80 (95% CI: 0.69–0.94)).

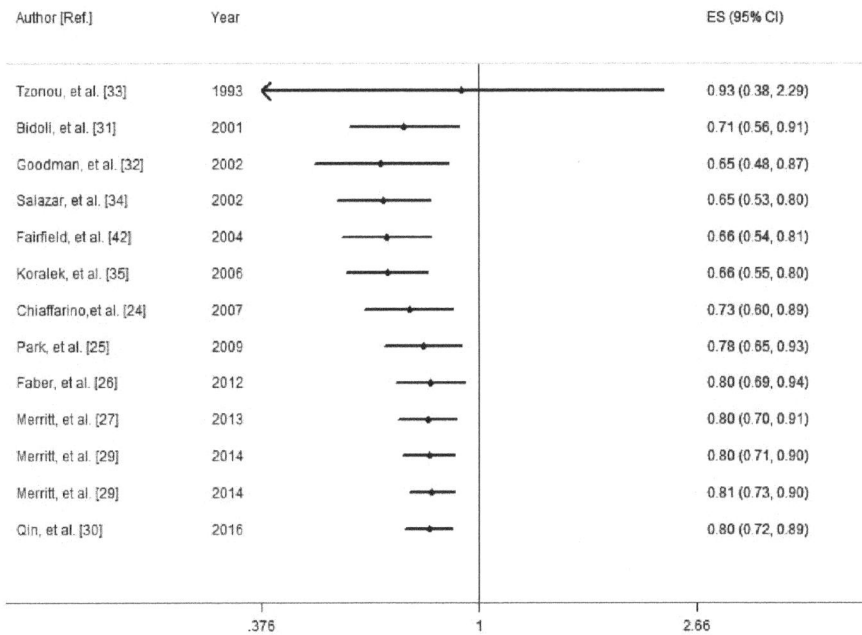

Author [Ref.]	Year		ES (95% CI)
Tzonou, et al. [33]	1993		0.93 (0.38, 2.29)
Bidoli, et al. [31]	2001		0.71 (0.56, 0.91)
Goodman, et al. [32]	2002		0.65 (0.48, 0.87)
Salazar, et al. [34]	2002		0.65 (0.53, 0.80)
Fairfield, et al. [42]	2004		0.66 (0.54, 0.81)
Koralek, et al. [35]	2006		0.66 (0.55, 0.80)
Chiaffarino, et al. [24]	2007		0.73 (0.60, 0.89)
Park, et al. [25]	2009		0.78 (0.65, 0.93)
Faber, et al. [26]	2012		0.80 (0.69, 0.94)
Merritt, et al. [27]	2013		0.80 (0.70, 0.91)
Merritt, et al. [29]	2014		0.80 (0.71, 0.90)
Merritt, et al. [29]	2014		0.81 (0.73, 0.90)
Qin, et al. [30]	2016		0.80 (0.72, 0.89)

.376   1   2.66

Figure 3. Cumulative meta-analysis of the association between dietary calcium intake and ovarian cancer risk. Open circle indicates the pooled relative risks, horizontal line represents the 95% confidence intervals.

3.4. Meta-Regression and Influence Analysis

Univariate meta-regression with covariates was conducted to explore the source of heterogeneity. In analysis of dietary calcium with risk of ovarian cancer, we performed univariate meta-regression with the covariates of sample size ($p = 0.162$), continent ($p = 0.296$), study design ($p = 0.394$), whether adjusted for energy intake ($p = 0.319$), parity ($p = 0.584$), oral contraceptive use ($p = 0.896$), tubal ligation ($p = 0.196$) and dietary assessment method for calcium intake ($p = 0.033$). The results showed that the dietary assessment method contributed to the between-study heterogeneity.

In analysis of dietary plus supplemental calcium with risk of ovarian cancer, we performed univariate meta-regression with the covariates of sample size ($p = 0.150$), study design ($p = 0.029$), dietary assessment method ($p = 0.190$) and whether adjusted for parity ($p = 0.874$), oral contraceptive use ($p = 0.190$) and tubal ligation ($p = 0.401$). The results showed that the study design contributed to the between-study heterogeneity.

In an influence analysis excluding one study at a time, no individual study had an excessive influence on the above-mentioned pooled effects (Supplementary Material Figures S3 and S4).

3.5. Small-Study Effect Evaluation

Egger's test showed no evidence of a significant small-study effect for the analyses between the consumption of dietary calcium ($p = 0.095$), dietary plus supplemental calcium ($p = 0.501$) and the risk of ovarian cancer. The funnel plot of the analysis of dietary calcium and the risk of ovarian cancer is shown in the Figure 4.

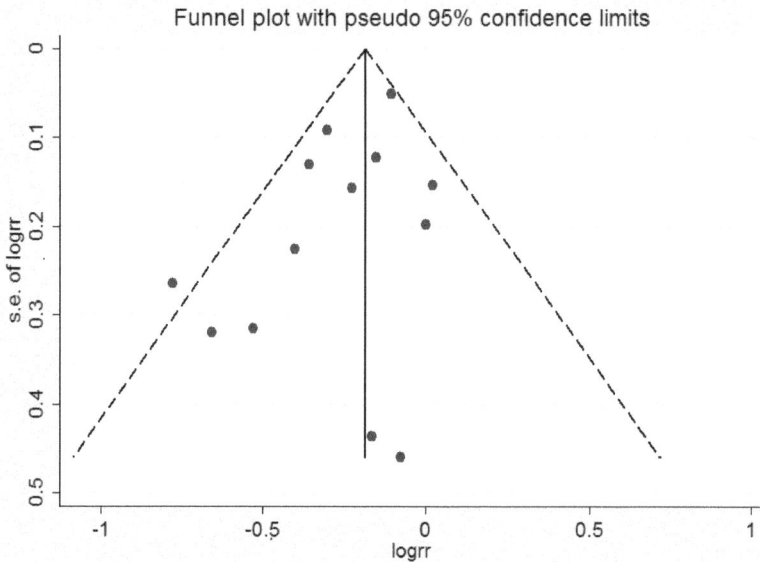

Figure 4. Funnel plot for the analysis of dietary calcium intake and ovarian cancer risk. Each dot represents a different study.

4. Discussion

This meta-analysis evaluated associations between the intake of dietary calcium, dietary plus supplemental calcium and dairy calcium and the risk of ovarian cancer, respectively. A total of 15 studies with 493,415 participants and 7453 cases were included. The results indicated that there were inverse associations between the intake of dietary calcium, dairy calcium and the risk of ovarian cancer, respectively. In subgroup analyses, there was a significant inverse association between dietary calcium and the risk of ovarian cancer for studies carried out in North America and Europe. The association was also significant among results in cohort studies and case-control studies. In cumulative meta-analysis, the above-mentioned significant association was first observed after adding one study in 2001, and the result tended to be stable since 2012. However, a pooled analysis of 12 cohort studies in 2006 indicated that intake of dairy calcium was not associated with ovarian cancer risk. In contrast to our study, such inconsistencies may be due in part to the different sources of calcium intake. The sources of dietary calcium are not only dairy products but also other sources including shrimp, broccoli, leafy green vegetables, etc. In addition, the absorption of calcium from the dairy and other diet is affected by different factors. The association of dietary plus supplemental calcium with ovarian cancer risk was not statistically significant. Presumably, the dose of dietary plus supplemental calcium was relatively high and different in the control group across studies, which could influence the effect of the result. Moreover, the number of studies for dietary plus supplemental calcium was relatively small and this could also affect the final result.

The relatively insufficient sample size and dietary measurement error of individual study could be likely to contribute to the inconsistency, thus we conducted the present meta-analysis to increase the sample size and improve the study power. In addition, considering the recall and select bias of case-control study, we conducted subgroup analysis stratified by the study design, but the results were not substantially affected.

The exact biological mechanisms underlying calcium intake and risk of ovarian cancer are still not completely determined. One underlying explanation for our findings is that a higher level of calcium might be inversely related to ovarian cancer risk via down-regulation of circulating parathyroid hormone (PTH) [21,22]. The reduction of PTH could decrease hepatic and osteoblastic synthesis of insulin-like growth factor-1 (IGF-1) [22,43]. IGF-1 may exert a direct effect by increasing cell proliferation and inhibition of apoptosis [44], and experimental studies have indeed shown that malignant transformation of ovarian epithelial cells (the cells from which ovarian cancer is believed to originate) can be induced by overexpression of the IGF-1 receptor [45]. These mitogenic and anti-apoptotic effects of IGF-I might be particularly relevant during ovulation related tissue remodeling of the surface epithelium [46]. The reduction of IGF-1 would weaken mitogenic effects on the pathogenesis of ovarian cancer [47,48]. In addition, PTH may be a tumour promoter acting as a co-mitogen and anti-apoptotic factor directly [22,49].

Between-study heterogeneity is common in meta-analysis [50], and it is essential to explore the potential sources of between-study heterogeneity. Diversity in population stratification, measurement of calcium intake and variation of the covariates might be the source of between-study heterogeneity. High between-study heterogeneity was found in the analysis of dietary plus supplemental calcium and risk of ovarian cancer. In meta-regression, we found that the study design contributed to between-study heterogeneity. In subgroup analysis by study design, the heterogeneity decreased to 44.8% ($P_{heterogeneity} = 0.124$) for cohort studies and 0% ($P_{heterogeneity} = 0.508$) for case-control studies, respectively. Additionally, low between-study heterogeneity was found in the analysis of dietary calcium and risk of ovarian cancer. In meta-regression, we found that the dietary assessment method was the contributor to between-study heterogeneity. In subgroup analysis by studies adjusted for dietary assessment method or not, the heterogeneity decreased to 20.5% ($P_{heterogeneity} = 0.254$) and 0% ($P_{heterogeneity} = 0.875$), respectively. The results were also consistent with the overall pooled RR, indicating that our results were stable and reliable.

There are several strengths in present meta-analysis. First of all, this study included a large number of participants and cases, allowing a much great possibility of reaching reasonable conclusions. Second, most of the studies had adjusted for potential confounders, such as age, energy and oral contraceptives, strengthening the credibility of the results. Third, most of the included studies used validated FFQs, ensuring the accuracy of dietary assessment. Fourth, a statistically significant inverse association between dietary calcium and ovarian cancer risk was found in cohort studies, indicating a potential causal relationship between them. Fifth, in cumulative meta-analysis by publication year, the significant result persisted and the CI became increasingly narrower.

However, several limitations of the study should also be considered. First, potential confounders adjusted for in each study were different and it might affect the results to some extent. For example, parity and tubal ligation were adjusted for in some studies, while they not adjusted for in other studies. In addition, residual confounding should be of concern. Second, most studies just used a complete dietary assessment, and it could not reflect change in diet for a long time. Third, the standards of lowest calcium intake were inconsistent among studies, which might influence the result. Fourth, case-control studies, which are prone to recall and select biases, were included in our meta-analysis, and the results would be partly affected. Fifth, the number of included studies for dairy calcium was too small (only four studies). Although the result of dairy calcium with risk of ovarian cancer was statistically significant, it was different from the result reported by Genkinger et al. in 2006 [28]. Sixth, we were unable to explore the dose–response relationship between the intake of calcium and the risk of ovarian cancer because of the limited data.

5. Conclusions

In summary, this meta-analysis revealed that dietary calcium and dairy calcium, but not dietary plus supplemental calcium, may reduce the risk of ovarian cancer. Increasing intake of dietary calcium should be advocated for the primary prevention of ovarian cancer. Better designed prospective cohort studies are needed to explore the association between calcium intake and ovarian cancer risk.

Supplementary Materials: The following are available online at www.mdpi.com/2072-6643/9/7/679/s1, Table S1: Quality assessment of studies included in the meta-analysis, Figure S1: Meta-analysis of the association between dietary plus supplemental calcium intake and ovarian cancer risk, Figure S2: Meta-analysis of the association between dairy calcium intake and ovarian cancer risk. Figure S3: Influence analysis of an individual study on the pooled estimate for studies on the association between dietary calcium intake and ovarian cancer risk, Figure S4: Influence analysis of an individual study on the pooled estimate for studies on the association between dietary plus supplemental calcium intake and ovarian cancer risk.

Author Contributions: Xingxing Song designed the research, collected the data, carried out the statistical analysis and drafted the manuscript. Zongyao Li and Xinqiang Ji collected the data and carried out the statistical analysis. Dongfeng Zhang designed the research, drafted the manuscript and made critical revision of the manuscript. All authors reviewed and approved the manuscript.

Conflicts of Interest: The authors declare no conflict of interest.

Abbreviations

RR	relative risk
CI	confidence interval
REM	random effect model
EOC	epithelial ovarian cancer
FFQs	food frequency questionnaires
PTH	parathyroid hormone
IGF-1	insulin-like growth factor-1
US	United States

References

1. Davidson, B.; Trope, C.G. Ovarian cancer: Diagnostic, biological and prognostic aspects. *Womens Health (Lond.)* **2014**, *10*, 519–533. [CrossRef] [PubMed]
2. Hankinson, S.E.; Danforth, K.N. Ovarian cancer. In *Cancer Epidemiology and Prevention*, 3rd ed.; Schottenfeld, D., Fraumeni, J., Eds.; Oxford University Press: New York, NY, USA, 2006; pp. 1013–1026.
3. Jemal, A.; Bray, F.; Center, M.M.; Ferlay, J.; Ward, E.; Forman, D. Global cancer statistics. *CA Cancer J. Clin.* **2011**, *61*, 69–90. [CrossRef] [PubMed]
4. Siegel, R.L.; Miller, K.D.; Jemal, A. Cancer statistics, 2016. *CA Cancer J. Clin.* **2016**, *66*, 7–30. [CrossRef] [PubMed]
5. Holschneider, C.H.; Berek, J.S. Ovarian cancer: Epidemiology, biology, and prognostic factors. *Semin. Surg. Oncol.* **2000**, *19*, 3–10. [CrossRef]
6. Webb, P.M.; Purdie, D.M.; Grover, S.; Jordan, S.; Dick, M.L.; Green, A.C. Symptoms and diagnosis of borderline, early and advanced epithelial ovarian cancer. *Gynecol. Oncol.* **2004**, *92*, 232–239. [CrossRef] [PubMed]
7. Goff, B.A.; Mandel, L.; Muntz, H.G.; Melancon, C.H. Ovarian carcinoma diagnosis. *Cancer* **2000**, *89*, 2068–2075. [CrossRef]
8. Pu, D.; Jiang, S.W.; Wu, J. Association between MTHFR gene polymorphism and the risk of ovarian cancer: A meta-analysis of the literature. *Curr. Pharm. Des.* **2014**, *20*, 1632–1638. [CrossRef] [PubMed]
9. Aune, D.; Navarro Rosenblatt, D.A.; Chan, D.S.; Abar, L.; Vingeliene, S.; Vieira, A.R.; Greenwood, D.C.; Norat, T. Anthropometric factors and ovarian cancer risk: A systematic review and nonlinear dose-response meta-analysis of prospective studies. *Int. J. Cancer* **2015**, *136*, 1888–1898. [CrossRef] [PubMed]
10. Poole, E.M.; Merritt, M.A.; Jordan, S.J.; Yang, H.P.; Hankinson, S.E.; Park, Y.; Rosner, B.; Webb, P.M.; Cramer, D.W.; Wentzensen, N.; et al. Hormonal and reproductive risk factors for epithelial ovarian cancer by tumor aggressiveness. *Cancer Epidemiol. Biomark. Prev.* **2013**, *22*, 429–437. [CrossRef] [PubMed]
11. Crane, T.E.; Khulpateea, B.R.; Alberts, D.S.; Basen-Engquist, K.; Thomson, C.A. Dietary intake and ovarian cancer risk: A systematic review. *Cancer Epidemiol. Biomark. Prev.* **2014**, *23*, 255–273. [CrossRef] [PubMed]

12. Larsson, S.C.; Orsini, N.; Wolk, A. Milk, milk products and lactose intake and ovarian cancer risk: A meta-analysis of epidemiological studies. *Int. J. Cancer* **2006**, *118*, 431–441. [CrossRef] [PubMed]

13. Zeng, S.T.; Guo, L.; Liu, S.K.; Wang, D.H.; Xi, J.; Huang, P.; Liu, D.T.; Gao, J.F.; Feng, J.; Zhang, L. Egg consumption is associated with increased risk of ovarian cancer: Evidence from a meta-analysis of observational studies. *Clin. Nutr.* **2015**, *34*, 635–641. [CrossRef] [PubMed]

14. Kolahdooz, F.; van der Pols, J.C.; Bain, C.J.; Marks, G.C.; Hughes, M.C.; Whiteman, D.C.; Webb, P.M. Meat, fish, and ovarian cancer risk: Results from 2 Australian case-control studies, a systematic review, and meta-analysis. *Am. J. Clin. Nutr.* **2010**, *91*, 1752–1763. [CrossRef] [PubMed]

15. Myung, S.K.; Ju, W.; Choi, H.J.; Kim, S.C. Soy intake and risk of endocrine-related gynaecological cancer: A meta-analysis. *BJOG* **2009**, *116*, 1697–1705. [CrossRef] [PubMed]

16. Hu, J.; Hu, Y.; Hu, Y.; Zheng, S. Intake of cruciferous vegetables is associated with reduced risk of ovarian cancer: A meta-analysis. *Asia Pac. J. Clin. Nutr.* **2015**, *24*, 101–109. [PubMed]

17. Asemi, Z.; Saneei, P.; Sabihi, S.S.; Feizi, A.; Esmaillzadeh, A. Total, dietary, and supplemental calcium intake and mortality from all-causes, cardiovascular disease, and cancer: A meta-analysis of observational studies. *Nutr. Metab. Cardiovasc. Dis.* **2015**, *25*, 623–634. [CrossRef] [PubMed]

18. Larsson, S.C.; Orsini, N.; Wolk, A. Dietary calcium intake and risk of stroke: A dose-response meta-analysis. *Am. J. Clin. Nutr.* **2013**, *97*, 951–957. [CrossRef] [PubMed]

19. Hong, Z.; Tian, C.; Zhang, X. Dietary calcium intake, vitamin D levels, and breast cancer risk: A dose-response analysis of observational studies. *Breast Cancer Res. Treat.* **2012**, *136*, 309–312. [CrossRef] [PubMed]

20. Toriola, A.T.; Surcel, H.M.; Calypse, A.; Grankvist, K.; Luostarinen, T.; Lukanova, A.; Pukkala, E.; Lehtinen, M. Independent and joint effects of serum 25-hydroxyvitamin D and calcium on ovarian cancer risk: A prospective nested case-control study. *Eur. J. Cancer* **2010**, *46*, 2799–2805. [CrossRef] [PubMed]

21. Goodman, M.T.; Wu, A.H.; Tung, K.H.; McDuffie, K.; Cramer, D.W.; Wilkens, L.R.; Terada, K.; Reichardt, J.K.; Ng, W.G. Association of galactose-1-phosphate uridyltransferase activity and N314D genotype with the risk of ovarian cancer. *Am. J. Epidemiol.* **2002**, *156*, 693–701. [CrossRef] [PubMed]

22. McCarty, M.F. Parathyroid hormone may be a cancer promoter—An explanation for the decrease in cancer risk associated with ultraviolet light, calcium, and vitamin D. *Med. Hypotheses* **2000**, *54*, 475–482. [CrossRef] [PubMed]

23. Chang, E.T.; Lee, V.S.; Canchola, A.J.; Clarke, C.A.; Purdie, D.M.; Reynolds, P.; Anton-Culver, H.; Bernstein, L.; Deapen, D.; Peel, D.; et al. Diet and risk of ovarian cancer in the California Teachers Study cohort. *Am. J. Epidemiol.* **2007**, *165*, 802–813. [CrossRef] [PubMed]

24. Chiaffarino, F.; Parazzini, F.; Bosetti, C.; Franceschi, S.; Talamini, R.; Canzonieri, V.; Montella, M.; Ramazzotti, V.; Franceschi, S.; La Vecchia, C. Risk factors for ovarian cancer histotypes. *Eur. J. Cancer* **2007**, *43*, 1208–1213. [CrossRef] [PubMed]

25. Park, Y.; Leitzmann, M.F.; Subar, A.F.; Hollenbeck, A.; Schatzkin, A. Dairy food, calcium, and risk of cancer in the NIH-AARP Diet and Health Study. *Arch. Intern. Med.* **2009**, *169*, 391–401. [CrossRef] [PubMed]

26. Faber, M.T.; Jensen, A.; Sogaard, M.; Hogdall, E.; Hogdall, C.; Blaakaer, J.; Kjaer, S.K. Use of dairy products, lactose, and calcium and risk of ovarian cancer—Results from a Danish case-control study. *Acta Oncol.* **2012**, *51*, 454–464. [CrossRef] [PubMed]

27. Merritt, M.A.; Cramer, D.W.; Vitonis, A.F.; Titus, L.J.; Terry, K.L. Dairy foods and nutrients in relation to risk of ovarian cancer and major histological subtypes. *Int. J. Cancer* **2013**, *132*, 1114–1124. [CrossRef] [PubMed]

28. Genkinger, J.M.; Hunter, D.J.; Spiegelman, D.; Anderson, K.E.; Arslan, A.; Beeson, W.L.; Buring, J.E.; Fraser, G.E.; Freudenheim, J.L.; Goldbohm, R.A.; et al. Dairy products and ovarian cancer: A pooled analysis of 12 cohort studies. *Cancer Epidemiol. Biomark. Prev.* **2006**, *15*, 364–372. [CrossRef] [PubMed]

29. Merritt, M.A.; Poole, E.M.; Hankinson, S.E.; Willett, W.C.; Tworoger, S.S. Dairy food and nutrient intake in different life periods in relation to risk of ovarian cancer. *Cancer Causes Control* **2014**, *25*, 795–808. [CrossRef] [PubMed]

30. Qin, B.; Moorman, P.G.; Alberg, A.J.; Barnholtz-Sloan, J.S.; Bondy, M.; Cote, M.L.; Funkhouser, E.; Peters, E.S.; Schwartz, A.G.; Terry, P.; et al. Dairy, calcium, vitamin D and ovarian cancer risk in African-American women. *Br. J. Cancer* **2016**, *115*, 1122–1130. [CrossRef] [PubMed]

31. Bidoli, E.; La Vecchia, C.; Talamini, R.; Negri, E.; Parpinel, M.; Conti, E.; Montella, M.; Carbone, M.A.; Franceschi, S. Micronutrients and ovarian cancer: A case-control study in Italy. *Ann. Oncol.* **2001**, *12*, 1589–1593. [CrossRef]

32. Goodman, M.T.; Wu, A.H.; Tung, K.H.; McDuffie, K.; Kolonel, L.N.; Nomura, A.M.; Terada, K.; Wilkens, L.R.; Murphy, S.; Hankin, J.H. Association of dairy products, lactose, and calcium with the risk of ovarian cancer. *Am. J. Epidemiol.* **2002**, *156*, 148–157. [CrossRef] [PubMed]

33. Tzonou, A.; Hsieh, C.C.; Polychronopoulou, A.; Kaprinis, G.; Toupadaki, N.; Trichopoulou, A.; Karakatsani, A.; Trichopoulos, D. Diet and ovarian cancer: A case-control study in Greece. *Int. J. Cancer* **1993**, *55*, 411–414. [CrossRef] [PubMed]

34. Salazar-Martinez, E.; Lazcano-Ponce, E.C.; Gonzalez Lira-Lira, G.; Escudero-De los Rios, P.; Hernandez-Avila, M. Nutritional determinants of epithelial ovarian cancer risk: A case-control study in Mexico. *Oncology* **2002**, *63*, 151–157. [CrossRef] [PubMed]

35. Koralek, D.O.; Bertone-Johnson, E.R.; Leitzmann, M.F.; Sturgeon, S.R.; Lacey, J.V., Jr.; Schairer, C.; Schatzkin, A. Relationship between calcium, lactose, vitamin D, and dairy products and ovarian cancer. *Nutr. Cancer* **2006**, *56*, 22–30. [CrossRef] [PubMed]

36. Moher, D.; Shamseer, L.; Clarke, M.; Ghersi, D.; Liberati, A.; Petticrew, M.; Shekelle, P.; Stewart, L.A. Preferred reporting items for systematic review and meta-analysis protocols (PRISMA-P) 2015 statement. *Syst. Rev.* **2015**, *4*, 1. [CrossRef] [PubMed]

37. Higgins, J.P.; Thompson, S.G.; Deeks, J.J.; Altman, D.G. Measuring inconsistency in meta-analyses. *BMJ* **2003**, *327*, 557–560. [CrossRef] [PubMed]

38. Higgins, J.P.; Thompson, S.G. Quantifying heterogeneity in a meta-analysis. *Stat. Med.* **2002**, *21*, 1539–1558. [CrossRef] [PubMed]

39. Tobias, A. Assessing the influence of a single study in the meta-analysis estimate. *Stata Tech. Bull.* **1999**, *47*, 15–17.

40. Egger, M.; Davey Smith, G.; Schneider, M.; Minder, C. Bias in meta-analysis detected by a simple, graphical test. *BMJ* **1997**, *315*, 629–634. [CrossRef] [PubMed]

41. Kushi, L.H.; Mink, P.J.; Folsom, A.R.; Anderson, K.E.; Zheng, W.; Lazovich, D.; Sellers, T.A. Prospective study of diet and ovarian cancer. *Am. J. Epidemiol.* **1999**, *149*, 21–31. [CrossRef] [PubMed]

42. Broadus, A.E.; Mangin, M.; Ikeda, K.; Insogna, K.L.; Weir, E.C.; Burtis, W.J.; Stewart, A.F. Humoral hypercalcemia of cancer. Identification of a novel parathyroid hormone-like peptide. *N. Engl. J. Med.* **1988**, *319*, 556–563. [PubMed]

43. Coxam, V.; Davicco, M.J.; Durand, D.; Bauchart, D.; Lefaivre, J.; Barlet, J.P. The influence of parathyroid hormone-related protein on hepatic IGF-1 production. *Acta Endocrinol. (Copenh.)* **1992**, *126*, 430–433. [CrossRef] [PubMed]

44. Khandwala, H.M.; McCutcheon, I.E.; Flyvbjerg, A.; Friend, K.E. The effects of insulin-like growth factors on tumorigenesis and neoplastic growth. *Endocr. Rev.* **2000**, *21*, 215–244. [CrossRef] [PubMed]

45. Coppola, D.; Saunders, B.; Fu, L.; Mao, W.; Nicosia, S.V. The insulin-like growth factor 1 receptor induces transformation and tumorigenicity of ovarian mesothelial cells and down-regulates their Fas-receptor expression. *Cancer Res.* **1999**, *59*, 3264–3270. [PubMed]

46. Lund, P.K. Insulin-like growth factors: Gene structure and regulation. In *Hormonal Control of Growth*, 1st ed.; Kostyo, J.L., Goodman, H.M., Eds.; Oxford University Press: New York, NY, USA, 1999; pp. 537–571.

47. Lukanova, A.; Lundin, E.; Toniolo, P.; Micheli, A.; Akhmedkhanov, A.; Rinaldi, S.; Muti, P.; Lenner, P.; Biessy, C.; Krogh, V.; et al. Circulating levels of insulin-like growth factor-I and risk of ovarian cancer. *Int. J. Cancer* **2002**, *101*, 549–554. [CrossRef] [PubMed]

48. Renehan, A.G.; Zwahlen, M.; Minder, C.; O'Dwyer, S.T.; Shalet, S.M.; Egger, M. Insulin-like growth factor (IGF)-I, IGF binding protein-3, and cancer risk: Systematic review and meta-regression analysis. *Lancet* **2004**, *363*, 1346–1353. [CrossRef]

49. Ramasamy, I. Recent advances in physiological calcium homeostasis. *Clin. Chem. Lab. Med.* **2006**, *44*, 237–273. [CrossRef] [PubMed]

50. Munafo, M.R.; Flint, J. Meta-analysis of genetic association studies. *Trends Genet.* **2004**, *20*, 439–444. [CrossRef] [PubMed]

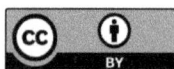

nutrients

MDPI

Review

Gene–Dairy Food Interactions and Health Outcomes: A Review of Nutrigenetic Studies

Kevin B. Comerford *and Gonca Pasin

California Dairy Research Foundation (CDRF), 501 G Street, Ste. 203, Davis, CA 95616, USA; pasin@cdrf.org
* Correspondence: kbcomerford@cdrf.org; Tel.: +1-530-753-0681

Received: 18 May 2017; Accepted: 3 July 2017; Published: 6 July 2017

Abstract: Each person differs from the next by an average of over 3 million genetic variations in their DNA. This genetic diversity is responsible for many of the interindividual differences in food preferences, nutritional needs, and dietary responses between humans. The field of nutrigenetics aims to utilize this type of genetic information in order to personalize diets for optimal health. One of the most well-studied genetic variants affecting human dietary patterns and health is the lactase persistence mutation, which enables an individual to digest milk sugar into adulthood. Lactase persistence is one of the most influential Mendelian factors affecting human dietary patterns to occur since the beginning of the Neolithic Revolution. However, the lactase persistence mutation is only one of many mutations that can influence the relationship between dairy intake and disease risk. The purpose of this review is to summarize the available nutrigenetic literature investigating the relationships between genetics, dairy intake, and health outcomes. Nonetheless, the understanding of an individual's nutrigenetic responses is just one component of personalized nutrition. In addition to nutrigenetic responses, future studies should also take into account nutrigenomic responses (epigenomic, transcriptomic, proteomic, metabolomic), and phenotypic/characteristic traits (age, gender, activity level, disease status, etc.), as these factors all interact with diet to influence health.

Keywords: nutrigenetics; gene–diet interactions; precision nutrition; polymorphisms; inter-individual response; dairy; milk; lactase persistence; obesity; cardiometabolic disease

1. Introduction

The fields of nutrigenetics and nutrigenomics both aim to elucidate how the genome interacts with nutrition to influence health. They differ in that nutrigenetics focuses on how gene variants influence responses to diet, while nutrigenomics focuses on how diet affects gene expression. The intended end goals of these sciences, which both fall under the umbrella of nutritional genomics, are to improve health through the application of personalized nutrition [1]. At present, most of the well-studied nutritional genomic relationships are nutrigenetic. More specifically, the most well-known examples can all be classified as monogenic relationships, consisting of the interactions between a single gene mutation and single dietary component. For example, a mutation in the gene coding for the enzyme phenylalanine hydroxylase leads to an inability to properly metabolize the amino acid phenylalanine, resulting in the life-threatening disease phenylketonuria (PKU) [2]. A mutation in the alcohol dehydrogenase gene leads to a reduced ability to process alcohol and has been associated with addiction [3]. Mutations in the 5,10-methylene tetrahydrofolate reductase (MTHFR) gene affect folate metabolism and are linked to increased risk for birth defects and chronic diseases including cardiovascular disease (CVD) and cancer [4]. Mutations in the lactase gene (LCT) can result in lactase persistence (LP), which is the extended ability to produce the lactase enzyme into adulthood. Lactase assists in the breakdown of milk sugar in the small intestine and is associated with a variety of complex health and disease outcomes in different populations [5,6].

The vast majority of genetic variants that have nutrigenetic consequences are loss of function mutations in which the ability to properly digest or metabolize dietary compounds are diminished. LP stands apart from the majority of monogenic mutations in that it is a gain of function mutation in which the ability to break down lactose into adulthood is gained. Nutrigenetic loss of function mutations tend to restrict or reduce dietary options, but LP does the opposite and increases the available number of dietary options that can be digested. This ability has resulted in LP becoming one of the strongest positive selective pressures in human history [7], reinforcing the importance of gene–dairy food interactions in relation to human reproductive success and survival [8].

LP polymorphisms have occurred independently in Northern Europe, Africa and the Middle East. This dominant trait provided these populations with the ability to greatly expand their cuisines and improve their access to energy, nutrients, and dietary sources of potable water [9,10]. LP gene variants have also dramatically influenced gene–culture co-evolution between humans and cattle through the practices of dairy herding, domestication, and farming [7,11]. Many of the implications of these interrelationships have yet to be discovered. While LP mutations have been advantageous for the survival of certain populations over the last several millennia, only recently have the scientific tools become available to investigate how the nutrigenetic relationships between gene variants and dairy intake affect human health. The purpose of this review is to summarize the available nutrigenetic literature investigating the relationships between genetics, dairy intake, and health outcomes in order to further explore the concept of personalized nutrition. The PubMed database was searched through the end of April 2017 for studies that examined the relationships between genetic variants, dairy intake, and health outcomes. We only included studies that reported at least one measure of dairy intake. Seventeen studies on LP polymorphisms and nine studies on metabolic and hormonal gene variants were included in the review and summarized in table form.

2. Lactase Persistence, Dairy Intake, and Health Outcomes

The LCT-13910 C > T single nucleotide polymorphism (SNP) at intron 13 is the most prevalent and most studied LP polymorphism. Traditionally, a person with two CC alleles is considered to be lactose intolerant, also known as lactase non-persistent (lactase activity <10 units/g protein) [12]. A majority of humans, especially those without Northern European ancestry, have the CC genotype. A person with one or more T alleles (CT or TT) is considered to be lactose tolerant, also known as lactase persistent (lactase activity ≥10 units/g protein). Recent evidence suggests that there is a stepwise relationship between the number of LP dominant T alleles a person inherits and their ability to digest lactose [13]. However, the LCT-13910 gene variant is not the only variant that can confer LP. Several mutations at different loci on the lactase gene (i.e., A-22018, C-14010, G-13907, and G-13915) result in an LP phenotype [14]. It is currently unclear as to if and how these different gene variants affect lactase form and function. Future research on how different LP variants, LP genotypes, and LP haplotypes interact with dairy intake patterns and health outcomes would contribute greatly to the basic understanding of gene–dairy interactions. However, at present, the available nutrigenetic research on LP, dairy intake, and health is still in the early stages and limited in its ability to inform personalized dietary advice (Table 1).

Table 1. Nutrigenetic studies on lactase persistence, dairy intake, and health outcomes in adults.

Reference	Study Design	Population	Variables	Outcomes
Obesity and Cardiometabolic Disease				
Lehtimäki et al., 2008. [15]	Observational, longitudinal—participants followed for an average of 21 years	2109 young and healthy adults from Finland	Milk and Dairy Intake, Carotid intima-media thickness, carotid artery compliance, brachial artery flow-mediated dilation	No significant association between LP and carotid intima-media thickness, carotid artery compliance or brachial artery flow-mediated dilation were found after adjustment for the use dairy products.
Almon et al., 2012. [16]	Meta-analysis, observational, cross-sectional	551 adults of European descent from the Canary Islands Nutrition Survey (ENCA) in Spain	Milk Intake, BMI, obesity	LP was associated with higher BMI, while lactase non-persistence was not after adjustment for milk intake.
Almon et al., 2010. [17]	Meta-analysis, observational, cross-sectional	551 adults of European descent from the Canary Islands Nutrition Survey (ENCA) in Spain	Milk Intake, Metabolic Syndrome risk markers	LP was associated with a higher odds ratio for metabolic syndrome than lactase non-persistence after adjustment for milk intake. This relationship was stronger for women than men.
Corella et al., 2011. [18]	Observational, cross-sectional	940 elderly Spanish adults with high risk for CVD	Milk and Dairy Intake, BMI, obesity	LP was associated with obesity risk. These associations were found to be significant only among those consuming moderate or high lactose intakes.
Lamri et al., 2013. [19]	Observational, longitudinal—participants followed for an average of 9 years	3575 Caucasians born in mainland France	Dairy Intake, Metabolic Syndrome risk markers	LP was associated with higher BMI mainly in those consuming high amounts of dairy products. LP was associated with higher risk for metabolic syndrome, but this association disappeared after adjustment for BMI.
Bergholdt et al., 2015. [20]	Observational, cross-sectional and longitudinal—participants followed for an average of 5.5 years	97,811 adults from the Danish general population	Milk Intake, Overweight, obesity, T2D risk	High milk intake was not associated with risk of T2D or overweight-obesity, observationally or genetically via LP.
Bergholdt et al., 2015. [21]	Observational, cross-sectional and longitudinal—participants followed for an average of 5.4 years	98,529 adults of Danish descent	Milk Intake, Ischemic heart disease, myocardial infarction	LP was not associated with plasma levels of total cholesterol, low-density lipoprotein cholesterol, high-density lipoprotein cholesterol, triglycerides or glucose, nor with blood pressure. Milk intake was not associated with risk of ischemic heart disease or myocardial infarction, observationally or genetically.
Hartwig et al., 2016. [22]	Meta-analysis, observational, longitudinal—participants followed for an average of 30 years	2843 adults from the 1982 Pelotas (Southern Brazil) Birth Cohort	Milk Intake, BMI, obesity, systolic and diastolic blood pressure	LP was associated with higher BMI and higher odds of overweight-obesity. Milk intake was not consistently associated with changes in blood pressure.
Smith et al., 2016. [23]	Meta-analysis, multiple study designs included	20,089 adults of American (Hispanics, African-Americans and Whites) and Mediterranean descent	Milk Intake, CVD biomarkers, mortality	Milk intake was not associated with CVD biomarkers, CVD or mortality either generally or in sub-groups. Lactase persistence was inconsistently associated with glucose and lipids, and not associated with CVD or total mortality in the whole population. LP was associated with higher CVD and mortality risk in women but not in men.

Table 1. *Cont.*

Reference	Study Design	Population	Variables	Outcomes
Ding et al., 2017. [24]	Meta-analysis, multiple study designs included	197,322 adults from Europe, the US, and Australia	Dairy Intake Systolic blood pressure, hypertension	LP was not associated with systolic blood pressure or risk of hypertension. No associations were found between dairy intake and blood pressure.
Colorectal, Prostate, and Renal Cell Cancer				
Szilagyi et al., 2006. [25]	Meta-analysis, observational, cohort and case-control	Data from 80 studies (27 cohort and 53 case-control reports)	Dairy Intake Colorectal cancer	The highest level of dairy food consumption protects subjects in both high and low lactase non-persistence regions, but not in regions with significant mixed LP and non-persistent populations.
Torniainen et al., 2007. [12]	Observational, case-control	LP study: 4153 Finnish and Swedish patients and 2315 controls. Milk intake study: 1499 Swedish prostate cancer patients and 1130 controls	Milk Intake Prostate cancer	LP showed no association with prostate cancer risk. High intake of low-fat milk was associated with a significantly increased relative risk of prostate cancer, whereas no association was observed between dietary intakes of total milk, high-fat milk, all dairy products, or dairy products high or low in lactose and risk of prostate cancer.
Timpson et al., 2010. [26]	Observational, case-control	915 cases and 2346 controls from adults of Eastern Europe and Russian descent	Milk Intake Renal cell carcinoma	In cancer cases, LP was associated with higher milk intake, but was not associated with renal cell carcinoma. In controls, milk consumption was associated with confounding factors, including smoking and education.
Travis et al., 2013. [13]	Observational, case-control	630 European men with prostate cancer and 873 matched controls	Milk and Dairy Intake Prostate cancer	LP was associated with greater milk intake, but was not significantly associated with prostate cancer risk.
Bone Density, Fractures, and Osteoporosis				
Obermayer-Pietsch et al., 2004. [27]	Observational, cross-sectional	258 postmenopausal women from Austria	Milk Intake Bone mineral density and bone fractures	LP was associated with higher milk intake, fewer bone fractures, and higher bone mineral density at the hip and the lumbar spine compared to lactase non-persistence.
Enattah et al., 2005. [28]	Observational, cross-sectional, case-control	453 elderly Finnish women. 52 elderly Finnish women with osteoporotic fractures. 59 controls without osteoporosis	Dairy Intake Osteoporosis, bone mineral density, and fractures	Lactose mal-digestion and lactose intolerance were not risk factors for osteoporosis, if calcium intake from diet and/or supplements remained sufficient.
Yang et al., 2017. [29]	Meta-analysis, observational, mixed design	Five studies of 102,750 adults of mixed descent	Milk and Dairy Intake Osteoporosis, ischemic heart disease, T2D	LP and milk consumption were not clearly associated with bone mineral density, ischemic heart disease, or T2D.

Abbreviations: Lactase Persistence (LP), Cardiovascular Disease (CVD), Type 2 Diabetes (T2D), Body Mass Index (BMI).

2.1. Body Mass Index (BMI), Overweight, Obesity

The study of nutrigenetics is expanding rapidly as researchers are now investigating the polygenic nature of several disease states. In fact, only a small percentage of obesity cases have been shown to be monogenic [30]. Rather, inherited predispositions to obesity are primarily polygenic and involve both dietary and non-dietary factors [30,31]. However, if a researcher decided to select only a single gene mutation to study in relation to body weight, the LP mutation might be a good candidate to interrogate due to its strong selective advantage and frequency of occurrence in countries with high obesity rates. In fact, several studies have found correlations between LP and higher body mass index (BMI) [32,33]. However, many of these studies use LP as a proxy for dairy intake rather than actually measuring or recording dairy intake. At first glance, using LP as a proxy for milk or dairy intake appears to be a common and reasonable assumption to make for European populations. Yet, this proxy may not actually represent what any particular individual in the population is consuming since dairy intake and LP prevalence both vary considerably from one European country to the next [13]. Furthermore, LP may not be an accurate proxy for overall dairy intake in most countries since many low-lactose and fermented dairy products are consumed by individuals who are lactose intolerant [34]. For this research paper, we have chosen to focus on studies that have included both LP genotype data and milk or dairy intake data, rather than rely solely on data that used LP as a proxy milk or dairy intake.

In agreement with the epidemiological data, several nutrigenetic studies of mixed design which did measure dairy intake also found the LCT-13910 C > T SNP to be correlated with higher dairy intake and BMI [16,18,19,22]. Most of these studies were relatively small, ranging in size from 551 to 3575 participants. In contrast to these findings, a recent Mendelian randomization study consisting of over 97,000 participants found no evidence linking the LP mutation and dairy intake to overweight or obesity measures [20]. These conflicting results on LP, dairy intake, and body weight offer further evidence that there are many additional variables, such as other gene variants, other dietary components, lifestyle factors, and environmental factors that may interact to influence the relationship between LP and body weight. Although a single gene mutation resulting in a phenotype such as LP can have significant effects on dietary patterns, the nutrigenetic effects of that mutation will differ considerably based on the types, amounts, frequencies, and combinations of foods consumed. Dairy is a complex food group, which contains many products that differ in their macronutrient, micronutrient, and bioactive compound composition. Several of these nutrients and bioactives may protect against chronic disease independently of any effects on body weight [35,36]. Additionally, the lactose content of dairy foods differs considerably depending on the product consumed. A closer look at how different dairy foods interact with different genetic mutations is the logical next step in better understanding the relationships between genetics, dairy intake, and body weight.

2.2. Cardiometabolic Disease

Overweight and obesity increase the risk for cardiometabolic disorders such as metabolic syndrome, CVD, and type 2 diabetes (T2D). The majority of dairy intake studies have consistently provided evidence of neutral or protective associations related to metabolic syndrome risk factors (e.g., glucose intolerance, dyslipidemia, and hypertension) and chronic diseases such as CVD and T2D [37–41]. These findings suggest that dairy intake may favorably affect cardiometabolic risk in certain populations despite augmenting BMI, or possibly, that dairy-associated gains in BMI may also involve gains in lean mass or alterations to gut bacteria that are associated with reduced cardiometabolic risk factors [42–44].

A study of 551 participants of European descent found that the LCT-13910 C > T polymorphism in combination with higher dairy intake could increase the risk for metabolic syndrome, but only in women [17]. These findings suggest that other major genetic factors such as gender can moderate the relationships between dietary intake and cardiometabolic risk factors to greater extent than LP. Research on over 2100 healthy adults from Finland found no associations between LP, dairy intake, and multiple measures of coronary artery disease (carotid intima-media thickness, carotid artery compliance, and brachial artery flow-mediated dilation) [15]. The findings did not differ based on gender, but the subjects who were lactose intolerant consumed significantly more alcohol (and less milk) than those who were lactose tolerant, suggesting that non-dairy factors (e.g., alcohol consumption) which can affect health may also be influenced by LP status. Moderate alcohol intake can beneficially influence cardiovascular health, but excessive intake is linked to an array of cardiovascular disease states [45].

A Mendelian randomization study of over 20,000 participants from multiple racial and ethnic groups including American (Hispanics, African-American and Whites) and Spanish populations assessed the relationship between a different and less commonly studied LP polymorphism (the MCM6-rs3754686 polymorphism at intron 15). The researchers found no associations between LP and CVD or total mortality rates [23]. The researchers also reported a lack of associations between milk intake and lipid levels, CVD, or mortality rates. A Mendelian randomization meta-analysis of 32 studies involving over 197,000 adults from Europe, the US, and Australia found that LP genotype and dairy consumption were not associated with systolic blood pressure or risk of hypertension [24]. Observational studies from this meta-analysis did show that each additional serving of dairy per day was associated with lower systolic blood pressure, but these findings were not confirmed by the intervention studies included in the report, which showed no relationship between dairy intake and systolic blood pressure or hypertension. Similarly, a Mendelian randomization study of over 98,000 Danish adults which followed its participants for over five years, found no associations between the LCT-13910 C > T polymorphism or milk intake with ischemic heart disease, myocardial infarction, or any major cardiovascular risk factor measured (i.e., total cholesterol, LDL, HDL, triglycerides, or blood pressure) [21]. The same researchers also did not find any associations between the LCT-13910 C > T polymorphism or milk intake with T2D [20]. However, the researchers did note that LP subjects who did not consume milk had a slightly higher risk for T2D compared to those LP subjects who habitually consumed milk, suggesting that an LP genotype may be able to affect health independently of dairy intake. No mechanistic explanations were reported for this finding; rather the researchers suggested the relationship between abstinence from milk intake, LP status, and T2D could be potentially explained by selection bias in the study instead of biological differences between the study participants. Another Mendelian randomization study which meta-analyzed genetic data from several studies comprised of mixed populations also investigated the relationship between the LCT-13910 C > T polymorphism, milk intake, and cardiometabolic disease [29]. This study confirmed the results from earlier studies, in that the researchers reported a lack of associations between LP status, milk intake, and cardiometabolic disease (i.e., ischemic heart disease and T2D).

2.3. Cancer

Epidemiological studies have provided mixed results regarding dairy intake and cancer risk [46–50], but these relationships begin to become clearer when specific dairy products, LP gene variants, and different types of cancer are considered. For example, colorectal cancer is one of the types of cancer most heavily influenced by dietary patterns since colorectal tissue comes into direct and prolonged contact with dietary components and products of digestion on a consistent basis. The colon also contains the majority of the gut microbiota that can modulate colonic exposure to carcinogenic toxins.

Large prospective cohort studies and meta-analyses provide evidence for protective associations of dairy intake on colorectal cancer that often depend on the type and amount of dairy products consumed [49,51,52]; however, these types of studies do not usually take into account LP status. Importantly, LP status is a major factor determining the type and amount of dairy products consumed as well as the dairy-derived end-products that are exposed to the colorectal tissue (i.e., lactose moves into the large intestine in lactose intolerant individuals, while lactose is broken down to glucose and galactose and absorbed in the small intestine in lactose tolerant individuals). A nutrigenetic meta-analysis of 80 studies regarding dairy intake and colorectal cancer showed key differences are dependent on dairy intake amount and LP status [25]. In fact, the researchers reported a protective role of higher dairy intake in both high LP prevalent and high non-LP prevalent populations. In other words, this research suggests that the potential anti-colorectal cancer benefits associated with dairy intake may not be limited to those who can digest lactose. Rather, higher lactose intakes in lactose intolerant individuals may lead to the production of favorable substrates that can be used by protective colonic microflora.

Prostate cancer is one of the most common cancers in men [12]. In contrast to the colorectal tissues, the prostate does not come into direct contact with the gut microbiota or gastrointestinal contents. Several indirect mechanisms have been proposed for how diet can affect cell replication and cancer risk. One hypothesis is that the circulating lactose breakdown products glucose and galactose, which are generally higher in LP dairy consumers, may affect cancer development or progression in certain tissues [53,54]. A Swedish case-cohort study (1499 cases and 1130 controls) which tested the associations between LP status, overall dairy intake, and prostate carcinoma, reported no associations between these variables [12]. The researchers did find an association between low-fat milk intake and prostate cancer risk, but this relationship did not appear to be influenced by LP status. When LP status, dairy intake, and prostate cancer risk were assessed in the European Prospective Investigation into Cancer and Nutrition (EPIC) study, the researchers found that both LP genotypes (CT and TT) and higher dairy intake were not associated with prostate cancer risk [13].

Relatively few nutrigenetic studies have been conducted on LP status, dairy intake, and cancer types residing outside of the digestive or reproductive systems. A recent study in nearly 23,000 Swedish adults with lactose intolerance found a decreased risk of lung, breast, and ovarian cancers compared to individuals who were lactose tolerant [55]. The authors of this research hypothesize that the decreased cancer risk in lactose intolerant individuals could be associated with lower intakes of: (1) lactose or lactose-containing products; (2) various non-lactose components of dairy, and/or (3) other protective foods and beverages consumed in place of dairy foods. Unfortunately, dietary intakes were not recorded for this study, so it is not possible to determine their effects on cancer risk. Furthermore, the study design used symptomology rather than genotype to diagnose lactose intolerance, so it is also not clear as to what percentage of individuals in this study were genetically considered lactase non-persistent. A Mendelian randomization study of nearly 1100 Eastern European and Russian adults that did take into account milk intake and LP genotype found that milk intake was associated with a slightly higher risk for renal cell carcinoma, but LP genotype was not [26]. The researchers of this study concluded that it is wise to exercise caution when interpreting observational associations between milk consumption and cancer risk since any perceived relationships between the two may be due to confounding by other dietary and lifestyle factors.

2.4. Bone Health

Total dairy intake [56], dairy protein intake [57,58], and dairy mineral intake [59–61] are all associated with bone health markers such as bone mineral density (BMD) and bone turnover. The relationship between lactose intake and bone health is a little less clear. Lactose intake has not been directly associated with bone strength or structure, but the ability to digest lactose is associated with higher intake of overall dairy intake, dairy protein intake, and dairy mineral intake—all factors consistently linked to improvements in BMD and reduced bone turnover. In agreement with this concept, lactose intolerance can increase the risk for osteoporosis and bone fractures in certain populations [62].

Researchers investigating the relationships between milk intake, LP status, and bone health in 258 postmenopausal women from Austria found that LP genotype influenced BMD and bone fractures [27]. The CC genotype, which is associated with lactose intolerance/lactase non-persistence was associated with the lowest hip and spine BMD measures and highest fracture rate. The CT genotype, which confers an intermediate level of lactose tolerance/lactase persistence, was associated with lower BMD scores compared to the TT genotype (which confers the greatest level of lactose tolerance/lactase persistence). The researchers suggested that the improved bone integrity found in LP individuals was not due to higher calcium intake alone, but rather due to the additive effects of calcium and other dairy components such as dairy proteins. In contrast to these findings, a cross-sectional study of two postmenopausal cohorts from Northern Europe found no differences in adjusted BMD or in fracture incidence between lactose tolerant and lactose intolerant women [28]. The researchers of this study came to very different conclusions, suggesting that there were no differences between these post-menopausal populations as long as the non-dairy consumers got enough calcium from other foods and supplements. A recent Mendelian randomization meta-analysis investigating the relationship between the Northern European LCT-13910 C > T gene variant, milk intake, and bone health also reported a lack of associations between the LP mutation and bone mineral density [29]. These researchers also cast doubt on the ability of dietary calcium to improve bone health by itself, and implied that there are additional factors (e.g., protein intake and vitamin D fortification) that need to be considered in relation to dairy intake and bone health.

Recent investigations into the associations between LP status, dairy intake, and health outcomes have provided nuanced findings that are moderated by factors including LP genotype, the type and amount of dairy product consumed, age, gender, body weight, and the specific pathology of the disease being assessed. Additionally, numerous other variables such as mutations in non-LP genes, whole dietary patterns, and environmental factors affect the nutrigenetic relationship between lactase persistence, dairy intake, and health. The science of nutrigenetics is quickly moving beyond the single candidate gene approach, and it is becoming clear that LP mutations are not the only mutations that have the potential to moderate the relationships between dairy intake and disease.

3. Metabolic and Hormonal Gene Variants, Dairy Intake, and Health Outcomes

In addition to lactose, dairy products contain a diverse set of constituents (i.e., proteins, fats, vitamins, minerals, and bioactives) that can affect human health. The digestion, metabolism, transport, and excretion of these compounds are all dependent on gene products (i.e., RNAs, and proteins such as enzymes, receptors, peptide hormones, binding proteins, and transport proteins). Therefore, genetic variants that result in altered metabolic and hormonal gene products may influence the relationship between dairy intake and disease risk. The gene variants that have been studied so far in relation to dairy intake include polymorphisms in genes related to lipid metabolism, hormone receptor function, and vitamin D receptor function (Table 2).

Table 2. Nutrigenetic studies on non-lactase polymorphisms, dairy intake, and health outcomes in adults.

Reference	Study Design	Population	Gene Variants	Variables	Outcomes
Lipid Metabolism SNPs					
Smith CE et al., 2013. [10]	Observational, cross-sectional	955 adults from the Boston Puerto Rican Health Study and 1116 adults from the Genetics of Lipid Lowering Drugs and Diet Network study	APOA2-265 T > C (rs5082)	Total dairy, higher-fat dairy (>1%), and low-fat dairy (≤1%) BMI, Body Weight	There was a significant interaction between the APOA2-265 T > C polymorphism and dairy food intake. Individuals with the CC genotype who consumed more higher-fat dairy products had a higher BMI compared with those consuming less higher-fat dairy products.
Loria-Kohen et al., 2014. [63]	Intervention, randomized trial (1 year)	161 middle-aged Spanish adults	14 SNPs in 9 genes related to lipid metabolism were examined	500 mL per day of skimmed or semi-skimmed milk for 1 year in addition to their usual diets. CVD risk markers	A TT genotype for PPARA rs135549 was associated with a reduction in the total cholesterol/HDL and LDL/HDL ratios after 1 year of skimmed milk intake. No differences were observed after consuming either skimmed or semi-skimmed milk in the C allele carriers.

Table 2. *Cont.*

Reference	Study Design	Population	Gene Variants	Variables	Outcomes
Abdullah et al., 2016. [64]	Intervention, RCT (4 weeks)	101 middle-aged Canadian adults	ABCG5, CYP7A1, DHCR7	3 servings per day of dairy or energy-matched control on background of a prudent diet. Serum lipids	Genetic variations in ABCG5, CYP7A1, and DHCR7 may contribute to differing responses of serum cholesterol to dairy intake among healthy adults.
Vitamin D Receptor SNPs					
Hubner et al., 2008. [65]	Sub-study of an RCT using aspirin and folate for the prevention of colorectal adenoma recurrence	480 participants in the United Kingdom Colorectal Adenoma Prevention trial	Cdx2, FokI, BsmI, ApaI and TaqI	Milk and Dairy Product Intake Colorectal cancer	VDR polymorphism genotypes and haplotypes did not directly alter colorectal cancer recurrence risk, but the reduction in risk associated with high dairy product intake was confined to individuals with ApaI aA/AA genotype.
Neyestani et al., 2013. [66]	Intervention, RCT (12 weeks)	140 middle-aged Iranian adults with T2D	FokI	500 mL yogurt drink (doogh) per day fortified with 1000 IU vitamin D T2D; glycemic status, lipid profiles, inflammatory biomarkers	The FF genotype group had the largest decrease of C-reactive protein and interleukin-6 compared with the Ff and ff groups. The vitamin D response of the ff genotype group was the lowest after consuming the vitamin D fortified doogh.
Shab-Bidar et al., 2015. [67]	Intervention, RCT (12 weeks)	140 middle-aged Iranian adults with T2D	FokI	500 mL yogurt drink (doogh) per day fortified with 1000 IU vitamin D or control yogurt drink with no vitamin D Oxidative stress biomarkers	No significant association between FokI genotypes and oxidative stress biomarkers, but the the ff variant subgroup showed the weakest response to vitamin D fortified doogh.
Shab-Bidar et al., 2015. [68]	Intervention, RCT (12 weeks)	60 middle-aged Iranian adults with T2D	Cdx2	500 mL yogurt drink (doogh) per day fortified with 1000 IU vitamin D or control yogurt drink with no vitamin D T2D, glycemic and adiposity biomarkers	Daily intake of vitamin D fortified doogh for 12 weeks improved the central obesity indices in T2D subjects, and the improvement was more pronounced in the carriers of the AA genotype of VDR-Cdx2.
Hormone and Hormone Receptor SNPs					
Sotos-Prieto et al., 2010. [69]	Observational, cross-sectional	945 high-CVD risk older subjects participating in the PREDIMED–Valencia Study	rs1466113 G > C in SSTR2	All food groups, including dairy BMI, obesity	Homozygous subjects for the C allele had significantly lower BMI and odds ratio for obesity than G-allele carriers. There were also significant differences in dairy product and protein intakes between CC- and G-allele carriers.
InterAct Consortium 2016. [70]	Observational, case-cohort, average follow up of 12.5 years	18,638 middle-aged, normal weight adults from EPIC-InterAct study	TCF7L2 rs12255372, TCF7L2 rs7903146, KCNQ1 rs163171, KCNQ1 rs163184, KCNQ1 rs2237892, GIPR rs10423928, WFS1 rs10010131	Intake of whey-containing dairy products T2D risk, incretins	No significant differences between any of the possible genotypes investigated and risk of T2D per one serving per day increment of Whey-containing dairy (150 g/day).

Abbreviations: Single Nucleotide Polymorphism (SNP), Randomized Controlled Trial (RCT), Body Mass Index (BMI), Cardiovascular Disease (CVD), Type 2 Diabetes (T2D), High-Density Lipoprotein (HDL), Low-Density Lipoprotein (LDL), Vitamin D Receptor (VDR), Somatostatin Receptor 2 (SSTR2), Peroxisome Proliferator-Activated Receptor Alpha (PPARA), Apolipoprotein A2 (APOA2), Cholesterol 7α-Hydroxylase (CYP7A1), ATP-Binding Cassette Subfamily G, Member 5 (ABCG5), 7-Dehydrocholesterol Reductase (DHCR7),Transcription Factor 7-like 2 (TCF7L2), Gastric Inhibitory Polypeptide Receptor (GIPR), Potassium Voltage-Gated Channel Subfamily Q Member 1 (KCNQ1), Wolframin ER Transmembrane Glycoprotein (WFS1).

3.1. Lipid Metabolism SNPs

Saturated fat is one of the most commonly studied dietary compounds in relation to genetic polymorphisms and health, primarily having to do with cholesterol levels and CVD risk [10]. Saturated fat is also one of the main compounds that differ considerably between dairy products, with commonly consumed products ranging from <1% saturated fat (fat-free milk) to over 50% saturated fat (butter). For decades, nutrition studies have provided mixed results regarding the health effects of saturated fats. These inconclusive results have often been attributed to factors such as study design, researcher bias, and the specific type of saturated fats consumed [64]. Until recently, another major factor has often been omitted from these studies, and that is the genetic predispositions of the subjects being studied. The recent advances in nutrigenetic research show that genetic inter-individual variability in how humans respond to dietary fats could help explain why hundreds of past studies have failed to provide a consensus understanding on the effects of saturated fat intake on human health.

A gene-candidate study involving 2000 ethnically diverse participants (Americans of Northern European ancestry and Americans of Puerto Rican origin) was conducted to determine the interactions between an apolipoprotein A2 gene (APOA2) gene variant, dairy product intake, and BMI [10]. In this study, a CC genotype was associated with a higher BMI, but only in those subjects consuming the highest amount of dairy fat. On the other hand, greater dairy fat intake was not associated with a higher BMI in subjects with a CT or TT genotype. Upon further analysis, females with the CC genotype from the American section of the study were also shown to have a higher BMI when consuming the lowest amount of low-fat dairy products. These findings reinforce the idea that the dairy intake and BMI relationship is not solely dependent on any single dietary or genetic factor. Rather, several variables including ethnicity and gender play key roles in how individuals respond to dietary patterns.

A year-long randomized trial of 161 Spanish adults investigated the relationship between dairy fat intake and 14 SNPs within nine different candidate lipid metabolism genes [63]. The participants were randomly assigned to ingest either 500 mL per day of skimmed milk (1 g of saturated fat) daily, or an equivalent amount of semi-skimmed milk (6.7 g of saturated fat) along with their normal diets. The results showed no differences in lipid biomarkers between the different groups even though the groups consumed a difference of more than 5 g/day of saturated dairy fat. When the different SNPs were assessed and corrections were made for multiple testing, only one of the 14 SNPs tested showed an association with dairy fat intake. The TT genotype for peroxisome proliferator-activated receptor alpha (PPARA) rs135549 correlated with reduced total cholesterol/HDL and LDL/HDL-C ratios, while CC and CT genotypes did not. A more recent assessment of dairy intake and candidate SNPs in cholesterol-related genes was performed in 101 Canadian adults [64]. This randomized crossover study assigned participants to consume a prudent diet for four weeks along with either three daily servings of dairy foods (low-fat milk, low-fat yogurt, and cheese) or a non-dairy control matched for total energy but lower in saturated fat. The researchers found multiple SNPs associated with varying lipid responses to the different diets. The GG genotype for the ATP-binding cassette subfamily G, member 5 (ABCG5) rs6720173 was associated with higher total cholesterol and LDL levels compared to CG and CC genotypes. GG and GT genotypes for cholesterol 7α-hydroxylase (CYP7A1) rs3808607 were associated with higher total cholesterol and LDL levels compared to the TT genotype. AA and AG genotypes for 7-dehydrocholesterol reductase (DHCR7) rs760241 were associated with higher LDL levels compared to subjects with the GG genotype. When considered all together, these studies show that individuals with mutations in particular lipid metabolism genes (e.g., APOA2 rs5082, PPARA rs135549, ABCG5 rs6720173, CYP7A1 rs3808607, DHCR7 rs760241) may show differential sensitivity to the health effects of dairy food intake, especially when it comes to the intake of products with different levels of saturated fats.

3.2. Hormone and Hormone Receptor SNPs

In addition to lipid metabolism SNPs, hormone and hormone receptor SNPs have also been studied in the context of dairy intake and health outcomes. Researchers from the InterAct Consortium investigated the relationships between incretin hormone SNPs, whey-containing dairy intake, and risk for T2D in 18,638 European adults [70]. Whey-containing dairy foods were chosen for this analysis since whey protein has been shown to influence the secretion of the incretins glucagon-like peptide-1 (GLP-1) and glucose-dependent insulinotropic peptide (GIP) to a greater degree than other protein sources. After more than 12 years of follow-up, the researchers found no associations between any of the seven incretin gene variants, whey-containing dairy servings, and T2D risk. A genetic risk score assessment was conducted on the participants from this study and also showed no interactions between the incretin gene variants, whey-containing dairy intake, and T2D risk. In simpler terms, a single serving per day of whey-containing dairy foods did not affect T2D risk even in the subjects who had the highest number of incretin-related allele SNPs.

A gene-candidate study involving 945 European adults at high risk for CVD from the PREDIMED-Valencia Study was conducted to determine if a particular genetic polymorphism in the somatostatin receptor 2 (SSTR2) gene interacts with dietary or anthropometric variables [69]. Among other functions, the somatostatin system (which includes its receptors) can inhibit the secretion of growth hormone, gut hormones, and pancreatic hormones; affecting cell growth, pituitary gland function, body weight regulation, and neuro-endocrine function [69,71]. The PREDIMED-Valencia study results showed that the rs1466113 C > G polymorphism tracked with both dairy intake and obesity. Individuals with one or more dominant G alleles tended to have a higher BMI and consumed a greater amount of dairy, while those with the CC genotype had a lower BMI, a lower odds ratio for obesity, and consumed a smaller amount of dairy. In addition to consuming less dairy, the CC group also consumed less total protein, meat, and legumes on a daily basis, suggesting that this particular gene might be associated with regulating protein intake, and that this particular SNP could influence several aspects of dietary intake and body weight beyond that of dairy consumption.

3.3. Vitamin D Receptor SNPs

Studies on vitamin D receptor (VDR) polymorphisms and dairy intake have provided key insights into how different polymorphisms in the same gene interact with diet to influence health outcomes. Indeed, while one VDR polymorphism might affect receptor-binding activity, another might pertain to receptor binding strength or substrate affinity. These differences can affect how the receptors will interact with dietary constituents, and in turn will affect how those dietary constituents are absorbed, transported, metabolized, and excreted.

A 12-week long intervention study investigated the relationships between VDR FokI polymorphism, vitamin D fortified dairy intake, and inflammatory and antioxidative markers in 140 Iranian subjects with T2D [66,67]. Subjects were assigned to ingest either 500 mL of vitamin D fortified yogurt per day (1000 IU of vitamin D), or a control yogurt beverage that was not fortified with vitamin D. The subjects who consumed the fortified yogurt had higher vitamin D levels and lower inflammatory markers (high-sensitivity C-reactive protein, interleukin-4, and interleukin-6) [66], and higher antioxidative markers (glutathione and total antioxidant capacity) [67], compared to subjects who consumed the plain yogurt. When genotype was assessed, subjects with the FF genotype had higher vitamin D levels than the ff genotype, and those with a FF genotype also had the greatest reduction in high-sensitivity C-reactive protein and interleukin-6 compared to both the Ff and ff genotypes. These findings suggest that FokI gene variants may influence the ability to utilize vitamin D from dairy foods and could thereby ameliorate the inflammatory response in diabetic subjects.

A similar 12-week long study was conducted by the same researchers to determine the relationships between a different VDR polymorphism (Cdx2 polymorphism), vitamin D fortified yogurt intake, and central obesity in 60 Iranian subjects with T2D [68]. The subjects were randomly assigned to consume either 500 mL of 1000 IU vitamin D fortified yogurt per day or the same amount of an unfortified control yogurt. At the end of the study, all subjects who consumed the fortified yogurt had higher vitamin D levels and reduced central adiposity measures compared to those who consumed the unfortified yogurt. When the Cdx2 genotype (AA, AG, GG) was assessed, circulating vitamin D levels were increased and central adiposity measures were decreased to a greater degree in the AA group, compared to the G-allele carriers. Overall, these results suggest that vitamin D fortification improves the health benefits of dairy products when consumed by type 2 diabetic subjects, but these effects appear to be moderated by specific genetic variants in the vitamin D receptors.

When multiple VDR polymorphism (FokI, Cdx2, ApaI, BsmI, TaqI) and dairy intake were investigated in relation to colorectal cancer recurrence in 480 subjects from the United Kingdom [65], only certain ApaI genotypes appeared to interact with dairy intake and health outcomes. The AA and Aa ApaI genotypes interacted with higher dairy product consumption to reduce colorectal cancer recurrence, but the aa genotype did not. Many of dairy's effects on colorectal cancer recurrence in this study were dependent on the type of dairy product consumed, with milk being more protective than other dairy products. Interestingly, these effects also appear limited to dairy-derived vitamin D, with intake of vitamin D from food and/or supplements not showing the same beneficial influence on colorectal cancer recurrence reduction.

In combination with the findings from LP and dairy intake studies, studies on non-LP gene variants and dairy intake provide convincing evidence that an array of gene variants are responsible for significant interindividual variations in dietary intake patterns and metabolic responses. Many of these gene–diet interactions converge to influence body weight, cardiometabolic disease risks, cancer risk and bone health. Further findings from the investigations of gene–dairy–disease interactions will contribute greatly to the development of more genetically informed and personalized recommendations regarding dairy product intake and disease risk management.

4. Conclusions

A major aim of personalized nutrition is to turn a person's nutrigenetic and nutrigenomic information into highly specific dietary advice that can be used to improve or maintain health. This type of dietary advice has the potential to revolutionize the fields of nutrition and healthcare. However, at present, the science of personalized nutrition is just scratching the surface of its potential, and we must be careful not to label it a panacea before proving its efficacy. While this review of nutrigenetic studies has focused solely on one food group and a few select genetic mutations, it has clearly shown the complexities of understanding and utilizing the information gathered from studies of gene–diet interactions. Nutrigenetic studies that have included data on dairy intake provide mixed results on health outcomes. Many of these studies show that LP is associated with higher dairy intake and BMI, but they also tend to show that LP and higher dairy intake are not consistently associated with cardiometabolic disease risk, certain types of cancer occurrence, or bone health. Nutrigenetic studies investigating the effects of polymorphisms in genes related to lipid metabolism, hormone receptor function, and vitamin D receptor function also show mixed results and the potential for differential sensitivity between genotypes to the health effects of dairy food intake. More research is necessary on polygenic and multifactorial relationships in the context of diet and disease. In the end, these nutrigenetic relationships are likely dependent on many other factors besides the individual SNPs tested, such as the type and amount of dairy product consumed, gender, age, ethnicity, and other genetic mutations that affect the metabolism, transport, or storage of nutrients in the body.

The interindividual variation between humans is on the magnitude of millions of SNPs, so the insights gained from a limited focus on a few SNPs having to do with dairy intake reveal only a small part of a person's nutrigenetic story. Furthermore, additional research is needed on the relationships between different gene variants and their abilities to interact and influence each other in antagonistic, additive, or synergistic ways. In summary, nutrigenetic research which is focused on the relationships between single SNPs (of which there are millions) and single food groups (which may be comprised of a diverse array of products with varying combinations and amounts of nutrients and bioactives), may provide great insights into improving the science of personalized nutrition. However, this type of research is only part of the personalized nutrition equation. Nutrigenomic responses (epigenomics, transcriptomics, proteomics, metabolomics) to different types and amounts of dairy products, along with microbiome data, and phenotypic/characteristic traits (age, gender, activity level, disease status, etc.) must also be accounted for, since these factors can all interact with the diet to influence health.

Acknowledgments: All authors have read and approved the final manuscript. This research was funded by the California Dairy Research Foundation.

Author Contributions: Kevin B. Comerford drafted the manuscript. Gonca Pasin provided expert guidance, review, and feedback throughout the manuscript development process.

Conflicts of Interest: Gonca Pasin is the executive director of the California Dairy Research Foundation. Kevin B. Comerford received consulting fees from the California Dairy Research Foundation. All conclusions are the work of the authors.

Abbreviation

LCT	Lactase Gene
LP	Lactase Persistence
SNP	Single Nucleotide Polymorphism
PKU	Phenylketonuria
MTHFR	5,10-Methylene Tetrahydrofolate Reductase
BMI	Body Mass Index
CVD	Cardiovascular Disease
T2DM	Type 2 Diabetes Mellitus
BMD	Bone Mineral Density
VDR	Vitamin D Receptor
APOA2	Apolipoprotein A2
ABCG5	ATP-Binding Cassette Subfamily G, Member 5
CYP7A1	Cholesterol 7α-Hydroxylase
DHCR7	7-Dehydrocholesterol Reductase
PPARA	Peroxisome Proliferator-Activated Receptor Alpha
SSTR2	Somatostatin Receptor 2
GLP-1	Glucagon-Like Peptide-1
GIP	Glucose-Dependent Insulinotropic Peptide

References

1. Ferguson, L.R.; De Caterina, R.; Gorman, U.; Allayee, H.; Kohlmeier, M.; Prasad, C.; Choi, M.S.; Curi, R.; de Luis, D.A.; Gil, A.; et al. Guide and Position of the International Society of Nutrigenetics/Nutrigenomics on Personalised Nutrition: Part 1—Fields of Precision Nutrition. *J. Nutrigenet. Nutrigenom.* **2016**, *9*, 12–27. [CrossRef] [PubMed]

2. Neeha, V.S.; Kinth, P. Nutrigenomics Research: A Review. *J. Food Sci. Technol.* **2013**, *50*, 415–428. [CrossRef] [PubMed]

3. Blum, K.; Downs, B.W.; Dushaj, K.; Li, M.; Braverman, E.R.; Fried, L.; Waite, R.; Demotrovics, Z.; Badgaiyan, R.D. The Benefits of Customized DNA Directed Nutrition to Balance the Brain Reward Circuitry and Reduce Addictive Behaviors. *Precis. Med.* **2016**, *1*, 18–33.

4. Liew, S.C.; Gupta, E.D. Methylenetetrahydrofolate Reductase (Mthfr) C677t Polymorphism: Epidemiology, Metabolism and the Associated Diseases. *Eur. J. Med. Genet.* **2015**, *58*, 1–10. [CrossRef] [PubMed]

5. Smith, G.D.; Lawlor, D.A.; Timpson, N.J.; Baban, J.; Kiessling, M.; Day, I.N.; Ebrahim, S. Lactase Persistence-Related Genetic Variant: Population Substructure and Health Outcomes. *Eur. J. Hum. Genet.* **2009**, *17*, 357–367. [CrossRef] [PubMed]

6. Szilagyi, A.; Leighton, H.; Burstein, B.; Xue, X. Latitude, Sunshine, and Human Lactase Phenotype Distributions May Contribute to Geographic Patterns of Modern Disease: The Inflammatory Bowel Disease Model. *Clin. Epidemiol.* **2014**, *6*, 183–198. [CrossRef] [PubMed]

7. Gerbault, P.; Liebert, A.; Itan, Y.; Powell, A.; Currat, M.; Burger, J.; Swallow, D.M.; Thomas, M.G. Evolution of Lactase Persistence: An Example of Human Niche Construction. *Philos. Trans. R. Soc. Lond. B Biol. Sci.* **2011**, *366*, 863–877. [CrossRef] [PubMed]

8. Bersaglieri, T.; Sabeti, P.C.; Patterson, N.; Vanderploeg, T.; Schaffner, S.F.; Drake, J.A.; Rhodes, M.; Reich, D.E.; Hirschhorn, J.N. Genetic Signatures of Strong Recent Positive Selection at the Lactase Gene. *Am. J. Hum. Genet.* **2004**, *74*, 1111–1120. [CrossRef] [PubMed]

9. Szilagyi, A. Adaptation to Lactose in Lactase Non Persistent People: Effects on Intolerance and the Relationship between Dairy Food Consumption and Evaluation of Diseases. *Nutrients* **2015**, *7*, 6751–6779. [CrossRef] [PubMed]

10. Smith, C.E.; Tucker, K.L.; Arnett, D.K.; Noel, S.E.; Corella, D.; Borecki, I.B.; Feitosa, M.F.; Aslibekyan, S.; Parnell, L.D.; Lai, C.Q.; et al. Apolipoprotein A2 Polymorphism Interacts with Intakes of Dairy Foods to Influence Body Weight in 2 U.S. Populations. *J. Nutr.* **2013**, *143*, 1865–1871. [CrossRef] [PubMed]

11. Beja-Pereira, A.; Luikart, G.; England, P.R.; Bradley, D.G.; Jann, O.C.; Bertorelle, G.; Chamberlain, A.T.; Nunes, T.P.; Metodiev, S.; Ferrand, N.; et al. Gene-Culture Coevolution between Cattle Milk Protein Genes and Human Lactase Genes. *Nat. Genet.* **2003**, *35*, 311–313. [CrossRef] [PubMed]

12. Torniainen, S.; Hedelin, M.; Autio, V.; Rasinpera, H.; Balter, K.A.; Klint, A.; Bellocco, R.; Wiklund, F.; Stattin, P.; Ikonen, T.; et al. Lactase Persistence, Dietary Intake of Milk, and the Risk for Prostate Cancer in Sweden and Finland. *Cancer Epidemiol. Prev. Biomark.* **2007**, *16*, 956–961. [CrossRef] [PubMed]

13. Travis, R.C.; Appleby, P.N.; Siddiq, A.; Allen, N.E.; Kaaks, R.; Canzian, F.; Feller, S.; Tjonneland, A.; Fons Johnsen, N.; Overvad, K.; et al. Genetic Variation in the Lactase Gene, Dairy Product Intake and Risk for Prostate Cancer in the European Prospective Investigation into Cancer and Nutrition. *Int. J. Cancer* **2013**, *132*, 1901–1910. [CrossRef] [PubMed]

14. Lukito, W.; Malik, S.G.; Surono, I.S.; Wahlqvist, M.L. From 'Lactose Intolerance' to 'Lactose Nutrition'. *Asia Pac. J. Clin. Nutr.* **2015**, *24*, S1–S8. [PubMed]

15. Lehtimaki, T.; Hutri-Kahonen, N.; Kahonen, M.; Hemminki, J.; Mikkila, V.; Laaksonen, M.; Rasanen, L.; Mononen, N.; Juonala, M.; Marniemi, J.; et al. Adult-Type Hypolactasia Is Not a Predisposing Factor for the Early Functional and Structural Changes of Atherosclerosis: The Cardiovascular Risk in Young Finns Study. *Clin. Sci. (Lond.)* **2008**, *115*, 265–271. [CrossRef] [PubMed]

16. Almon, R.; Alvarez-Leon, E.E.; Serra-Majem, L. Association of the European Lactase Persistence Variant (Lct-13910 C > T Polymorphism) with Obesity in the Canary Islands. *PLoS ONE* **2012**, *7*, e43978. [CrossRef] [PubMed]

17. Almon, R.; Alvarez-Leon, E.E.; Engfeldt, P.; Serra-Majem, L.; Magnuson, A.; Nilsson, T.K. Associations between Lactase Persistence and the Metabolic Syndrome in a Cross-Sectional Study in the Canary Islands. *Eur. J. Nutr.* **2010**, *49*, 141–146. [CrossRef] [PubMed]

18. Corella, D.; Arregui, M.; Coltell, O.; Portoles, O.; Guillem-Saiz, P.; Carrasco, P.; Sorli, J.V.; Ortega-Azorin, C.; Gonzalez, J.I.; Ordovas, J.M. Association of the Lct-13910c > T Polymorphism with Obesity and Its Modulation by Dairy Products in a Mediterranean Population. *Obesity* **2011**, *19*, 1707–1714. [CrossRef] [PubMed]

19. Lamri, A.; Poli, A.; Emery, N.; Bellili, N.; Velho, G.; Lantieri, O.; Balkau, B.; Marre, M.; Fumeron, F. The Lactase Persistence Genotype Is Associated with Body Mass Index and Dairy Consumption in the D.E.S.I.R. Study. *Metabolism* **2013**, *62*, 1323–1329. [CrossRef] [PubMed]

20. Bergholdt, H.K.; Nordestgaard, B.G.; Ellervik, C. Milk Intake Is Not Associated with Low Risk of Diabetes or Overweight-Obesity: A Mendelian Randomization Study in 97,811 Danish Individuals. *Am. J. Clin. Nutr.* **2015**, *102*, 487–496. [CrossRef] [PubMed]

21. Bergholdt, H.K.; Nordestgaard, B.G.; Varbo, A.; Ellervik, C. Milk Intake Is Not Associated with Ischaemic Heart Disease in Observational or Mendelian Randomization Analyses in 98,529 Danish Adults. *Int. J. Epidemiol.* **2015**, *44*, 587–603. [CrossRef] [PubMed]

22. Hartwig, F.P.; Horta, B.L.; Smith, G.D.; de Mola, C.L.; Victora, C.G. Association of Lactase Persistence Genotype with Milk Consumption, Obesity and Blood Pressure: A Mendelian Randomization Study in the 1982 Pelotas (Brazil) Birth Cohort, with a Systematic Review and Meta-Analysis. *Int. J. Epidemiol.* **2016**, *45*, 1573–1587. [CrossRef] [PubMed]

23. Smith, C.E.; Coltell, O.; Sorli, J.V.; Estruch, R.; Martinez-Gonzalez, M.A.; Salas-Salvado, J.; Fito, M.; Aros, F.; Dashti, H.S.; Lai, C.Q.; et al. Associations of the Mcm6-Rs3754686 Proxy for Milk Intake in Mediterranean and American Populations with Cardiovascular Biomarkers, Disease and Mortality: Mendelian Randomization. *Sci. Rep.* **2016**, *6*, 33188. [CrossRef] [PubMed]

24. Ding, M.; Huang, T.; Bergholdt, H.K.; Nordestgaard, B.G.; Ellervik, C.; Qi, L.; Consortium, C. Dairy Consumption, Systolic Blood Pressure, and Risk of Hypertension: Mendelian Randomization Study. *BMJ* **2017**, *356*, j1000. [CrossRef] [PubMed]

25. Szilagyi, A.; Nathwani, U.; Vinokuroff, C.; Correa, J.A.; Shrier, I. The Effect of Lactose Maldigestion on the Relationship between Dairy Food Intake and Colorectal Cancer: A Systematic Review. *Nutr. Cancer* **2006**, *55*, 141–150. [CrossRef] [PubMed]

26. Timpson, N.J.; Brennan, P.; Gaborieau, V.; Moore, L.; Zaridze, D.; Matveev, V.; Szeszenia-Dabrowska, N.; Lissowska, J.; Mates, D.; Bencko, V.; et al. Can Lactase Persistence Genotype Be Used to Reassess the Relationship between Renal Cell Carcinoma and Milk Drinking? Potentials and Problems in the Application of Mendelian Randomization. *Cancer Epidemiol. Prev. Biomark.* **2010**, *19*, 1341–1348. [CrossRef] [PubMed]

27. Obermayer-Pietsch, B.M.; Bonelli, C.M.; Walter, D.E.; Kuhn, R.J.; Fahrleitner-Pammer, A.; Berghold, A.; Goessler, W.; Stepan, V.; Dobnig, H.; Leb, G.; et al. Genetic Predisposition for Adult Lactose Intolerance and Relation to Diet, Bone Density, and Bone Fractures. *J. Bone Miner. Res.* **2004**, *19*, 42–47. [CrossRef] [PubMed]

28. Enattah, N.; Pekkarinen, T.; Valimaki, M.J.; Loyttyniemi, E.; Jarvela, I. Genetically Defined Adult-Type Hypolactasia and Self-Reported Lactose Intolerance as Risk Factors of Osteoporosis in Finnish Postmenopausal Women. *Eur. J. Clin. Nutr.* **2005**, *59*, 1105–1111. [CrossRef] [PubMed]

29. Yang, Q.; Lin, S.L.; Au Yeung, S.L.; Kwok, M.K.; Xu, L.; Leung, G.M.; Schooling, C.M. Genetically Predicted Milk Consumption and Bone Health, Ischemic Heart Disease and Type 2 Diabetes: A Mendelian Randomization Study. *Eur. J. Clin. Nutr.* **2017**. [CrossRef] [PubMed]

30. Hinney, A.; Vogel, C.I.; Hebebrand, J. From Monogenic to Polygenic Obesity: Recent Advances. *Eur. Child Adolesc. Psychiatry* **2010**, *19*, 297–310. [CrossRef] [PubMed]

31. Stein, Q.P.; Mroch, A.R.; De Berg, K.L.; Flanagan, J.D. The Influential Role of Genes in Obesity. *South Dak. Med.* **2011**, 12–15, 17.

32. Kettunen, J.; Silander, K.; Saarela, O.; Amin, N.; Muller, M.; Timpson, N.; Surakka, I.; Ripatti, S.; Laitinen, J.; Hartikainen, A.L.; et al. European Lactase Persistence Genotype Shows Evidence of Association with Increase in Body Mass Index. *Hum. Mol. Genet.* **2010**, *19*, 1129–1136. [CrossRef] [PubMed]

33. Manco, L.; Dias, H.; Muc, M.; Padez, C. The Lactase-13910 C > T Polymorphism (Rs4988235) Is Associated with Overweight/Obesity and Obesity-Related Variables in a Population Sample of Portuguese Young Adults. *Eur. J. Clin. Nutr.* **2017**, *71*, 21–24. [CrossRef] [PubMed]

34. Savaiano, D.A.; Levitt, M.D. Milk Intolerance and Microbe-Containing Dairy Foods. *J. Dairy Sci.* **1987**, *70*, 397–406. [CrossRef]

35. Phelan, M.; Kerins, D. The Potential Role of Milk-Derived Peptides in Cardiovascular Disease. *Food Funct.* **2011**, *2*, 153–167. [CrossRef] [PubMed]

36. Meisel, H. Multifunctional Peptides Encrypted in Milk Proteins. *Biofactors* **2004**, *21*, 55–61. [CrossRef] [PubMed]

37. Sluijs, I.; Forouhi, N.G.; Beulens, J.W.; van der Schouw, Y.T.; Agnoli, C.; Arriola, L.; Balkau, B.; Barricarte, A.; Boeing, H.; Bueno-de-Mesquita, H.B.; et al. The Amount and Type of Dairy Product Intake and Incident Type 2 Diabetes: Results from the EPIC-Interact Study. *Am. J. Clin. Nutr.* **2012**, *96*, 382–390. [CrossRef] [PubMed]

38. Talaei, M.; Pan, A.; Yuan, J.M.; Koh, W.P. Dairy Intake and Risk of Type 2 Diabetes. *Clin. Nutr.* **2017**. [CrossRef] [PubMed]

39. Drouin-Chartier, J.P.; Cote, J.A.; Labonte, M.E.; Brassard, D.; Tessier-Grenier, M.; Desroches, S.; Couture, P.; Lamarche, B. Comprehensive Review of the Impact of Dairy Foods and Dairy Fat on Cardiometabolic Risk. *Adv. Nutr.* **2016**, *7*, 1041–1051. [CrossRef] [PubMed]

40. Astrup, A. Yogurt and Dairy Product Consumption to Prevent Cardiometabolic Diseases: Epidemiologic and Experimental Studies. *Am. J. Clin. Nutr.* **2014**, *99*, 1235S–1242S. [CrossRef] [PubMed]

41. Drouin-Chartier, J.P.; Brassard, D.; Tessier-Grenier, M.; Cote, J.A.; Labonte, M.E.; Desroches, S.; Couture, P.; Lamarche, B. Systematic Review of the Association between Dairy Product Consumption and Risk of Cardiovascular-Related Clinical Outcomes. *Adv. Nutr.* **2016**, *7*, 1026–1040. [CrossRef] [PubMed]

42. Pasiakos, S.M. Metabolic Advantages of Higher Protein Diets and Benefits of Dairy Foods on Weight Management, Glycemic Regulation, and Bone. *J. Food Sci.* **2015**, *80*, A2–A7. [CrossRef] [PubMed]

43. McGregor, R.A.; Poppitt, S.D. Milk Protein for Improved Metabolic Health: A Review of the Evidence. *Nutr. Metab. (Lond.)* **2013**, *10*, 46. [CrossRef] [PubMed]

44. Bourrie, B.C.; Willing, B.P.; Cotter, P.D. The Microbiota and Health Promoting Characteristics of the Fermented Beverage Kefir. *Front. Microbiol.* **2016**, *7*, 647. [CrossRef] [PubMed]

45. Bell, S.; Daskalopoulou, M.; Rapsomaniki, E.; George, J.; Britton, A.; Bobak, M.; Casas, J.P.; Dale, C.E.; Denaxas, S.; Shah, A.D.; et al. Association between Clinically Recorded Alcohol Consumption and Initial Presentation of 12 Cardiovascular Diseases: Population Based Cohort Study Using Linked Health Records. *BMJ* **2017**, *356*, j909. [CrossRef] [PubMed]

46. Yang, Y.; Wang, X.; Yao, Q.; Qin, L.; Xu, C. Dairy Product, Calcium Intake and Lung Cancer Risk: A Systematic Review with Meta-Analysis. *Sci. Rep.* **2016**, *6*, 20624. [CrossRef] [PubMed]

47. Zang, J.; Shen, M.; Du, S.; Chen, T.; Zou, S. The Association between Dairy Intake and Breast Cancer in Western and Asian Populations: A Systematic Review and Meta-Analysis. *J. Breast Cancer* **2015**, *18*, 313–322. [CrossRef] [PubMed]

48. Aune, D.; Navarro Rosenblatt, D.A.; Chan, D.S.; Vieira, A.R.; Vieira, R.; Greenwood, D.C.; Vatten, L.J.; Norat, T. Dairy Products, Calcium, and Prostate Cancer Risk: A Systematic Review and Meta-Analysis of Cohort Studies. *Am. J. Clin. Nutr.* **2015**, *101*, 87–117. [CrossRef] [PubMed]

49. Aune, D.; Lau, R.; Chan, D.S.; Vieira, R.; Greenwood, D.C.; Kampman, E.; Norat, T. Dairy Products and Colorectal Cancer Risk: A Systematic Review and Meta-Analysis of Cohort Studies. *Ann. Oncol.* **2012**, *23*, 37–45. [CrossRef] [PubMed]

50. Genkinger, J.M.; Hunter, D.J.; Spiegelman, D.; Anderson, K.E.; Arslan, A.; Beeson, W.L.; Buring, J.E.; Fraser, G.E.; Freudenheim, J.L.; Goldbohm, R.A.; et al. Dairy Products and Ovarian Cancer: A Pooled Analysis of 12 Cohort Studies. *Cancer Epidemiol. Prev. Biomark.* **2006**, *15*, 364–372. [CrossRef] [PubMed]

51. Murphy, N.; Norat, T.; Ferrari, P.; Jenab, M.; Bueno-de-Mesquita, B.; Skeie, G.; Olsen, A.; Tjonneland, A.; Dahm, C.C.; Overvad, K.; et al. Consumption of Dairy Products and Colorectal Cancer in the European Prospective Investigation into Cancer and Nutrition (EPIC). *PLoS ONE* **2013**, *8*, e72715. [CrossRef] [PubMed]

52. Huncharek, M.; Muscat, J.; Kupelnick, B. Colorectal Cancer Risk and Dietary Intake of Calcium, Vitamin D, and Dairy Products: A Meta-Analysis of 26,335 Cases from 60 Observational Studies. *Nutr. Cancer* **2009**, *61*, 47–69. [CrossRef] [PubMed]

53. Singh, G.; Lakkis, C.L.; Laucirica, R.; Epner, D.E. Regulation of Prostate Cancer Cell Division by Glucose. *J. Cell. Physiol.* **1999**, *180*, 431–438. [CrossRef]

54. Rock, C.L. Milk and the Risk and Progression of Cancer. *Nestle Nutr. Workshop Ser. Pediatr. Program.* **2011**, *67*, 173–185. [PubMed]

55. Ji, J.; Sundquist, J.; Sundquist, K. Lactose Intolerance and Risk of Lung, Breast and Ovarian Cancers: Aetiological Clues from a Population-Based Study in Sweden. *Br. J. Cancer* **2015**, *112*, 149–152. [CrossRef] [PubMed]

56. Fardellone, P.; Sejourne, A.; Blain, H.; Cortet, B.; Thomas, T.; Committee, G.S. Osteoporosis: Is Milk a Kindness or a Curse? *Jt. Bone Spine* **2016**, *84*, 275–281. [CrossRef] [PubMed]

57. Durosier-Izart, C.; Biver, E.; Merminod, F.; van Rietbergen, B.; Chevalley, T.; Herrmann, F.R.; Ferrari, S.L.; Rizzoli, R. Peripheral Skeleton Bone Strength Is Positively Correlated with Total and Dairy Protein Intakes in Healthy Postmenopausal Women. *Am. J. Clin. Nutr.* **2017**, *105*, 513–525. [CrossRef] [PubMed]

58. Bowen, J.; Noakes, M.; Clifton, P.M. A High Dairy Protein, High-Calcium Diet Minimizes Bone Turnover in Overweight Adults During Weight Loss. *J. Nutr.* **2004**, *134*, 568–573. [PubMed]

59. Wlodarek, D.; Glabska, D.; Kolota, A.; Adamczyk, P.; Czekajlo, A.; Grzeszczak, W.; Drozdzowska, B.; Pluskiewicz, W. Calcium Intake and Osteoporosis: The Influence of Calcium Intake from Dairy Products on Hip Bone Mineral Density and Fracture Incidence—A Population-Based Study in Women over 55 Years of Age. *Public Health Nutr.* **2014**, *17*, 383–389. [CrossRef] [PubMed]

60. Wadolowska, L.; Sobas, K.; Szczepanska, J.W.; Slowinska, M.A.; Czlapka-Matyasik, M.; Niedzwiedzka, E. Dairy Products, Dietary Calcium and Bone Health: Possibility of Prevention of Osteoporosis in Women: The Polish Experience. *Nutrients* **2013**, *5*, 2684–2707. [CrossRef] [PubMed]

61. Martin Jimenez, J.A.; Consuegra Moya, B.; Martin Jimenez, M.T. Nutritional Factors in Preventing Osteoporosis. *Nutr. Hosp.* **2015**, *32*, 49–55. [PubMed]

62. Buzas, G.M. Lactose Intolerance: Past and Present. Part II. *Orvosi Hetil.* **2015**, *156*, 1741–1749.

63. Loria-Kohen, V.; Espinosa-Salinas, I.; Ramirez de Molina, A.; Casas-Agustench, P.; Herranz, J.; Molina, S.; Fonolla, J.; Olivares, M.; Lara-Villoslada, F.; Reglero, G.; et al. A Genetic Variant of PPARA Modulates Cardiovascular Risk Biomarkers after Milk Consumption. *Nutrition* **2014**, *30*, 1144–1150. [CrossRef] [PubMed]

64. Abdullah, M.M.; Cyr, A.; Lepine, M.C.; Eck, P.K.; Couture, P.; Lamarche, B.; Jones, P.J. Common Variants in Cholesterol Synthesis- and Transport-Related Genes Associate with Circulating Cholesterol Responses to Intakes of Conventional Dairy Products in Healthy Individuals. *J. Nutr.* **2016**, *146*, 1008–1016. [CrossRef] [PubMed]

65. Hubner, R.A.; Muir, K.R.; Liu, J.F.; Logan, R.F.; Grainge, M.J.; Houlston, R.S.; Members of UKCAP Consortium. Dairy Products, Polymorphisms in the Vitamin D Receptor Gene and Colorectal Adenoma Recurrence. *Int. J. Cancer* **2008**, *123*, 586–593. [CrossRef] [PubMed]

66. Neyestani, T.R.; Djazayery, A.; Shab-Bidar, S.; Eshraghian, M.R.; Kalayi, A.; Shariatzadeh, N.; Khalaji, N.; Zahedirad, M.; Gharavi, A.; Houshiarrad, A.; et al. Vitamin D Receptor Fok-I Polymorphism Modulates Diabetic Host Response to Vitamin D Intake: Need for a Nutrigenetic Approach. *Diabetes Care* **2013**, *36*, 550–556. [CrossRef] [PubMed]

67. Shab-Bidar, S.; Neyestani, T.R.; Djazayery, A. The Interactive Effect of Improvement of Vitamin D Status and VDR Foki Variants on Oxidative Stress in Type 2 Diabetic Subjects: A Randomized Controlled Trial. *Eur. J. Clin. Nutr.* **2015**, *69*, 216–222. [CrossRef] [PubMed]

68. Shab-Bidar, S.; Neyestani, T.R.; Djazayery, A. Vitamin D Receptor Cdx-2-Dependent Response of Central Obesity to Vitamin D Intake in the Subjects with Type 2 Diabetes: A Randomised Clinical Trial. *Br. J. Nutr.* **2015**, *114*, 1375–1384. [CrossRef] [PubMed]

69. Sotos-Prieto, M.; Guillen, M.; Guillem-Saiz, P.; Portoles, O.; Corella, D. The Rs1466113 Polymorphism in the Somatostatin Receptor 2 Gene Is Associated with Obesity and Food Intake in a Mediterranean Population. *Ann. Nutr. Metab.* **2010**, *57*, 124–131. [CrossRef] [PubMed]

70. InterAct, C. Investigation of Gene-Diet Interactions in the Incretin System and Risk of Type 2 Diabetes: The EPIC-Interact Study. *Diabetologia* **2016**, *59*, 2613–2621.

71. Eigler, T.; Ben-Shlomo, A. Somatostatin System: Molecular Mechanisms Regulating Anterior Pituitary Hormones. *J. Mol. Endocrinol.* **2014**, *53*, R1–R19. [CrossRef] [PubMed]

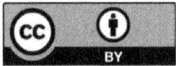

nutrients

MDPI

Article

Influence of Genetic Variations in Selenoprotein Genes on the Pattern of Gene Expression after Supplementation with Brazil Nuts

Janaina L. S. Donadio [1,*], Marcelo M. Rogero [2], Simon Cockell [3], John Hesketh [3] and Silvia M. F. Cozzolino [1]

[1] Department of Food and Experimental Nutrition, Faculty of Pharmaceutical Sciences, University of São Paulo, São Paulo 05508-900, Brazil; smfcozzo@usp.br

[2] Department of Nutrition, Faculty of Public Health, University of São Paulo, São Paulo 01246-904, Brazil; mmrogero@usp.br

[3] Institute for Cell and Molecular Biosciences, Faculty of Medical Sciences, Newcastle University, Newcastle upon Tyne NE2 4HH, UK; simon.cockell@newcastle.ac.uk (S.C.); j.e.hesketh@newcastle.ac.uk (J.H.)

* Correspondance: janainadonadio@gmail.com; Tel.: +55-11-30913625

Received: 31 May 2017; Accepted: 9 June 2017; Published: 11 July 2017

Abstract: Selenium (Se) is an essential micronutrient for human health. Its beneficial effects are exerted by selenoproteins, which can be quantified in blood and used as molecular biomarkers of Se status. We hypothesize that the presence of genetic polymorphisms in selenoprotein genes may: (1) influence the gene expression of specific selenoproteins and (2) influence the pattern of global gene expression after Brazil nut supplementation. The study was conducted with 130 healthy volunteers in Sao Paulo, Brazil, who consumed one Brazil nut (300 μg/Se) a day for eight weeks. Gene expression of *GPX1* and *SELENOP* and genotyping were measured by real-time PCR using TaqMan Assays. Global gene expression was assessed by microarray using Illumina HumanHT-12 v4 BeadChips. Brazil nut supplementation significantly increased *GPX1* mRNA expression only in subjects with CC genotype at rs1050450 ($p < 0.05$). *SELENOP* mRNA expression was significantly higher in A-carriers at rs7579 either before or after supplementation ($p < 0.05$). Genotype for rs713041 in *GPX4* affected the pattern of blood cell global gene expression. Genetic variations in selenoprotein genes modulated both *GPX1* and *SELENOP* selenoprotein gene expression and global gene expression in response to Brazil nut supplementation.

Keywords: SNPs; polymorphisms; microarray; transcriptomics; micronutrient

1. Introduction

There is a considerable evidence to indicate that nuts are an important component of a healthy diet and this is thought to be at least partly due to their fatty acid composition and micronutrient content [1–3]. Brazil nuts (*Bertholletia excelsa*, family Lecythidaceae) are unique in also containing a high level of the micronutrient selenium (Se), and its use as a dietary supplement was able to increase the concentrations of biomarkers of Se status in different populations [4–7]. Se is an essential trace element that has an important role in human biology. There are 25 genes encoding selenoproteins with a wide range of functions, including antioxidant defense, redox function, thyroid hormone metabolism, immune function, reproduction and fertility [8,9]. Unlikely in most minerals that interact as cofactors in the active site of enzymes, Se is inserted as the amino acid selenocysteine (Sec) during translation. This process involves recoding the stop codon UGA to insert Sec and requires the presence of a stem-loop structure in the 3′untranslated region (3′UTR) of selenoprotein mRNAs (Sec Insertion Sequence or SECIS) and a specific tRNA for Sec (tRNA[Ser]Sec) [10].

Selenoprotein expression is regulated by Se supply, but different selenoproteins respond differently to available Se, depending on the specific tissue and the specific selenoprotein. As a result, there is a hierarchy in the response of selenoproteins to Se supply. For example, under Se-deficient conditions, Se is directed to the brain and endocrine tissues rather than to liver and kidneys [11]. Within the same tissue, some proteins have a preference for synthesis when the Se supply is limiting. This difference in regulation of selenoprotein expression reflects their physiological importance, and during deficiency states, the ones ranked high in the hierarchy have preference for synthesis [11].

The concept of hierarchy in the regulation of selenoprotein expression raises the possible use of molecular biomarkers of Se status in supplementation studies using humans and rodents. In mouse models, nine selenoprotein genes had reduced mRNA expression in the liver during Se-deficiency, including *GPX1*, *SELENOH*, *SELENOW*, *TXNRD1*, *TXNRD2*, *DIO1*, and *SELENOF*. This reduction ranked them low in the hierarchy and made them a possible target for use as molecular biomarkers in rodents [12]. Nevertheless, several human studies have failed to demonstrate an association of Se status and selenoproteins transcripts [13–15]. Only two studies have observed a positive relationship between Se supplementation and increased selenoprotein expression [16,17].

Genetic polymorphisms are an important source of inter-individual variation in response to nutritional supplementation [18]. Several single nucleotide polymorphisms (SNPs) in selenoproteins genes have been shown to be functionally significant and to affect the response of biomarkers of Se status to Se supplementation [19–22]. In particular, rs1050540 in *GPX1*, rs713041 in *GPX4* and rs7579 in the Selenoprotein P gene (*SELENOP*) are known to affect the expression of the respective selenoproteins. In the case of rs713041, the variant is a C > T substitution located in the 3'UTR of the *GPX4* gene and it affects Se incorporation in a cell culture model [23] and the response to Se supplementation in healthy adults [20]. It should be highlighted that rs713041 can modulate GPx4 activity by altering Sec insertion and protein binding to the 3'UTR [20]. rs7579 is a change G > A present in the 3'UTR of *SELENOP* and has been shown to affect Selenoprotein P (SePP) concentrations to Se supplementation in both European Americans and South Asians (12).

However, although Brazil nuts are a rich source of Se and therefore it is expected that Brazil nut supplementation would affect selenoprotein expression, no studies have investigated the influence of genetic polymorphisms on response to Brazil nut supplementation in healthy adults. In addition, none of the studies investigating the effect of either Se or Brazil nut Se supplementation in humans have considered the effect of genetic variants on the pattern of global gene expression. Therefore, the aims of the present study were twofold: firstly, to investigate the influence of three functional SNPs in selenoprotein genes (rs1050540, rs713041 and rs7579) on the expression of selenoproteins in response to Brazil nut supplementation, and secondly to use microarray analysis to assess the influence of rs713041, a well-characterized functional SNP in *GPX4*, on the pattern of global gene expression after Brazil nut supplementation in healthy adults.

2. Materials and Methods

2.1. Brazil Nut Supplementation and Blood Sampling

The present study involved 130 unrelated healthy volunteers with a mean age of 29.8 years old and a BMI of 23.3 kg/m^2, who took part of the Supplementation with Brazil Nuts study (SU.BRA.NUT) described previously [24]. Volunteers taking multivitamins and mineral supplements, anti-inflammatory drugs, with excessive alcohol consumption, athletes, obese (BMI > 30) and with chronic diseases such as cancer, diabetes and cardiovascular disease were not included in the study. At the beginning of the study (baseline), 20 mL venous blood samples were drawn, and, subsequently, the volunteers took a daily supplement of one Brazil nut for eight weeks. At the end of four (4-week intervention) and eight weeks (8-week intervention) of supplementation, another 20 mL blood sample was taken, and then two more blood samples were taken after a further four (4-week washout) and eight weeks without intervention (8-week washout) (see Figure 1). Volunteers were asked to complete a control calendar and mark with an "x" when they consumed each nut throughout the intervention period. Written informed consent was signed by all volunteers before blood sampling. The protocol was approved by the Faculty of Pharmaceutical Sciences Ethical Committee (CAE: 00961112.3.0000.0067) and was conducted according to the Declaration of Helsinki. The study was registered at clinicaltrials.gov under the number NCT03111355.

2.2. Genotyping

Total genomic DNA was extracted from whole blood using a Purelink Genomic DNA Minikit (Invitrogen, Thermo Scientific, Carlsbad, CA, USA) and the final DNA concentration and purity were measured by spectrophotometry at 260 and 280 nm (NanoDrop ND 1000, Thermo Scientific, Wilmington, DE, USA). Genotyping was carried out by real-time PCR using the StepOne Plus Real Time system with Taqman SNP Genotyping Assays (Applied Biosystems, Thermo Scientific, Fostercity, CA, USA). The allelic discrimination was obtained by performing an endpoint read. The SNPs selected were located in the *GPX1* gene (rs1050450), the *GPX4* gene (rs713041), the *SELENOP* gene (rs3877899 and rs7579), the *SELENOS* gene (rs34713741) and the *SELENOF* gene (rs5845).

2.3. Selenoprotein Gene Expression

Total RNA was extracted from whole blood using a Ribopure Blood Kit (Ambion, Thermo Scientific, Austin, TX, USA) and final concentration and purity were measured spectrometrically in a NanoDrop ND 1000 spectrophotometer (NanoDrop ND 1000, Thermo Scientific, Wilmington, DE, USA). cDNA was synthesized by reverse trancriptase PCR using a High Capacity Reverse Transcriptase kit (Applied Biosystems, Thermo Scientific, Fostercity, CA, USA). Analysis of gene expression was performed by real-time quantitative PCR (qPCR) in the QuantStudio 12K Real-Time PCR System using Taqman Gene Expression Assays for *GPX1*, *SELENOP*, *SELENOS* and *SELENOF* (Applied Biosystems, Thermo Scientific, Fostercity, CA, USA). Glyceraldehyde phosphate dehydrogenase (GAPDH) mRNA was used as a reference gene. Relative gene expression was calculated based on the $2^{-\Delta\Delta Cq}$ method [25].

2.4. Microarray Analysis

Microarray analysis was carried out to investigate the influence of rs713041 in *GPX4* on the pattern of global gene expression after Brazil nut supplementation. Total RNA was extracted before and after nut supplementation from the whole blood of 12 volunteers previously genotyped (see Figure 1): 6 with the common genotype CC and 6 with the rare genotype TT for rs713041. Total RNA was extracted from whole blood using a Purelink Blood MiniKit (Ambion, Thermo Scientific, Austin, TX, USA). The integrity of these samples was checked by capillary electrophoresis using Tape Station 2000 (Agilent Technologies, Santa Clara, CA, USA) with the Agilent RNA Nano kit. Samples with a RNA integrity number (RIN) of above seven were used for whole genome microarray analysis by Service XS (Leiden, The Netherlands) using the Illumina HumanHT-12 v4 BeadChip (Illumina, San Diego, CA, USA). RNA quality control measurements were confirmed by Service XS using an Agilent Bioanalyzer (Agilent Technologies, Santa Clara, CA, USA), and then RNA labeling, amplification, and hybridization were performed. Raw microarray scan files were exported using the Illumina Beadstudio program and loaded into R for downstream analysis using the BioConductor and specific packages for each step of the bioinformatics analysis [26]. Probes with signals that fulfilled the criteria of the Illumina probe detection *p*-value of 0.05 were considered different. The bioinformatics analysis was performed by the Bioinformatics Support Unit, Faculty of Medical Sciences, Newcastle University, Newcastle upon Tyne, England, UK.

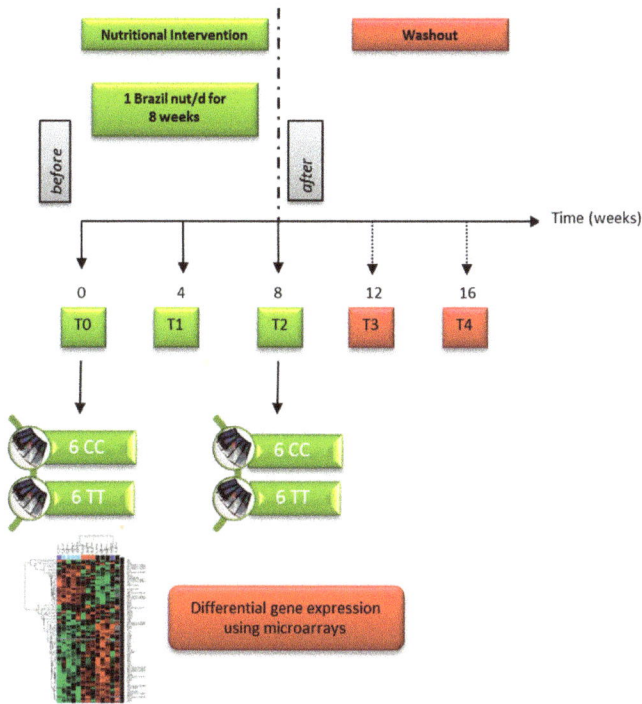

Figure 1. Intervention protocol of the Supplementation with Brazil Nuts study (SU.BRA.NUT) Biological sample collection for the microarray experiment is shown. CC indicates common genotype and TT indicates rare genotype for rs713041 in *GPX4* gene.

2.5. Gene Set Enrichment Analysis (GSEA)

The transcriptome data were analyzed by gene set enrichment analysis (GSEA), which ranks the genes in a list by their differential expression and tests for coordinated differences in a set of genes in response to a specific situation, rather than individual genes with increased or decreased expression in two conditions. One advantage of this integrated approach is the facility to interpret a large amount of data by identifying biological pathways and processes. In addition, GSEA considers the entire list of genes of the experiment, rather than only the ones that passed a fold-change cut-off. GSEA has been shown to be more sensitive than the traditional approach of single gene analyses [27]. The GSEA application from the Broad Institute, described previously [27], was used in the present work . Three files were created (dataset file.gct, phenotype file.cls and gene sets file.gmt) and loaded into the software. The dataset file contained the normalized microarray data, in our case with 19,835 probes and 23 arrays. The phenotype file contained the information about the experimental conditions, which were numbered. In this experiment, the genotypes for rs713041 and the supplementation were used. Therefore, four experimental conditions were created: 0 = CC_before, 1 = CC_after, 2 = TT_before and 3 = TT_after. The gene sets file was downloaded from the Molecular Signature Database v5.1 (MSigDB), an online collection of gene sets from different databases available for free to use with the GSEA application. The MSigDB has 8 different collections. Only two sets applicable to our context were used: C2, curated gene sets from online pathways databases and C5, Gene Ontology gene sets.

2.6. Statistical Analysis

Volunteers were selected for gene expression analysis based on their genotype that had been determined previously. For all statistical analysis, individuals who were homozygous and heterozygous for the rare alleles were combined together in one group, leaving the homozygous dominant in another category. Relative gene expression of each gene was normalized by the GAPDH reference gene using the $2^{-\Delta\Delta Cq}$ method. The final fold-change was used for statistical comparisons and submitted to normality tests using the Shapiro–Wilk test. The genotype effect before and after nuts was assessed by the Mann–Whitney test. The supplementation effect of each genotype was assessed by the Wilcoxon Test. Differences were considered significant if $p < 0.05$.

3. Results

The Supplementation with Brazil Nuts study (SU.BRA.NUT) was carried out to investigate the influence of genetic variations on the response to Brazil nut supplementation in biochemical and molecular biomarkers of Se status in healthy Brazilians. The study was conducted with 130 healthy adults, of which 66 were selected according to their genotype for analysis of gene expression of four selenoproteins and 12 were selected based on their genotype for rs713041 for microarray analysis. The mean ± standard deviation for Se content of the four batches used for the supplementation was 100.4 ± 5.3 µg/g. The average weight of the nuts was from 3 to 4 g, therefore each nut provided approximately 300 µg of Se, which is approximately five times higher than the Recommended Dietary Allowance (RDA) for adults of 55 µg/day.

3.1. Selenoprotein Gene Expression

Gene expression of two selenoprotein genes (*GPX1* and *SELENOP*) is shown in Figure 2. *GPX1* mRNA expression was affected by genotype for rs1050450 with the increase in *GPX1* expression after supplementation observed only in CC individuals but not in CT or TT individuals ($p = 0.026$). After Brazil nut consumption, *GPX1* expression was lower in T-carriers compared to CC individuals (Figure 2a). rs7579 in *SELENOP* affected *SELENOP* expression before and after nut supplementation: *SELENOP* mRNA expression was higher in carriers of the rare allele A compared to GG individuals either before or after supplementation (Figure 2b, $p < 0.05$). No differences were observed for SELENOS and SELENOF mRNA expression in response to Brazil nut supplementation (results not shown).

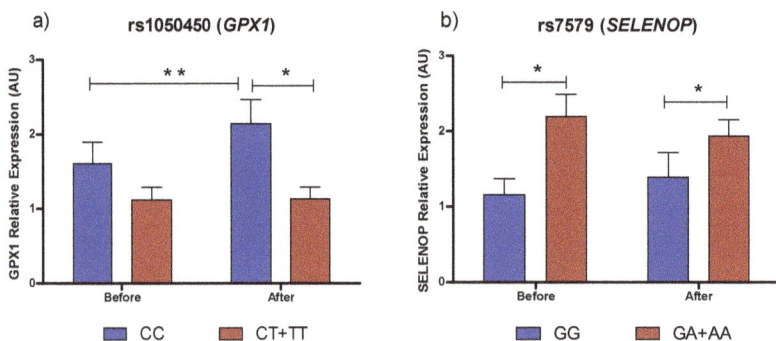

Figure 2. Selenoprotein expression in response to Brazil nut supplementation in previously genotyped volunteers. (**a**) GPX1 mRNA expression as a function of genotype for rs1050450; (**b**) SELENOP mRNA expression as a function of genotype for rs7579. * $p < 0.05$, Mann–Whitney test. ** $p < 0.05$, Wilcoxon test.

3.2. Global Gene Expression

The overall pattern of differential gene expression before and after nut supplementation and as a function of genotype for rs713041 is shown in Figure 3. Before supplementation, as illustrated by Volcano plots, there was no effect of genotype on gene expression (Figure 3a). On the contrary, after supplementation, there was some evidence of genes differentially expressed comparing both genotypes, using a fold change of 1.0 and a *p*-value of 0.05 (Figure 3b). The pattern of differentially expressed genes before and after supplementation in CC and TT individuals is shown in Figure 3c,d. The effect of Brazil nut supplementation was significant only in individuals with the CC genotype (Figure 3c). No effect was observed for individuals with the less common TT genotype (Figure 3d). The heatmap in Figure 4 illustrates the gene expression pattern after supplementation comparing CC and TT individuals (referent to volcano plot 3b), and shows an opposite pattern of response of individuals with the different genotypes. Genes that were downregulated in TT individuals after nuts were upregulated in CC individuals.

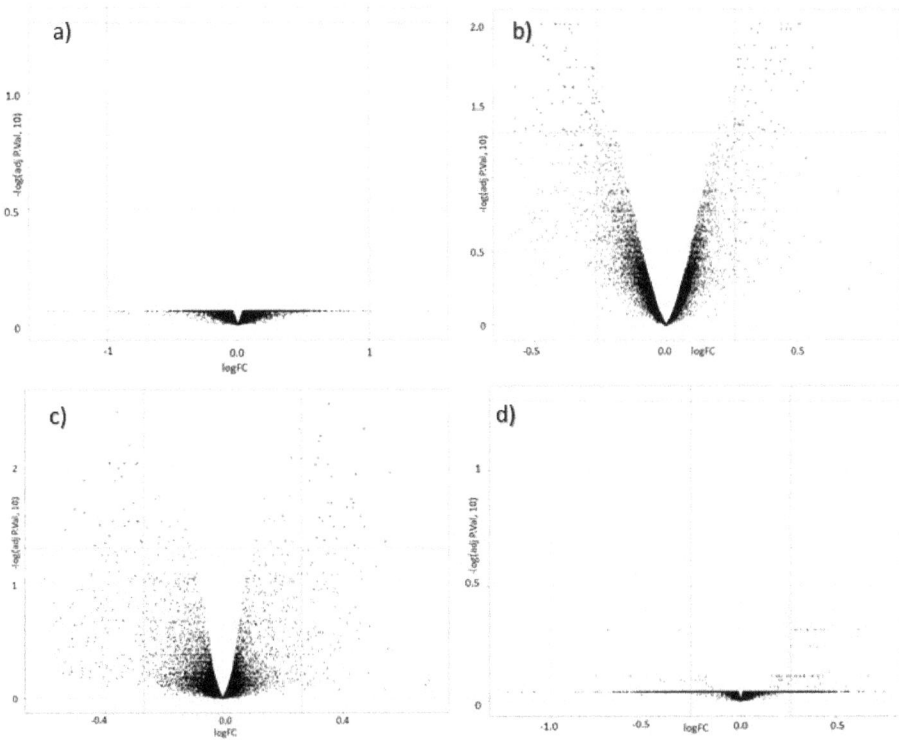

Figure 3. Volcano plots for the four experimental conditions investigated in the SU.BRA.NUT study. (**a**) Before supplementation comparing the genotypes CC × TT; (**b**) after supplementation comparing the genotypes CC × TT; (**c**) effect of the supplementation in the CC genotype and (**d**) effect of the supplementation in TT genotype.

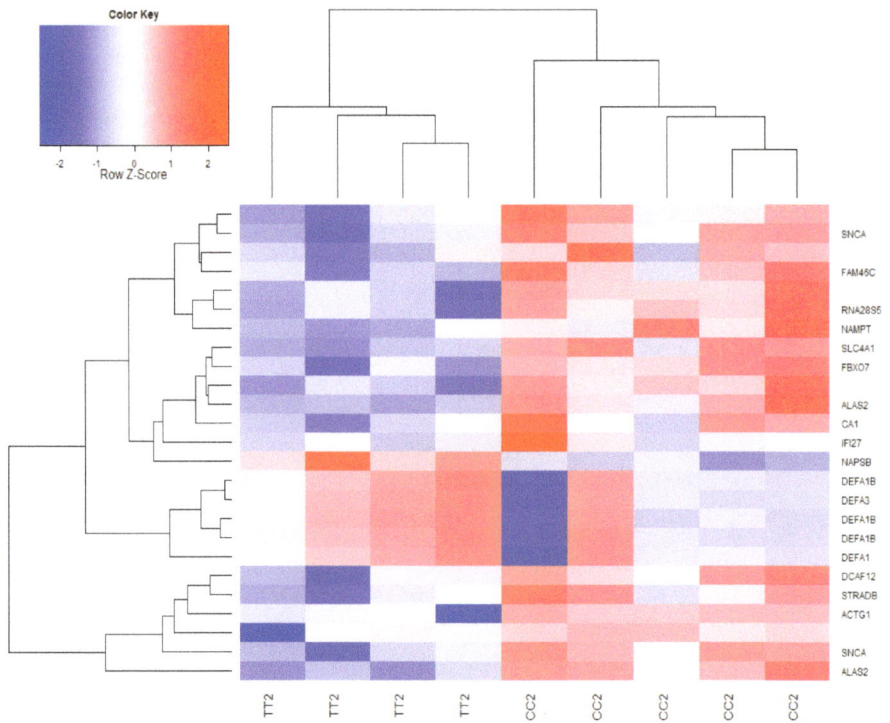

Figure 4. Heatmap showing patterns of differential expression in TT and CC genotype after Brazil nut supplementation. Red indicates genes with higher expression levels and blue genes with lower expression levels.

Gene set enrichment analysis was carried out using 19,835 probes and 23 arrays. Both genotypes and the supplementation were used as conditions for the comparisons. The collection of gene sets available in the Molecular Signatures Database (MSigDB) as C2, curated gene sets from online pathways databases, and C5, Gene Ontology gene sets, were tested. No gene sets from C2 pathways were enriched either in CC individuals before and after nuts or in between CC and TT genotypes after nuts. However, 13 gene sets from the Cellular Component list from Gene Ontology (C5) related to ribosomes, Endoplasmatic Reticulum (ER) and Golgi compartments, and mitochondria were found to be enriched in TT individuals after nuts (Table 1). This effect of rs713041 in *GPX4* may reflect the importance of GPX4 in mitochondrial function [28]

Table 1. Enriched gene sets from Gene Ontology (C5) in TT individuals for rs713041 in a GPX4 gene after supplementation with Brazil nuts compared with CC individuals. Gene sets were considered to be enriched at an (FDR) cut-off of 25%.

Name	Size	ES	NES	NOM *p*-Value	FDR *q*-Value
Cellular component					
Organellar ribosome	22	−0.69	−1.56	0.035	1.000
Mitochondrial ribosome	22	−0.69	−1.56	0.035	0.571
Early endosome	15	−0.74	−1.53	0.012	0.582
ER Golgi Intermediate compartment	20	−0.52	−1.52	0.004	0.496
Microtubule cytoskeleton	101	−0.41	−1.51	0.025	0.397
Ribosomal subunit	20	−0.66	−1.51	0.076	0.332
Intrinsic to endoplasmic reticulum membrane	23	−0.58	−1.50	0.035	0.320
Integral to endoplasmic reticulum membrane	23	−0.58	−1.50	0.035	0.280
Mitochondrial matrix	44	−0.55	−1.49	0.066	0.289
Mitochondrial lumen	44	−0.55	−1.49	0.066	0.260
Replication fork	16	−0.61	−1.48	0.014	0.242
Nuclear chromosome part	25	−0.55	−1.48	0.036	0.223
Golgi apparatus	166	−0.37	−1.45	0.008	0.280

ER: Endoplasmatic reticulum; ES: Enrichment Score; NES: Negative Enrichment Score; FDR: False Discovery Rate.

4. Discussion

Previous works have investigated possible associations between Se supplementation and molecular biomarkers of Se status such as transcripts of selenoproteins in white blood cells in human studies [13–16]. These studies were not able to find an association between plasma Se biomarkers and selenoprotein expression after Se supplementation, except for one study conducted with healthy adults in the UK, which could observe the upregulation of some selenoprotein genes after Se supplementation [16]. The present study demonstrated that three genetic variants in selenoprotein genes (rs1050450, rs7579 and rs713041) affected the response to supplementation with Se-rich Brazil nuts at the transcriptional level. Furthermore, the results indicate that the SNP rs713041 in *GPX4* gene could modulate the pattern of global gene expression. This transcriptomic approach to investigating the response to Brazil nut supplementation based on the genetic profile has not been observed before.

The supplementation with one unit of Brazil nut in other populations significantly increased blood selenium levels [6,7], indicating that indeed the Brazil nuts are a rich source of dietary selenium. In our study, *GPX1* mRNA expression in whole blood was also increased by the nut supplementation. This result was different from three previous human studies that have investigated if Se supplementation affects selenoprotein transcript levels. A small study conducted in Denmark found no association of Se supplementation as Se-enriched milk, yeast or selenate for one week with *GPX1* mRNA expression [13]. Similarly, the five-year long PRECISE study and a longitudinal study conducted in the UK also found no association [14,15]. Nevertheless, two studies are in agreement with our results. One study conducted with healthy adults in the UK observed that the supplementation with 100 µg/day with sodium selenite for six weeks increased the expression of Selenoprotein K (*SELENOK*) and Selenoprotein 15 (*SELENOF*), showing that these selenoproteins are sensible to alterations of Se status [16]. A second study conducted with Alzheimer's patients also found an increase in *GPX1* mRNA expression after supplementation with one unit of Brazil nuts for six months [17]. Possible explanations for this variation in response to Se supplementation could be either the presence of genetic variants, which most of the aforementioned works have not considered, the baseline Se status of the populations or the high level of Se provided by Brazil nuts.

Interestingly, the increase in *GPX1* mRNA expression observed in our study was dependent on the presence of genetic polymorphisms. The increase in *GPX1* mRNA expression was significant only for individuals with the common CC genotype. No difference was observed in T-carriers. This genetic variation was associated with increased *GPX1* mRNA expression in other Brazilian work conducted with Alzheimer's patients, but the authors found an increase in T-carriers instead of CC [17]. Although some studies have investigated the association of this SNP with differences in GPx1 activity [22,29,30], few studies have associated this variation with *GPX1* mRNA expression.

The presence of SNPs in *SELENOP* gene influenced its mRNA expression. The presence of the less common allele A for rs7579 was associated with an increase in *SELENOP* expression at baseline and after supplementation. Previous works with humans have not found an association between Se supplementation and *SELENOP* mRNA expression in white blood cells [13,15]. SePP is known to have two different isoforms in human plasma, the 60 kDa and the 50 kDa, and the presence of SNPs in *SELENOP* gene was associated with different proportions of the isoforms [31]. The 60 kDa isoform is more abundant in plasma and is found in higher proportion in the presence of the less common allele A for rs7579 [31]. One hypothesis was that the increase in *SELENOP* mRNA expression found only in A-carriers for rs7579 in our study could be related to the 60 kDa isoform being expressed more in plasma. Further studies are needed to confirm this association of rs7579 on *SELENOP* mRNA expression and the proportion of the 60 kDa in plasma.

Our work also had the goal of determining if genetic variants would influence the pattern of global gene expression in response to a natural source of Se, such as Brazil nuts. The SNP rs713041 in the *GPX4* gene was selected to test this hypothesis, as there is evidence that this SNP is functional [20,23,32]. It was observed that, although not statistically significant, the heatmap and volcano plots suggested the opposite response to Brazil nut supplementation based on genotype. To our knowledge, the association of rs713041 genotypes with the profile of global gene expression has not been observed previously. Moreover, GSEA showed that the biological processes and cellular compartments altered by the supplementation were related to protein synthesis, mitochondria and endoplasmatic reticulum. This supports the findings of previous humans studies that used microarrays to investigate the effect of Se supplementation [16,33]. These studies observed that processes related to protein biosynthesis were upregulated after Se supplementation. This could be explained by the molecular biosynthesis of selenoproteins, which needs the synthesis of a specific tRNA[Ser]Sec for the amino acid selenocysteine, inserted in the proteins during translation. In addition, the effect of rs713041 in *GPX4* on mitochondrial pathways may reflect the importance of GPX4 in mitochondrial function [28]. One of the limitations of this study includes the small number of individuals to perform the analysis of the pattern of global gene expression, considering this a pilot study. Therefore, further work conducted with a higher sample size is needed to confirm our results.

5. Conclusions

In conclusion, the present study suggested that supplementation with Brazil nuts can modify the gene expression of some selenoproteins depending upon the presence of genetic polymorphisms. In addition, it has been demonstrated that the use of microarrays to investigate the pattern of global gene expression in response to a nutritional intervention with nuts is feasible, and that a genetic profile for a particular variant in *GPX4* (rs713041) possibly modulates global gene expression and is an important source of inter-individual variation. This could be relevant to direct future nutritional interventions for the use of molecular and biochemical biomarkers considering the interaction with the genetic variations.

Acknowledgments: The authors are very grateful to all volunteers who took part in this study. This work was supported by Brazilian grants from the São Paulo Research Foundation (Fundação de Amparo a Pesquisa do Estado de São Paulo, FAPESP processes: 2011/17720-0; 2013/03224-0).

Author Contributions: Janaina L. S. Donadio, Marcelo M. Rogero, John Hesketh and Silvia M. F. Cozzolino conceived and designed the study; Janaina L. S. Donadio performed all experiments; Simon Cockell and Janaina L. S. Donadio performed the bioinformatics analysis; Janaina L. S. Donadio performed the statistical analysis; Janaina L. S. Donadio, John Hesketh and Marcelo M. Rogero wrote the paper with input from all authors. All authors approved the final version of the manuscript for submission.

Conflicts of Interest: The authors declared no conflict of interests.

References

1. Bolling, B.W.; Chen, C.-Y.O.; McKay, D.L.; Blumberg, J.B. Tree nut phytochemicals: Composition, antioxidant capacity, bioactivity, impact factors. A systematic review of almonds, Brazils, cashews, hazelnuts, macadamias, pecans, pine nuts, pistachios and walnuts. *Nutr. Res. Rev.* **2011**, *24*, 244–275. [CrossRef] [PubMed]
2. Alasalvar, C.; Bolling, B.W. Review of nut phytochemicals, fat-soluble bioactives, antioxidant components and health effects. *Br. J. Nutr.* **2015**, *113*, S68–S78. [CrossRef] [PubMed]
3. O'Neil, C.E.; Fulgoni, V.L.; Nicklas, T.A. Tree Nut consumption is associated with better adiposity measures and cardiovascular and metabolic syndrome health risk factors in U.S. adults: NHANES 2005–2010. *Nutr. J.* **2015**, *14*, 64–71. [CrossRef] [PubMed]
4. Dumont, E.; De Pauw, L.; Vanhaecke, F.; Cornelis, R. Speciation of Se in Bertholletia excelsa (Brazil nut): A hard nut to crack? *Food Chem.* **2006**, *95*, 684–692. [CrossRef]
5. Thomson, C.D.; Chisholm, A.; Mclachlan, S.K.; Campbell, J.M. Brazil nuts: An effective way to improve selenium status. *Am. J. Clin. Nutr.* **2008**, *87*, 379–384. [PubMed]
6. Cardoso, B.R.; Apolinário, D.; Bandeira, V.S.; Busse, A.L.; Magaldi, R.M.; Jacob-Filho, W.; Cozzolino, S.M.F. Effects of Brazil nut consumption on selenium status and cognitive performance in older adults with mild-cognitive impairment: A randomized controlled pilot trial. *Eur. J. Nutr.* **2016**, *55*, 107–116. [CrossRef] [PubMed]
7. Cominetti, C.; de Bortoli, M.C.; Garrido, A.B.; Cozzolino, S.M.F. Brazilian nut consumption improves selenium status and glutathione peroxidase activity and reduces atherogenic risk in obese women. *Nutr. Res.* **2012**, *32*, 403–407. [CrossRef] [PubMed]
8. Kryukov, G.V.; Castellano, S.; Novoselov, S.V.; Lobanov, A.V.; Zehtab, O.; Guigó, R.; Gladyshev, V.N. Characterization of mammalian selenoproteomes. *Science* **2003**, *300*, 1439–1443. [CrossRef] [PubMed]
9. Rayman, M.P. Selenium and human health. *Lancet* **2012**, *379*, 1256–1268. [CrossRef]
10. Labunskyy, V.M.; Hatfield, D.L.; Gladyshev, V.N. Selenoproteins: Molecular Pathways and Physiological Roles. *Physiol. Rev.* **2014**, *94*, 739–777. [CrossRef] [PubMed]
11. Schomburg, L.; Schweizer, U. Hierarchical regulation of selenoprotein expression and sex-specific effects of selenium. *Biochim. Biophys. Acta* **2009**, *1790*, 1453–1462. [CrossRef] [PubMed]
12. Sunde, R.A.; Raines, A.M.; Barnes, K.M.; Evenson, J.K. Selenium status highly regulates selenoprotein mRNA levels for only a subset of the selenoproteins in the selenoproteome. *Biosci. Rep.* **2009**, *29*, 329–338. [CrossRef] [PubMed]
13. Ravn-Haren, G.; Bügel, S.; Krath, B.N.; Hoac, T.; Stagsted, J.; Jørgensen, K.; Bresson, J.R.; Larsen, E.H.; Dragsted, L.O. A short-term intervention trial with selenate, selenium-enriched yeast and selenium-enriched milk: Effects on oxidative defence regulation. *Br. J. Nutr.* **2008**, *99*, 883–892. [CrossRef] [PubMed]
14. Ravn-Haren, G.; Krath, B.N.; Overvad, K.; Cold, S.; Moesgaard, S.; Larsen, E.H.; Dragsted, L.O. Effect of long-term selenium yeast intervention on activity and gene expression of antioxidant and xenobiotic metabolising enzymes in healthy elderly volunteers from the Danish Prevention of Cancer by Intervention by Selenium (PRECISE) pilot study. *Br. J. Nutr.* **2008**, *99*, 1190–1198. [CrossRef] [PubMed]
15. Sunde, R.A.; Paterson, E.; Evenson, J.K.; Barnes, K.M.; Lovegrove, J.A.; Gordon, M.H. Longitudinal selenium status in healthy British adults: Assessment using biochemical and molecular biomarkers. *Br. J. Nutr.* **2008**, *99* (Suppl. 3), S37–S47. [CrossRef] [PubMed]
16. Pagmantidis, V.; Méplan, C.; Van Schothorst, E.M.; Keijer, J.; Hesketh, J.E. Supplementation of healthy volunteers with nutritionally relevant amounts of selenium increases the expression of lymphocyte protein biosynthesis genes. *Am. J. Clin. Nutr.* **2008**, *87*, 181–189. [PubMed]
17. Cardoso, B.R.; Busse, A.L.; Hare, D.J.; Cominetti, C.; Horst, M.A.; Mccoll, G.; Magaldi, R.M.; Jacob-Filho, W.; Cozzolino, S.M.F. Pro198Leu polymorphism affects the selenium status and GPx activity in response to Brazil nut intake. *Food Funct.* **2016**, *9*, 825–833. [CrossRef] [PubMed]
18. Hesketh, J.; Méplan, C. Transcriptomics and functional genetic polymorphisms as biomarkers of micronutrient function: Focus on selenium as an exemplar. *Proc. Nutr. Soc.* **2011**, *70*, 365–373. [CrossRef] [PubMed]

19. Méplan, C.; Crosley, L.K.; Nicol, F.; Beckett, G.J.; Howie, A.F.; Hill, K.E.; Horgan, G.; Mathers, J.C.; Arthur, J.R.; Hesketh, J.E. Genetic polymorphisms in the human selenoprotein P gene determine the response of selenoprotein markers to selenium supplementation in a gender-specific manner (the SELGEN study). *FASEB J.* **2007**, *21*, 3063–3074. [CrossRef] [PubMed]

20. Méplan, C.; Crosley, L.K.; Nicol, F.; Horgan, G.W.; Mathers, J.C.; Arthur, J.R.; Hesketh, J.E. Functional effects of a common single-nucleotide polymorphism (GPX4c718t) in the glutathione peroxidase 4 gene: Interaction with sex. *Am. J. Clin. Nutr.* **2008**, *87*, 1019–1027. [PubMed]

21. Combs, G.F.; Jackson, M.I.; Watts, J.C.; Johnson, L.K.; Zeng, H.; Idso, J.; Schomburg, L.; Hoeg, A.; Hoefig, C.S.; Chiang, E.C.; et al. Differential responses to selenomethionine supplementation by sex and genotype in healthy adults. *Br. J. Nutr.* **2012**, *107*, 1514–1525. [CrossRef] [PubMed]

22. Jablonska, E.; Gromadzinska, J.; Reszka, E.; Wasowicz, W.; Sobala, W.; Szeszenia-Dabrowska, N.; Boffetta, P. Association between GPx1 Pro198Leu polymorphism, GPx1 activity and plasma selenium concentration in humans. *Eur. J. Nutr.* **2009**, *48*, 383–386. [CrossRef] [PubMed]

23. Bermano, G.; Pagmantidis, V.; Holloway, N.; Kadri, S.; Mowat, N.A.G.; Shiel, R.S.; Arthur, J.R.; Mathers, J.C.; Daly, A.K.; Broom, J.; et al. Evidence that a polymorphism within the 3'UTR of glutathione peroxidase 4 is functional and is associated with susceptibility to colorectal cancer. *Genes Nutr.* **2007**, *2*, 225–232. [CrossRef] [PubMed]

24. Donadio, J.L.S.; Rogero, M.M.; Guerra-shinohara, E.M.; Desmarchelier, C.; Borel, P.; Cozzolino, S.M.F. SEPP1 polymorphisms modulate serum glucose and lipid response to Brazil nut supplementation. *Eur. J. Nutr.* **2017**, 1–10. [CrossRef] [PubMed]

25. Livak, K.J.; Schmittgen, T.D. Analysis of relative gene expression data using real-time quantitative PCR and the 2(-Delta Delta C(T)) Method. *Methods* **2001**, *25*, 402–408. [CrossRef] [PubMed]

26. Ritchie, M.E.; Dunning, M.J.; Smith, M.L.; Shi, W.; Lynch, A.G. BeadArray Expression Analysis Using Bioconductor. *PLoS Comput. Biol.* **2011**, *7*, e1002276. [CrossRef] [PubMed]

27. Subramanian, A.; Tamayo, P.; Mootha, V.K.; Mukherjee, S.; Ebert, B.L. Gene set enrichment analysis: A knowledge-based approach for interpreting genome-wide. *Proc. Natl. Acad. Sci. USA* **2005**, *102*, 15545–15550. [CrossRef] [PubMed]

28. Cole-Ezea, P.; Swan, D.; Shanley, D.; Hesketh, J. Glutathione peroxidase 4 has a major role in protecting mitochondria from oxidative damage and maintaining oxidative phosphorylation complexes in gut epithelial cells. *Free Radic. Biol. Med.* **2012**, *53*, 488–497. [CrossRef] [PubMed]

29. Hamanishi, T.; Furuta, H.; Kato, H.; Doi, A.; Tamai, M.; Shimomura, H.; Sakagashira, S.; Nishi, M.; Sasaki, H.; Sanke, T.; et al. Functional variants in the glutathione peroxidase-1 (GPx-1) gene are associated with increased intima-media thickness of carotid arteries and risk of macrovascular diseases in Japanese type 2 diabetic patients. *Diabetes* **2004**, *53*, 2455–2460. [CrossRef] [PubMed]

30. Hansen, R.D.; Krath, B.N.; Frederiksen, K.; Tjønneland, A.; Overvad, K.; Roswall, N.; Loft, S.; Dragsted, L.O.; Vogel, U.; Raaschou-Nielsen, O. GPX1 Pro198Leu polymorphism, erythrocyte GPX activity, interaction with alcohol consumption and smoking, and risk of colorectal cancer. *Mutat. Res.* **2009**, *664*, 13–19. [CrossRef] [PubMed]

31. Méplan, C.; Nicol, F.; Burtle, B.T.; Crosley, L.K.; Arthur, J.R.; Mathers, J.C.; Hesketh, J.E. Relative abundance of selenoprotein P isoforms in human plasma depends on genotype, se intake, and cancer status. *Antioxid. Redox Signal.* **2009**, *11*, 2631–2640. [CrossRef] [PubMed]

32. Crosley, L.K.; Bashir, S.; Nicol, F.; Arthur, J.R.; Hesketh, J.E.; Sneddon, A.A. The single-nucleotide polymorphism (GPX4c718t) in the glutathione peroxidase 4 gene influences endothelial cell function: Interaction with selenium and fatty acids. *Mol. Nutr. Food Res.* **2013**, *57*, 2185–2194. [CrossRef] [PubMed]

33. Hawkes, W.C.; Richter, D.; Alkan, Z. Dietary selenium supplementation and whole blood gene expression in healthy North American men. *Biol. Trace Elem. Res.* **2013**, *155*, 201–208. [CrossRef] [PubMed]

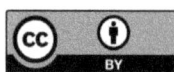

MDPI

St. Alban-Anlage 66

4052 Basel

Switzerland

Tel. +41 61 683 77 34

Fax +41 61 302 89 18

www.mdpi.com

Nutrients Editorial Office

E-mail: nutrients@mdpi.com

www.mdpi.com/journal/nutrients

www.ingramcontent.com/pod-product-compliance
Lightning Source LLC
Chambersburg PA
CBHW051839210326
41597CB00033B/5710